Roman Fever

ALSO BY BENJAMIN REILLY

Disaster and Human History: Case Studies in Nature, Society and Catastrophe, 2d ed. (McFarland, 2022)

Roman Fever

Malaria, Transalpine Travelers and the Eternal City

Benjamin Reilly

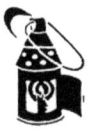

McFarland & Company, Inc., Publishers
Jefferson, North Carolina

ISBN (print) 978-1-4766-8655-4
ISBN (ebook) 978-1-4766-4395-3

LIBRARY OF CONGRESS AND BRITISH LIBRARY
CATALOGUING DATA ARE AVAILABLE

Library of Congress Control Number 2021060576

© 2022 Benjamin Reilly. All rights reserved

*No part of this book may be reproduced or transmitted in any form
or by any means, electronic or mechanical, including photocopying
or recording, or by any information storage and retrieval system,
without permission in writing from the publisher.*

Front cover image: Medieval illustration of a pilgrim with staff and scrip
(Gottfried Deppisch, *Geschichte und Wunder-Wercke des heiligen Colomanni
Königlichen Pilgers und Martyrers* [Vienna: Frantz André Kirchberger, 1743]);
background map from W. North, *Roman Fever* (London: Sampson Low,
Marston and Co., 1896), plate V.

Printed in the United States of America

*McFarland & Company, Inc., Publishers
Box 611, Jefferson, North Carolina 28640
www.mcfarlandpub.com*

Table of Contents

Preface vii

Introduction 1

Part I: Malaria and Rome

1. The Nature of the Beast   8
2. Romulus' Mistake   15
3. Assessing the Threat   25

Part II: Transalpine Europe and the *Caput Mundi*

4. Grave of Nations   36
5. To Roam/Rome   45
6. Dragon's Lair   55
7. The Christmas Crown   63
8. Brood of Vipers   78
9. Imperium's Price   93
10. Jubilee   103
11. Fullness of Power   115
12. From Scandal to Sack   125
13. The Scarlet Whore   139
14. Fork in the Road   147
15. Homecoming   157
16. Last Gasps   168

Conclusion   181

Chapter Notes   185

Bibliography   201

Index   209

Preface

Imagine for a moment that you are a celestial being who wishes to create a human civilization. This new polity, you decide, should have a clear capital: a single city serving as the source of political legitimacy, spiritual guidance, legal jurisprudence, and artistic inspiration. However, since you are a capricious deity, you play a cruel prank on the mortals below. Rather than placing that capital in the civilization's center, you decide to locate it instead on the geographic periphery—and in an exotic climate zone to boot. Worse yet, you position the capital within the range of a virulent disease against which few members of that civilization have any acquired or intrinsic immunity. Having set the trap, there is nothing left for you to do but to watch your dysfunctional civilization from above as generations upon generations of travelers are drawn to their deaths.

A fanciful scenario, to be sure. Nonetheless, it does capture an essential truth about the troubled historical relationship between the city of Rome and the various peoples of Europe, who looked at Rome with distant admiration but quite often did not survive up-close encounters with the Eternal City. I first became aware of the phenomenon while writing a 2009 textbook on natural disasters for McFarland. In my chapter on malaria I speculated, with perhaps more grandiloquence than the textbook genre normally allows, that "Rome played the role of the legendary will-o'-the-wisp, a shining light that lured nighttime travelers into deadly marshes."[1]

Over the course of the next ten years I returned repeatedly to different aspects of the topic, publishing various academic papers which sought to establish how many European travelers went to Rome, how many were there in the summer, how much of a risk malaria posed to those travelers, and how aware Europeans from across the Alps were of the risk that Roman Fever represented.[2] In this book, I will attempt to stitch these scraps together into a single, coherent narrative tapestry.

A historian is only as good as his or her sources, so I want to thank Theresa McGregor, Evangeline Castillo, Jasmine Kirby, Shaima Sheriff, and Fabeena Ummer on the CMU Qatar campus library. Similarly, my gratitude goes to Andrew Marshall of the main campus library, who handled my innumerable interlibrary loan requests with skill and patience. In addition, my sincere thanks to the generosity of the Qatar Foundation, whose SEED money grant was essential to the project, as well as to the overseers of those grants, including Meg Rogers in the research office, Dudley Reynolds of the Arts and Sciences faculty group, and Dean Michael Trick. My thanks as well to Supriya Sinha for her stalwart administrative assistance every step along the way.

In terms of intellectual influence on the project, I want to thank first and foremost Jörg Matthias Determann, who encouraged me to pursue this research when my last big project was winding down. I am also in debt to Lansine Kaba, who helped mentor me during his years at CMUQ—and whose own research speaks to the impact of malaria on historical affairs. My gratitude goes as well to Jon Robertson, who introduced me to the story of Daisy Miller, the archetypical victim of fever in the Eternal City. I would also like to thank the two anonymous reviewers who looked over previous versions of the manuscript and whose insights helped to shape the finished book, as well as to Matthew Romaniello who gave me valuable advice on preparing the text for critical review.

 My heartfelt thanks go to my wife Anita, who helped me hash out my thoughts and ideas about Rome, northern Europeans, and malaria over the course of many long conversations. Much the same is true of my sons, Will and especially AJ, who heard some of the arguments I make in this text over the course of numerous late-night walks. Best of luck to both of you as you head off to college

INTRODUCTION

For much of the past two millennia, Europeans regarded Rome as the *caput mundi*, the veritable head of the world. As the resting-place of the holy apostles, the sacred seat of both popes and emperors, and the capital of art and classical learning, Rome exerted an outsize pull on the mind of Europe. As one 19th-century author quipped, "what Paris is to France, what London is to England, Rome is to the universe."[1]

Yet Rome's attractions could prove deadly. Due to an accident of biology and geography Rome lies just within the northern limit of *P. falciparum*, the deadliest member of the malaria plasmodia family. As a result, generations upon generations of starry-eyed European visitors to Rome's fabled seven hills were putting themselves in mortal peril from "Roman Fever"—in other words, the endemic malaria plasmodia of the Eternal City. Culture and biology, therefore, worked in cruel conjunction throughout European history to kill countless unacclimated visitors from Britain, France, Germany, and other regions of the transalpine European north.

Fatal attractions of this sort are not entirely unprecedented in the historical record. During the 19th century, for example, the city of Mecca played a somewhat analogous role for Islamic civilization. In 1865 alone, one-sixth of the estimated 90,000 Muslims who descended upon Mecca for the Hajj pilgrimage never returned, succumbing to cholera due to contamination of the water supply. That year the holy city became a necropolis.[2] But Mecca's disease problems were acute, not chronic. Cholera was not native to Mecca and Western-imposed quarantine stations soon rendered Mecca safe for visitors once again. In contrast, Rome represented a chronic threat to transalpine travelers for an extraordinarily long period of time, from the founding of the city all the way into the early 20th century.

The central question central question of this book seeks to answer, then, is whether the interaction between Rome's attraction to European visitors and its resident malaria species exerted a significant impact upon European historical development. It is not entirely a new question. Scholars of the Medieval German Empire, for example, have long acknowledged that malaria was a major player in the dramatic Medieval clashes between empire and papacy, and some have even speculated that Germany's *Romegedanke*, or obsession with Rome, may have hindered German national development. By and large, however, the interplay between Roman malaria and unacclimated travelers from beyond the Alps has gone almost unnoticed by scholars despite its potential importance to European history. This book intends to fill that void in the current literature. It is not intended to be the definitive book about malaria in Roman history: Robert Sallares already wrote it, *Malaria and Rome*, in 2002. Rather, this book seeks to provide a general history of Europe's long engagement with the Eternal City, with a particular focus on the deadly interaction between Rome's resident malarial parasites and 40 generations of unacclimated travelers from over the Alps.

So *did* malaria play an important role in shaping European history? Based on the findings of this book, the overall answer was yes, though to various degrees at various times. Although Rome beguiled European visitors during all periods of European history, the magnitude of that attraction oscillated from century to century. It rose in the Medieval era with Northern Europe's conversion to Christianity, climbed still higher with the inauguration of German coronation trips to Rome, and climaxed with the development of the Jubilee pilgrimage tradition to Rome in 1300. By the 16th century, however, travel to Rome from some northern European countries fell sharply due to the Protestant Reformation, through it revived somewhat during the golden age of the Grand Tour in the 18th century before spiking once more in the subsequent era of steam transportation.

Motives for travel to Rome changed over time as well. During the Medieval era, pilgrimage and ecclesiastical business were the most important motives for visitors to Rome, but the winds of political circumstance also deposited large numbers of French, German, Hungarian, and other soldiers into the vicinity of the Eternal City. During the Renaissance, Rome became a center of both culture and the arts, attracting a growing number of scholars, painters, engravers, and collectors. The early modern era, in turn, saw the definitive rise of the tourist as well as the long-time expatriate resident of Italy. Finally, in the modern era, tourism continued to be the primary motive for European travel to Rome, but fickle fortune once again brought many soldiers into the habitat of Rome's malaria plasmodia, often with fatal results. What is more, Rome's malaria danger varied over time as well, from a relative low during the ancient period to a Medieval peak, after which it gradually diminished over the course of the early modern and modern era. Only in the 20th century was Italy's malaria problem definitively solved, much to the relief of would-be travelers to the Eternal City.

Although the relationship between European travelers, Rome, and malaria is varied and complex, two periods stand out in which malaria may have played the greatest role in shaping Europe's fortunes. First, during the Medieval era, malaria played an important but underappreciated role in the conflict between the papacy and the German Empire. In these centuries, the Bishop of Rome—better known today as the pope—sought to assert spiritual primacy over the entire Christian West. However, his power was challenged by German emperors who had universalist ambitions of their own inherited from the Caesars of Rome. The inevitable result was over five centuries of bitter clashes between popes and emperors, not just over money and power, but also over the inheritance of immortal Rome and thus the very soul of Western Christianity. As we shall see, malaria intervened repeatedly and decisively in these conflicts, and usually on the side of the home team, the Roman papacy.

Secondly, and more controversially, my research suggests that the relationship between malaria and the Protestant Reformation needs to be fundamentally re-examined. Malaria did not cause the Protestant Reformation, of course: Luther's 95 theses were directed against the fiscal parasitism of the Roman Curia, not the biological parasitism of Rome's resident plasmodia. However, by transforming the city of Rome from the cradle of culture into the seat of the Antichrist, the Protestant Reformation greatly reduced the number of British, German, Dutch, and other Protestant-region travelers to the Eternal City. As a consequence, far fewer travelers from Europe's north, where the Protestant movement was strongest and acquired malaria resistance was generally weakest, were exposed to Rome's fevers in the following decades.

What is more, from the standpoint of demographics and biology, the Protestant revolution occurred at a crucial time. During the era of the Reformation, Rome was still highly malarious. In addition, early modern Rome still routinely received a substantial number of visitors even in the dangerous summer fever season. The Reformation therefore almost certainly saved a great number of lives that centuries earlier would have been lost to the ravages of Rome's malarial fevers. If this is accepted, then the reduction of European traffic to Rome from the Protestant north must have had a significant and previously unacknowledged impact on the demographics of these states during the 16th and 17th centuries. True, Protestant Europeans would eventually rediscover the delights of Rome in the late 17th century and early 18th century, but medical advances, urban growth, improvements to the infrastructure, and growing popular knowledge about the seasonality of Rome's "bad air" combined to reduce the risk that these travelers faced from Rome's endemic malaria. Indeed, by the 19th century, Roman Fever was well on its way to becoming a local curiosity which no longer posed a mortal threat to voyagers to the Eternal City.

In terms of source materials, this study does not blaze new trails into unexplored archives or new-found letters. Nonetheless, I do use the existing materials rather differently from most previous scholars of the Roman/European connections. Historians traditionally create knowledge by conducting a close examination of a few key primary source documents, seeking to read between the lines for deep meanings and connections. My own approach has been rather different, and owes as much to newer techniques of digital humanities as it does to traditional historical scholarship. In order to derive data about general patterns of European travel to Rome, I searched a very large number of sources for selected pieces of quantitative data, such as places visited, months traveled, and references to disease; my main tool has not been the magnifying glass of an archival historian but the spreadsheet of an accountant. Rather than basing my findings largely on anecdotal accounts, I have tried as much as possible to build my arguments on percentages and hard numerical data.

What is more, when I was not able to find a body of existing data relevant to a research question, I did not hesitate to use unconventional approaches. For example, when seeking to determine the differential mortality between Italian and non–Italian visitors to Rome, I made heavy use of the historical death data of Catholic cardinals which I believe can serve as a useful proxy data set for differential mortality patterns over time. In a still more unorthodox move, when trying to quantify the impact that the Reformation had on the travel patterns of Protestant-majority states, I used the World Wide Web itself as a sort of meta-archive by using targeted keyword searches in multiple languages to compile a robust list of hundreds of names, dates, and ethnicities. As some of my more traditionally-minded historian colleagues are wont to remind me, this is not the ideal way to generate historical data. However, in the absence of systematic record-keeping, such methodologies often offer the only way forward—and in this endeavor, as with all things worth doing, we must not let the perfect become the enemy of the good.

While composing the 16 chapters of this book I tried to strike several balances. While I organized the material by theme and not by century, I did try to arrange the chapters in rough chronological order. As a result, the text occasionally backtracks and makes references to earlier events but overall keeps moving towards the present. I also tried to find a happy medium between focusing narrowly on malaria and providing the broader background knowledge a non-specialist reader needs in order to understand the historical context in which malaria acted.

The book is divided into two main sections. The first section, consisting of three chapters, is designed to set the stage for the story that follows. Chapter 1 outlines the biological underpinnings of Rome's malaria problems in terms of temperature, plasmodia species, and insect vectors. The second chapter goes on to consider the physical environment of Rome, focusing specifically on how the Tiber River both allowed Rome to become the metropolis of the Mediterranean while also predisposing Rome to malarial fevers. This section then concludes with a discussion that is central to the theme of this book: determining the relative vulnerability of transalpine Europeans to Rome's summer-season malarial infections. As we shall see, unacclimated visitors from outside of Italy were far more prone to serious malaria infection in the Eternal City than the resident Italians, and may have suffered three times the malaria mortality rates as the peninsula's native inhabitants.

With the stage now set, the second half of the book goes on to re-tell the story of Rome's various connections with European visitors from the standpoint of malaria. Chapter 4 covers the first encounter between unacclimated European invaders and Roman Fever by discussing the various Germanic invasions of Italy, culminating in three sacks of Rome and the establishment of various Germanic successor-states amidst the ruins of empire in the west. Chapter 5, in turn, examines the origins the Roman papacy, the institution that did the most to attract clerics and laymen from the far corners of Europe to the Eternal City in the centuries to come. Chapter 6 examines the Medieval European mindset about Rome through three key documents, the *Mirabilia*, the *Gesta Romanorum*, and the *Kaiserchronik*, all of which linked Rome to ancient empire—and to monstrous manifestations of malarial fevers. Chapters 7 through 9, in turn, focus primarily on the long conflict between the papacy and empire, arguing that the attraction of Rome served as a destabilizing force in Medieval German history. While the German connection to Rome and empire made sense from the standpoint of history and ideology, it proved to be a disastrous mistake from the standpoint of biology, as it propelled a constant flow of unacclimated imperial soldiers up a steep disease gradient into the malarial Italian south. Chapters 10 and 11, in turn, examine two further categories of European travelers into Rome and its environs, namely pilgrims to the threshold of the apostles and litigants before the papal curia, both of which arrived in Rome in astounding numbers during the later Middle Ages—much to the benefit of Rome's resident malaria plasmodia.

Turning now to the early modern era of European/Roman interaction, Chapter 12 chronicles the crisis of corruption that consumed the Catholic church after the end of the Middle Ages, gradually transforming the Roman Pope from the lieutenant of God into a mere prince of men, "more worldly than the world" in the words of Martin Luther. The result was the Protestation Reformation, which as will be seen in Chapter 13 severed a long-standing connection between parts of Europe, Rome, and malaria—and probably changed the trajectory of European history in the process. Travelers from Britain, Germany, and elsewhere in the Protestant north would eventually return to the Eternal City, as Chapters 14 and 15 will show, though malaria posed less of a threat to these visitors due to greater seasonality of travel and growing awareness of the fever danger that Rome posed to unacclimated foreign travelers. Finally, Chapter 16 explores French military intervention in Rome during the 19th century, partially for its own sake and partially for the light it shines on earlier German Imperial expeditions to the city. This chapter then brings the story to a close by discussing the eradication of malaria in the Italian peninsula as well as a dramatic last encounter between an invading army and Roman Fever.

Part I:
Malaria and Rome

1

The Nature of the Beast

In June of 1988, archeologists from the University of Arizona made a startling discovery while excavating a vast Roman villa ruin near Lugnano, a Tiber Valley hamlet in the modern Italian province of Umbria. Given the impressive scale of the villa remains, the archeologists no doubt expected to find artifacts mainly related to the comfortable lives of Rome's privileged elite. What they discovered instead was evidence of an ancient tragedy. The building, they realized, had been abandoned in the mid–3rd century CE due to fatal flaws in its foundation. For two hundred years afterwards, the site had lain unused. Then, in the 5th century, local farmers began to use crumbling vestiges of this already-derelict structure as a makeshift infant cemetery. In all, the archeological team extracted the grim remains of 47 children, most of whom were newborns or pre-term stillbirths, from the ruins of Lugnano.

While finding the infant burials was surprise enough, the real shock that awaited the archeologists at Lugnano was the bizarre manner in which the infants had been interred. At the lowest stratum of the excavated cemetery the burials were single, but at higher (more recent) levels mass graves became more common, with up to seven children being buried at once. What is more, the soil of the grave site was "loose and uncompacted," indicating that the burials were made in haste over a short period of time. For archeologist David Soren, the lesson from these graves was clear: the farmers of Lugnano must have fallen prey to some sort of escalating disease epidemic.[1] While no adult remains were found in the villa, the burial of so many newborn and aborted babies suggested considerable illness, and perhaps high mortality, among the adult population as well.

As excavations continued, researchers uncovered poignant testimony to the psychological distress of Lugnano's disease-afflicted farmers. One of the infants was weighted down with stones as if his afflicted corpse might rise up to threaten the living. A cooking pot was found filled with bone scraps and flipped upside-down, probably as a placatory offering to the gods of the underworld. Even more grotesquely, researchers discovered that the grave site was littered with the skeletons of 13 puppies, one of which had been cut in half, and all of which were missing their jaws, suggesting that the young dogs had been ritually sacrificed in order to ward off whatever malign force was besetting Lugnano. Most tellingly of all, a significant amount of *Lonicera carprifolia* honeysuckle was recovered from the gravesite, perhaps placed there in purification ceremonies designed to counter the pollution that ancient Romans associated with stillborn births. This was a crucial find, as *Lonicera carprifolia* only blooms in late July and early August. Lugnano's tragedy, therefore, must have unfolded during the dog days of summer.

On the basis of this information, David Soren thought he knew the identity of the killer at Lugnano. He considered but ultimately rejected *Brucella* and *Listeria* bacteria as well as *Toxoplasmi gondii* parasites, each of which could have explained the high number of aborted fetuses. The honeysuckle suggested a more convincing explanation: not only did it allow researchers to time the burials to high summer, it also suggested that some sort of fever was responsible, since ancient Roman medicine prescribed *Lonicera caprifolia* against both intermittent fever and the spleen enlargement that usually accompanied such infections. The most likely culprit for the Lugnano epidemic, therefore, was *P. falciparum* malaria, which generally peaked in the summer heat. Soren's hunch was later conformed forensically. After DNA analysis, one of the child burials found at Lugnano tested positive for *P. falciparum*.

Malaria and Man

What is *P. falciparum*, and how does it relate to, and differ from, other species of malaria? And what does it have to do with Rome? These are complex questions, so it is perhaps best to start from the beginning. Malaria is caused by plasmodia, unicellular life forms that survive by consuming the blood cell proteins of reptiles, birds, and mammals. In their quest to access the hemoglobin of these hosts, all plasmodia species rely on the assistance of some sort of blood-sucking insect vector, usually a species of mosquito, though some reptilian plasmodia are transmitted via sand flies. The plasmodia species that now afflict mankind first arose in Africa as parasites of primates and when human beings began to diverge genetically from the common genetic forebear that we share with the other higher primates, plasmodia tagged along. The first such species was probably *P. malariae*, a fairly mild form of the disease that can stay dormant within the human body for extended periods, perhaps as long as seven decades. This ability to bide its time in the infected host was necessary for the survival of the species, as was the mild nature of *P. malariae* infections: during the long hunter-gatherer stage of human history, our ancestors lived in small and scattered groups, so *Plasmodia malaria* parasites evolved in the direction of low grade but persistent infections that rarely kill their human carrier.[2]

When it did jump to a new host, *P. malariae* invariably enlisted the help of *Anopheles* mosquitoes. *Anopheles* means "good for nothing" in Greek, and while this description is true from the standpoint of humans it is entirely false from the perspective of the malaria plasmodia, which are dependent on *Anopheles* for transportation among their human victims. Indeed, the relationship between *Anopheles*, *Plasmodia*, and humans is both intimate and astonishingly complex. In order to colonize a new human victim, malaria parasites in mosquitoes must first develop into sporozoites (literally "seed animals"), which migrate into the mosquito salivary glands. When the mosquito feeds, it injects its prey with anticoagulant saliva; the primary purpose of this saliva is to prevent the mosquito proboscis from being clogged up by blood clotting agents, but the malaria plasmodia exploit this injection mechanism to spread to new human hosts. Once introduced, malaria sporozoites are carried by the bloodstream to the liver where they form schizonts, breeding factories for the parasite. When the swollen schizonts burst they release large numbers of merozoites, whose name in Greek translates roughly to "mid-stage life forms." These merozoites then return to the bloodstream and begin infiltrating human red blood cells.

The next stage of the process is where trouble begins for the plasmodia's unwilling human carriers. Once inside the red blood cells, the merozoites consume hemoglobin, create yet more schizonts, and eventually release a new waves of merozoites, rupturing the host blood cells in the process. These merozoites then seek fresh blood cells to colonize and the cycle continues. Since the merozoites and schizonts all follow similar timelines, the rupture of blood cells occurs at regular intervals, triggering predictable bouts of acute, intermittent fever. In the case of *P. malariae* the fevers occur and recur at three-day intervals, prompting ancient doctors to term them "quartan fevers," in other words, fevers which come back on the fourth day. The fever itself may be an inflammatory reaction of the human body to hemozoin, a waste product produced by the digestion of hemoglobin. This inflammatory reaction is compounded by the sudden and simultaneous loss of millions of red blood cells and their oxygen-carrying hemoglobin proteins, leading to deficient blood oxygen levels and corresponding bodily weakness.

At this point, malaria parasites are living large at the expense of their human carrier, but the clock is ticking, since the malaria victim will typically either fight off the infection or die trying. Thus, in order to find a new host, some portion of merozoites in the human body differentiate into male and female forms called gametocytes (in Greek, "reproductive cells"). When a mosquito bites an infected human malaria victim it ingests these gametocytes, which then combine sexually in the mosquito's stomach. The resulting zygote cells penetrate the mosquito's stomach wall and creates oocysts, Greek for "egg cell." Each oocyst eventually will release large numbers of sporozoites, which migrate to the mosquito salivary glands and begin the process anew.

Given the complexity of the malaria lifecycle, it seems almost miraculous that malaria infection occurs at all, and indeed scientists are now focusing on specific stages in this Rube Goldberg–esque process, such as the parasite's conversion of hemoglobin to hemozoin, in an attempt to break the chain for good. I should point out, though, that the text above, as detailed as it is, actually oversimplifies the malaria life cycle—I glossed over several intermediate stages of plasmodia development such as the trophozoite and ookinete phases. I should also point out that the process described here is valid only for *P. malariae*. As shall be seen, later species of malaria would add further stages or introduce further variants to an already-complex process in an effort to overcome human defenses.

The rivalry between malaria and mankind, therefore, has been both long and intimate. In his fascinating 2014 book on malaria in Ethiopia, James McCann likened this struggle to an "ever-changing dance" in which host and parasite constantly change their movements in response to each other's steps. Human beings, for example, have never been passive victims of malarial infection, and at-risk populations have long adopted cultural practices that reduce the dangers posed by their unwanted dance partner. In my own research on malaria in the pre-modern Arabian Peninsula, for example, I found that Arabs tended to associate some oases and drainage basins with *jinn*, potentially malevolent spirits who could possess visiting humans and afflict them with illness. These *jinn* were said to be most dangerous at around nightfall, which is not coincidentally the preferred feeding time for malaria's *Anopheles* insect carriers. Arabian Bedouins avoided some oases altogether during the most dangerous season: Yemeni camel-herders, for example, knew to avoid the "cloud-steaming lowlands" during the summer as "all who go there when the dates are in flower, fall ill with a fever and die."[3] Arabs also adapted to the malaria threat by employing large numbers of malaria-resistant African slaves as proxy farmers in Arabia's humid date oases rather than cultivating these oases themselves. In the era before modern medicine, such avoidance tactics were mankind's most reliable defense against malaria: if you can't out-dance your partner, you could at least stay clear of the dance floor, or perhaps have someone else dance in your place.

Unfortunately, malaria could learn new dance moves too. Sometime around 200,000 to 300,000 years ago a variant of malaria emerged that could break into red blood cells much more efficiently by exploiting certain proteins on the cellular wall. This malaria species, now called *P. vivax*, developed faster and probably killed more frequently than its *malariae* cousin. As a result, *vivax* epidemics probably burned like a wildfire through defenseless human populations. Human evolution soon responded with a new dance step of its own: the Duffy negative antigen, which causes red blood cells to discontinue producing precisely those vulnerable proteins that *vivax* uses to break into blood cells. Carriers of the Duffy negative antigen are somewhat more disposed to asthma and some other ailments than their Duffy positive counterparts but this disability is counterbalanced by their considerable resistance to *vivax* infection.

Vivax recovered from this setback by once again finding a way to change the rules of the dance. Unlike the less aggressive *P. malariae* parasite, *P. vivax* was long limited to tropical Africa since chains of *vivax* infection necessitated constant circulation between human hosts by mosquito vectors, making it impossible for *vivax* to sustain itself in areas where temperature was too low to maintain year-round mosquito activity. However, at some point within the last 10,000 years ago *vivax* developed the ability to lie dormant in the human body in the form of hypnozoites, a term that basically means "sleeper cells." Thanks to hypnozoites, *vivax* could now wait out the winter in the human liver and then emerge in the spring when mosquitos began to rouse from winter hibernation. As a result, the dance floor of *P. vivax* expanded dramatically. *P. vivax* is today the most world's most widespread form of malaria, and *vivax* epidemics have been recorded as far north as Ontario in Canada and Archangel on Russia's Arctic coast. Wherever it went, *vivax* made itself at home by evolving into a host of local variants, each of which times the latency period of its hypnozoite stage to match the weather conditions and mosquito breeding habits of specific geographic locations.[4]

One of those locations was almost certainly Lugnano, whose farmers were no strangers to *vivax* malaria. *Vivax* was present in Italy long before the founding of Rome, and Lugnano's farmers probably knew it as "spring fever," a seasonal affliction that set in from April through June. The mortality rate from *vivax* in Lugnano was probably fairly low, as *vivax* seems to have learned some manners as it moved northwards from Africa and infections by *vivax*, while certainly debilitating, are rarely deadly. Outside of Africa, the mortality rate for *vivax* among untreated victims is usually about 5 percent, and can be as low as 1 or 2 percent.[5] Although it is impossible to know for sure, Lugnano's farmers may have also enjoyed some degree of genetic protection against *vivax* infections. Although the Duffy Negative antigen is not very common in Italy, many Italians suffer from thalassemia, a blood disorder which leads to anemia but is protective against malaria.[6] So too is glucose-6-phosphate dehydrogenase deficiency, a mouthful of a malady, and one more commonly known as favism.[7] Carriers of two copies of this gene are normally asymptomatic but can be thrown into crisis by exposure to certain foods such as fava beans, triggering blood cell breakdown, anemia, and lethargy. Despite these disadvantages this negative trait persisted in Italy, and possibly in Lugnano, as it offered some defense against malarial infection.

P. falciparum *Joins the Dance*

In comparison to *vivax*, which has been dancing with our species for tens of thousands of years, *P. falciparum* arrived late to the ball. An ancient primate plasmodia species, *Falciparum* probably jumped to humans now and again during our long hunter-gathering apprenticeship, but never stuck. This is not because it was insufficiently infective—in fact, quite the opposite was true. While *P. malariae* and *P. vivax* only attacked about 1 percent and 2 percent of red blood cells respectively, *P. falciparum* is ferocious, attacking all red corpuscles indiscriminately to the point that up to 80 percent of a human victim's red blood cells may be invaded and destroyed. However, this very virulence, combined with *falciparum*'s inability to produce *vivax*-style hypnozoites, kept *falciparum* from switching species on a sustained basis. The high death toll that follows in the wake of a falciparum epidemic would have meant, paradoxically, that not enough human carriers remained to transmit the disease to a new round of *Anopheles* mosquitoes, breaking the chain of infection. Deprived of its dance partner, *falciparum* would have retreated back to the gorilla population reservoir from which it came.[8]

Falciparum finally got the chance to colonize mankind permanently around 10,000 to 5,000 years ago, and humans were themselves to blame. At that time, agriculture had begun to spread into equatorial Africa, triggering a wave of forest clearance. This set the stage for *falciparum* in two ways. First of all, deforestation created new habitats for *A. gambiae* mosquitoes, voracious year-round feeders that were strongly anthropophilic, meaning that they greatly preferred human over animal blood. Secondly, agriculture could sustain far higher population densities than hunter-gathering. Even if *falciparum* took a heavy annual toll on the health and the lives of the inhabitants of an equatorial African village, agriculture's bounty ensured that enough survivors remained to serve as carriers. Falciparum thus became an endemic disease in African farming populations, constantly burning within the population, and falling disproportionately on the young, who had the least previous exposure to the disease.[9]

As before, malaria's new dance moves provoked a human counterpoint, though this time our response smacked of desperation. Around 7,200 years ago, a girl was born with an abnormal copy of the gene that manufactures hemoglobin. When "Sickle-cell Eve" was attacked by *P. falciparum*, the hemoglobin in her cells fused with itself, morphing her blood cells from their normal doughnut shape into miniature croissants.[10] These blood stream gymnastics were highly protective against *falciparum* malaria, which cannot invade these altered red corpuscles, and as a result the carriers of the sickle-cell trait tend to suffer only one tenth the death rate from *falciparum* as those with normal hemoglobin.

Not surprisingly, the sickling trait spread rapidly throughout African tropical populations. However, the protection offered by the S-hemoglobin mutation comes at a terrible price. While carriers of only one copy of the sickle-cell gene are mostly unaffected by the trait, children with two copies suffer continual bouts of anemia, pain, swelling, vulnerability to bacterial infection, and stroke, since the malformed cells in their blood stream can get stuck in vein junctions and block the flow of blood. As a result, in the absence of modern medicine, most homozygous (two copy) carriers of the sickling trait do not survive childhood. One out of four children born to sickle-cell carriers, therefore, are doomed to a short and painful life.

As bad as the sickle-cell trait can be, it flourished in the human gene pool wherever *P. falciparum* was present due to *falciparum*'s ferocious assault on the human body. The most

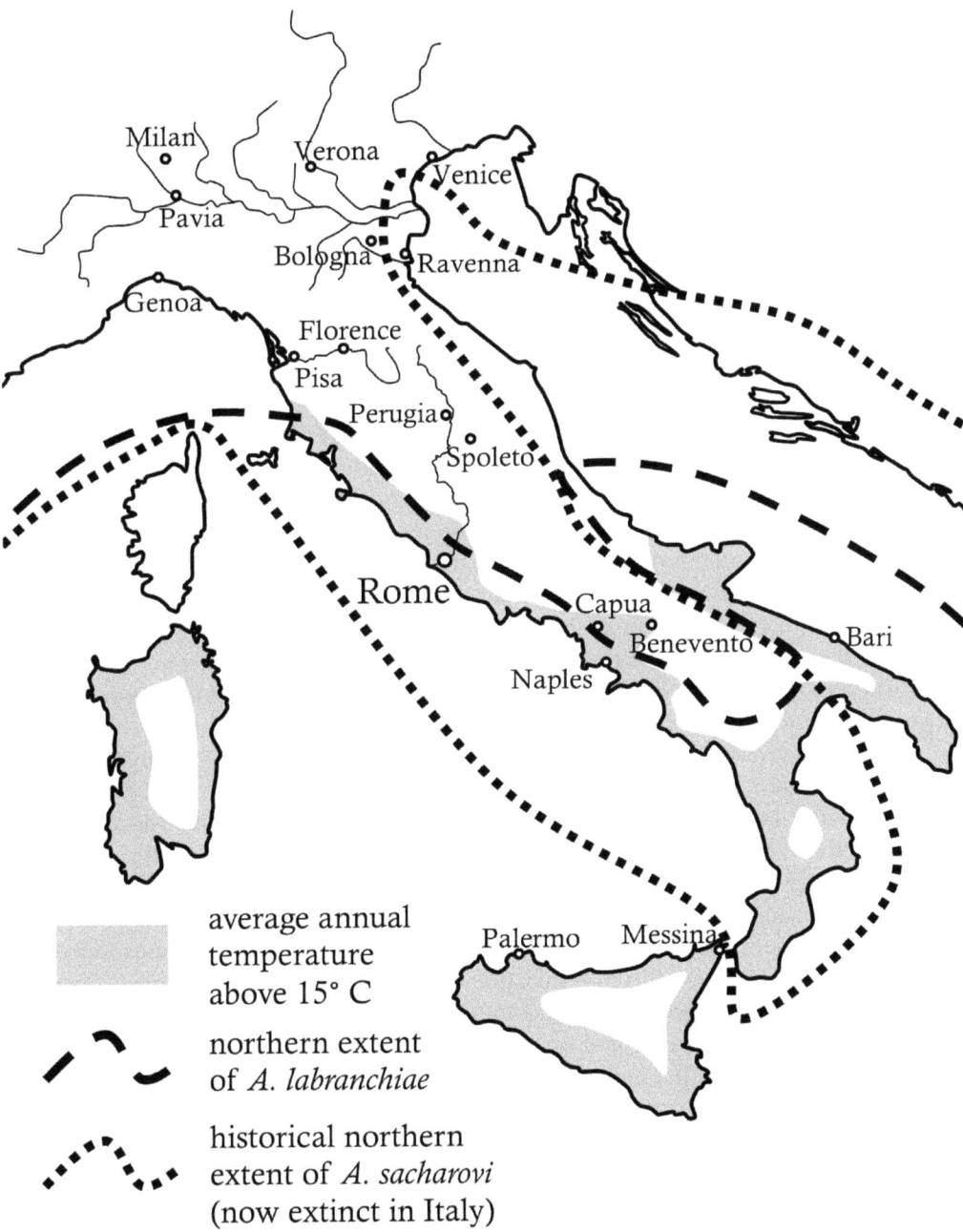

Italy, Average Annual Temperature Above 15° C and Northern Range of Malaria Vectors. Adapted from Benjamin James Reilly, "Cardinal Numbers: Changing Patterns of Malaria and Mortality in Rome, 494–1850," *Journal of Interdisciplinary History*, Vol. 49, no. 3 [2019], p. 399, © Massachusetts Institute of Technology and the Journal of Interdisciplinary History, Inc.

common symptom of *falciparum* infections is a high fever, usually tertian (recurring on the third day) as with *vivax* infection, though fevers caused by *falciparum* are sometimes continuous and unrelenting. Victims also suffer from chills, sweating, dizziness, pain, nausea, and diarrhea. As the mothers of Lugnano knew all too well, *P. falciparum* also complicates pregnancy, raising the rate of spontaneous abortion, stillbirths and premature labor. Worse yet, *falciparum* has a particularly dangerous dance step in its repertoire. In order to avoid being destroyed in the human liver, which constantly cleans the blood, *falciparum* schizonts induce their host cells to become sticky and adhere to blood cell walls. In the process, these cells can clog up the small vessels that serve the brain, leading to "cerebral malaria"—delirium, seizures, loss of consciousness, coma, and (frequently) death. As a result, the toll of death reaped by *falciparum* is typically much higher than that of *malariae* and *vivax*. Exact mortality rates are hard to come by, but *falciparum*'s death rate in unacclimated victims can be as high as 20 percent to 30 percent, and even with modern medical intervention death rates amongst *falciparum* patients with cerebral malaria range can reach 50 percent.[11]

Luckily for mankind, *falciparum* has an Achilles heel: it cannot dance in the cold. While *vivax* requires an ambient temperature of only about 15°C (59°F) to form sporozoites in mosquitos, *falciparum* cannot develop into an infective form in temperatures below 20°C (68°F), and develops optimally at temperatures above 30°C (86°F).[12] In addition, since *falciparum* cannot develop hypnospores, it depends on continuous transmission and re-transmission even through the winter, meaning that *falciparum* cannot survive in places where temperatures are too cold to allow for at least some winter-time mosquito activity. As a result, large parts of the world, including most of Europe, lie outside of *falciparum*'s effective reach.

These limitations would have been small comfort for the farmers of Lugnano, however, who had the misfortune to live just within the northern extent of *P. falciparum*'s range. Lugnano's average temperatures exceed 20°C in five months of the year, from May through October, and July and August temperatures peak at around 30°C, the butter zone for *falciparum* plasmodial development. Still worse, Lugnano is close to the range of *A. labranchiae* mosquitoes, which feed intermittently throughout region's mild winters and are nearly as efficient a vector for malaria as Africa's dreaded *A. gambiae* mosquitoes. *A. labranchiae* is also highly anthropophilic, preferring blood meals from humans over animals. This is crucially important because in order for plasmodia to spread to new hosts, mosquitos must bite humans at least twice: once to acquire the parasite, and once to transmit it to a further victim. If a mosquito prefers four-legged hosts, and only bites humans 1/20th of the time, the chance of any given mosquito transmitting malaria might be only about 1 in 400. For an anthropophilic mosquito like *labranchiae*, however, humans might make up half of all blood meals, so the comparable chance of transmission would be 1 in 4.[13] Since the chance of acquiring malaria rises exponentially with the rate at which mosquitos prefer human blood, the presence of *A. labranchiae* at Lugnano would no doubt have contributed enormously to the toll taken by malaria amongst infants and the unborn.

But so what? While the suffering that *A. labranchiae* and *P. falciparum* inflicted upon the farmers of Lugnano was tragic, it was a local tragedy, limited to a handful of rustics in an obscure corner of the Tiber Valley. What is more, Lugnano was not a common destination for foreign visitors, so it kept its misery to itself. Unfortunately for European travelers, however, the same biological and geographic realities that plagued Lugnano were equally present in another town which lay about 75 miles south along the same river. It is to Rome we now turn.

2

Romulus' Mistake

In late October 1739, after a meandering tour of Northern Italy, French traveler Charles de Brosses was finally approaching the outskirts of Rome. He was not impressed by what he saw. The hills south of Siena, he judged, were "not mountains, but skeletons, cemeteries of rocks, all covered up with debris of burned-up mountains, without a single twig of greenery."[1] Closer still to Rome was the "famous *campagna*" or field of Rome, which resembled a "prodigious and continuous quantity of sterile little hills, uncultivated, absolutely deserted, sad and horrible to the last. Romulus," he concluded, "must have been drunk when he dreamt of building a town upon such ugly terrain."[2]

Although de Brosses was fascinated by the contrast between the glory of Rome and the drear of Rome's *campagna*, he did not linger long to consider the matter. The *campagna*, he knew, was dangerous terrain, empoisoned by the "*intempérie* of the air," fatal miasmas which arose when the hot Italian sunshine interacted with the stagnant waters of the marshes.[3] As a result, de Brosses—like many transalpine travelers before and afterward—hurried through the uninhabited *campagna* to the comparative safety of the occupied districts of the city of Rome.

The Gifts of Tiburnus

So why *was* Rome founded amidst such an ugly and unhealthy landscape? The answer lies along the banks of Rome's river, the Tiber. While not the largest river in Italy—that honor belongs to the Po in the Northern Italian plain—the Tiber is a river of considerable size and length, arising in a beech forest on the flanks of Mount Fumaiolo in the Apennine Range of central Italy and then meandering 406 kilometers to the Mediterranean, draining in the process a territory larger than the state of Connecticut. On average, the Tiber's waters flow at an average rate of about 240 square meters per second, which admittedly is not an especially impressive volume of water. While the Tiber's discharge far surpasses that of London's Thames, which is more of a tidal estuary than a freshwater river in any case, Paris' Seine River contains over twice the Tiber's discharge volume, and the mighty Danube of Eastern Europe boasts over 30 times the Tiber's flow.

The modest current of the Tiber, however, has exerted a pull on Italian history entirely disproportional to its size. Indeed, the foundation legend of Rome itself begins with the waters of the Tiber. As the story goes, in ancient Latium lived the priestess Silvia, a virgin sworn to celibacy in the service of Vesta, the goddess of the hearth. While tending Vesta's ever-burning fires, the lovely Silvia caught the eye of the war-god Mars, who disregarded her vows and begat with her twin sons, Romulus and Remus. Regarding Silvia's pregnancy as an impious betrayal of her sacred office but fearing the displeasure of Silvia's divine lover, the King of Latium chose to eliminate the children indirectly by exposing them to the elements. The king therefore bundled the babes into a basket and dispatched one of his lackeys to toss the children into the Tiber. The man charged with the task, however, found the river swollen with winter rains, and due to the standing pools of floodwater on river's banks he was unable to reach the churning midstream flood. As a result, instead of being swept down river and out to sea the boys were deposited, like young Moses, safely in verdure of the riverbank.[4] Today, we would ascribe their salvation to an eddy current stirred up by the river's central torrent, but the ancient Romans attributed the boy's survival to the benevolence of the god Tibernus, who gave the river his name.

In addition to acting as an agent of divine providence, the river played a more prosaic role in the founding of Rome, since its lynchpin strategic location dictated that any city built on its banks would loom large in the history of Italy. While the mouth of the Tiber lies on the west coast of Italy, its headwaters lie far closer to the east coast, less than 70 kilometers as the crow flies from the Adriatic Sea. As a result, the Tiber effectively cuts Italy in half and poses a formidable barrier to north-south travel. Whoever controlled the crossing of the Tiber would have held considerable sway over central Italy, not only because they could control a choke-point of trade, but because they would have been at the center of a far-flung web of regional communication.

The founders of Rome, however, probably did not have these considerations in mind. Rather, they would have been initially attracted to Rome's hills. Today, the hills of Rome rise only modestly above the surrounding riverfront terrain, in large part because a thick layer of accumulated rubble and debris has softened their contours. In the ancient era, however, the hills were far steeper and thus offered their inhabitants some degree of protection. Farmers and shepherds clinging to these heights could have seen their enemies coming at a distance and would have held the high ground in a fight. The hills afforded some safety against non-human threats as well. The flocks of ancient Latium were probably prey to wolves—indeed, Romulus and Remus were initially suckled by a she-wolf before they were adopted by a kindly shepherd—and such shepherds probably herded their goats and sheep up the hillsides for defense each night. Small wonder, then, that these Tiber-side hills have been inhabited off and on for at least 14,000 years and have hosted permanent settlements since the 14th century BCE.

More to the point, Rome's hills also offered protection from a different sort of threat, the malarial fevers of the surrounding lowlands. We have precious little archeological or literary evidence concerning malaria in Rome at this early date—the first written references to intermittent fevers in Roman literature date only to the 2nd century BCE.[5] However, evidence from nearby Greece suggests that malaria, including the dreaded *P. falciparum*, had colonized the Mediterranean basin well before the founding of Rome. The *Iliad*, which was likely composed in the mid–8th century BCE, describes autumn as the season in which the sun's "burning breath taints the red air with fevers, plagues, and death."[6] By the 4th century BCE, Greek physician Hippocrates had already identified malaria as a distinct category of infections, distinguishing different strains according to their tertian, quartan, or quotidian (daily) recurrence. Taken together, Hippocrates argues, malarial infections were the "worst, most protracted and most painful of all the diseases then occurring."[7] There can be little doubt that the moist river valley of the Tiber, which reaches about the same summertime high temperatures as Athens, would have boasted similar seasonal afflictions.

2. Romulus' Mistake

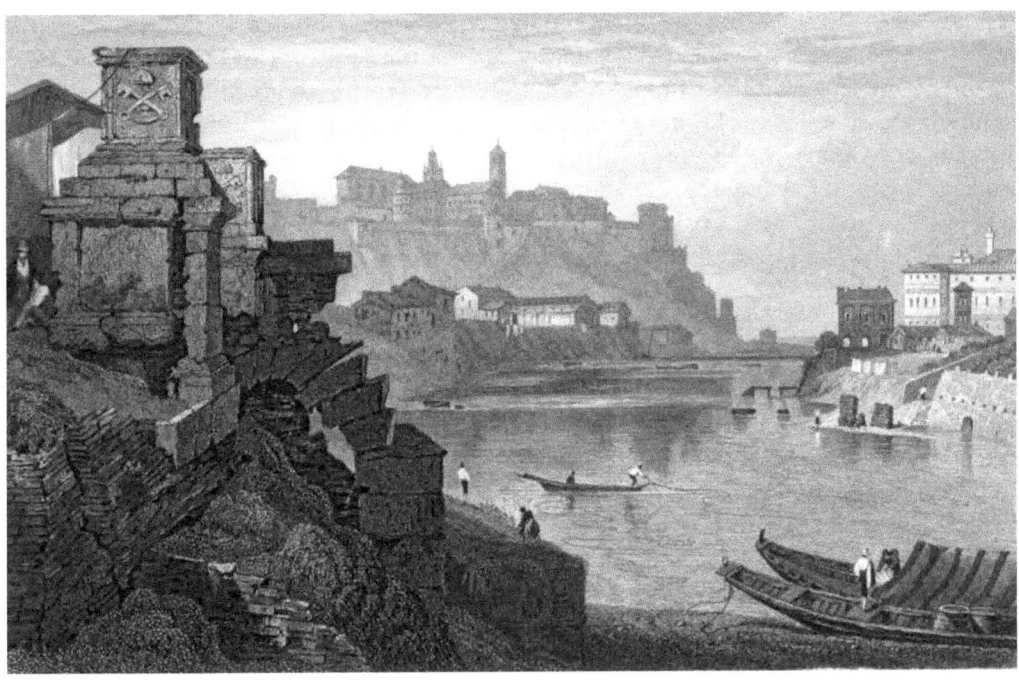

A somewhat idealized 19th-century view of Aventine Hill, preferred city-site of Romulus, looming over the Tiber River. Thomas Roscoe, *The Continental Tourist: Views of Cities and Scenery in Italy, France, and Switzerland, Series Two* [London: Peter Jackson, 1850], between pp. 64 and 65.

Given the strategic and health benefits of the heights above the Tiber, it was never in question that Rome would be founded upon a hill. The real question was *which* hill. According to legend, Remus preferred the Aventine, which looms steeply over the Tiber. Romulus, however, favored the centrally-located Palatine hill where the she-wolf Lupa had suckled them in infancy. Unable to agree, the brothers came to blows—they were sons of a war god, after all—and the argument was settled by Remus's death. After wiping his brother's blood from his hands, Romulus went on to personally establish most of the enduring institutions of Rome, including the urban tribes and their tribunes, the Senate and the patrician class, and the division of the army into "centuries" of a hundred men. Or so the story goes. In reality, the creation of Rome was probably not due to a one-time founding event but was instead the result of a slow process of fusion, with the largest village, the one atop the Palatine, gradually gaining ascendency over its near neighbors.

Rise of Rome

This town had a bright future ahead of it, but for the moment it was just a minor riverside outpost and a petty political player within Latium, which in turn was just one region of Italy among many. For the first two centuries, the Romans were ruled by kings, but the monarchy was broken in 509 when King Tarquin was driven from Rome after forcing himself upon the wife of a Roman nobleman. This act marked the birth of Rome's republican institutions, but the infant republic was almost stillborn. In the years that followed, Rome barely survived a pair of attacks, first the by powerful Etruscans and later by the Latin League, both of which sought to restore Tarquin to his Roman throne. More conflicts would follow, as Rome's growing power was challenged by its regional rivals, the Sabines, the Umbri, the Picentes, the Marsi, and above all the powerful Samnites of the central Apennines. Along the way, Rome slowly gobbled up the territory of the Etruscans, who were in decline after unsuccessfully challenging Greek colonists in the heel, toe, and instep of Italy. The Etruscans live on today only as a geographic expression: their former homeland is the modern province of Tuscany.

Rome's underdog success against these various foes was doubtless due to a number of factors. One important advantage that Rome possessed was its republican institutions. Now that Tarquin and his brood were gone, Romans competed amongst themselves for power and prestige, and warlike valor became a sure way to raise yourself above your rivals. However, geography still offers the most compelling explanations for Rome's rise to hegemony within Italy. Geographers classify Rome as a "bridge city," in other words a city built at the first upriver site where bridge construction is a practical possibility. Below Rome the Tiber is too wide and the banks too swampy for bridge building, at least with the techniques available to the ancients. At Rome, however, the banks of the Tiber are constrained by a series of low volcanic hills, most notably the Palatine, the Aventine, and the Capitoline, and these hills both narrow the Tiber and provide a firm bedrock footing for bridge construction. Rome also benefited from Tiber Island at the foot of Capitoline, allowing the early Romans to bridge the Tiber with two smaller and more cost-efficient spans. As a result, Rome became the natural conduit for all north-south coastal travel along the length of the Italian peninsula and the hub of a road network linking the Apennine interior to the Tuscan north and the plains to the south.[8] In its conflicts with its regional enemies, therefore, Rome enjoyed a decided transportation and communication advantage.

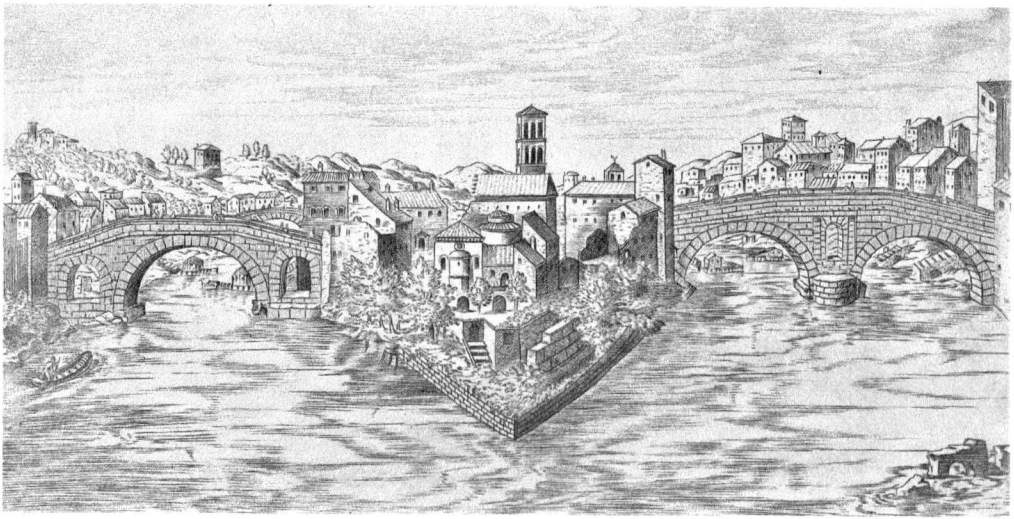

Tiber Island and its bridges as they appeared in the early 17th-century Etienne du Perac, *I Vestigi dell'Antichità di Roma: Raccolti et Ritratti in Perspettiva con Ogni Diligentia* [Rome, 1621], p. 39.

Thanks to these early military successes against its Italian neighbors, 3rd century Rome had the resources it needed to expand out of central Italy. Its first encounter with a non–Italian army was a near-disaster; following a dispute with the Greek city Tarentum on Italy's southern coast, the Tarantines appealed to the Greeks of Epirus for help, and the phalanxes and war elephants of the Epirite Greeks defeated Roman forces in two decisive battles. Luckily for Rome, these Greek victories came at such a high price that the Greek general Pyrrhus had to abandon the war and his name has been synonymous with too-costly victories ever since. Much the same drama played out when Rome challenged the Carthaginians, a North African city-state of Phoenician origins which dominated Sicily and the Iberian Peninsula. Pontic general Hannibal waged a punishing campaign against the Romans that culminated in a disastrous Roman defeat at the battle of Cannae. Nonetheless, Rome eventually prevailed by drawing on its deep pool of central Italian manpower and with its victory Rome supplanted Carthage as the dominant naval power of the Western Mediterranean. In the meantime, Rome annexed parts of Illyria in what is today Dalmatia in an attempt to subdue the Ardiaei pirates, bringing Rome into conflict with Greek Macedonia, to whom the Ardiaei appealed for help. The result was more than fifty years of conflict, and when the dust settled in the mid–2nd century the Roman Republic found itself in control over Greece, parts of Asia Minor, and the entire Western Adriatic Coast.

From Republic to Empire

These overseas conquests, however, put enormous strain on Rome's republican political institutions, designed for the governance of a single city rather than a sprawling, multinational state. As Rome expanded, successful generals were able to acquire an unconstitutional share of political power and influence, in part because such men were enriched by the spoils of war, but also thanks to the clientage relationships they enjoyed with their own military veterans. The breaking point finally came during the 1st century CE in the person of Julius Caesar, a Roman governor who achieved tremendous military success in France and Britain but ran afoul of the traditionalist party within the Senate. When that faction threatened to charge him with treason for waging unsanctioned wars and demanded his resignation, Caesar countered by taking his army across the Rubicon River, which marked the limit of his legal authority, and marching directly on Rome. Over the course of the next five years the industrious Julius defeated his domestic enemies in a civil war, fought successful military campaigns in Egypt and Asia Minor, reformed the Roman provincial system, issued coins decorated with his image, and intimidated the Senate into declaring him dictator for a ten-year term. He also demanded that the Senate bestow upon him the title of *imperator*, meaning "victorious commander." In some ways, this would be Caesar's greatest legacy: the term "emperor" was thereby introduced into the European vocabulary and the fantasy that there should be a single, sacred, and universal political authority over the entire world would haunt Europe's political thinking for the next two millennia.

Worried (and with good reason) that Rome was sliding back into monarchy, Caesar's enemies in the Senate assassinated him on the Ides of March in 44 BCE, but they proved unable to turn back the clock. Instead, Caesar's adopted son Octavian claimed the right to step into Caesar's shoes and after a short civil war Octavian ruled Rome as

Augustus Caesar for 41 years. Like Caesar before him, Augustus kept the framework of the old Roman republic mostly intact. However, Republican Rome's cherished institutions increasingly became a mere façade behind which Augustus transformed Rome into a centralized monarchy. What is more, not content to be merely the first among mortals, Augustus continued the process Julius Caesar had begun of transforming the *imperator* into a god. During his lifetime, Caesar had served as *pontifex maximus*, the high priest of the Roman state, and furthermore had claimed to be partially divine by virtue of his Julian ancestry, since the Julians traced their lineage to the loins of the goddess Venus. As Caesar's adopted son, Octavian demanded his own share of that that divinity, as epitomized by his chosen title of Augustus, meaning "majestic" or "venerable." Later emperors would follow this path even farther and over time temples to the cult of the *genius* (divine nature) of the emperor sprang up in most Roman cities. Even living emperors such as Domitian demanded that their subjects address them as "master and god." Rome was more than just a city, then: it was the earthly seat of celestial power.

In addition to transforming the Roman political system, Rome's foreign conquests fundamentally altered the layout of Rome itself. Thanks to the influx of overseas resources, Rome became a wealthy imperial capital. Its population ballooned, rising from just a few thousands in the 5th century BCE to over a half-million by the end of the Republican era and an apogee of over 1 million during the 1st century CE. These multitudes overwhelmed the provisioning capacity of the province of Latium, so Rome was forced to import much of its supplies, and in this endeavor the Tiber proved itself once again to be Rome's most invaluable ally. Since the Tiber is navigable south of Rome, some seagoing vessels could unload their cargoes directly into the wharves that sprung up south of the bridges over the Tiber. Alternatively, large vessels could dock at Ostia near the mouth of the Tiber and transship their produce to Rome cheaply on barges pulled up the Tiber by draft animals. If not for the lower Tiber, which opened a door to the resources of the Mediterranean basin, Rome could never have served as the capital city of an empire.

These naval imports into Rome were so large in scale that they have left an unexpected mark on the geography of the modern city. Just inland of the former wharf district in southern Rome rises Monte Testaccio, a 35-meter high artificial hill built entirely from the shards of an estimated 53 million olive oil amphorae. More astounding still is the fact almost all these amphorae originated in just one region, the Guadalquivir valley of Spain. Rome imported oil, wine, grain, and other provisions from elsewhere in the Mediterranean as well, but these other trade routes did not commemorate themselves upon the landscape of Rome with mountains of broken pottery. It is hypothesized that the amphorae and pottery vessels imported from elsewhere in the Mediterranean places were recycled or ground up to make cement, but that the Guadalquivir amphorae were unsuitable to those purposes either due to their shape or because of the insoluble fats that their oils contained.[9] Ironically, later Christian Romans did eventually find a creative way to re-use these amphorae. Until World War II, the Catholic Church used lonely Mount Testaccio each spring as a stand-in for Jerusalem's hill of Golgotha in its annual Good Friday re-enactment of the crucifixion.

Rome's population explosion transformed the city in other ways as well. Since the hills of Rome had few sources of water, Romans had long channeled distant hillside springs to Rome via aqueducts, and by the end of the Republican era Rome was served by at least four such structures. In the Imperial years that followed, another six aqueducts were built, in large part to supply water to the fountains, public baths, and other

2. Romulus' Mistake

edifices that emperors built as monuments to their memory. Even the aqueducts themselves bore the names of emperors, such as the *Aqua Claudia* of Claudius (41–54 CE) and the *Aqua Traiana* of the great soldier-emperor Trajan (98–117).[10] Rome's emperors were not just content to be gods in their lifetime—they wanted thirsty Romans to remember them fondly after their death.

However, these aqueducts could not solve a second problem faced by the growing city, namely the increasing overcrowding of Rome's hills, a problem exacerbated by the seizure of land on the heights by the emperors for palace construction. Plenty of flat land was available in the shadow of the hills, but the Romans had long reserved these malaria-prone lowlands for public functions.[11] The epitome of such spaces was the famous Forum, which lay on drained marshland between the Palatine and Capitoline hills and contained markets, law courts, public monuments, and ample space for political assembly. Similarly, the lowlands just southeast of the Forum became the site of the

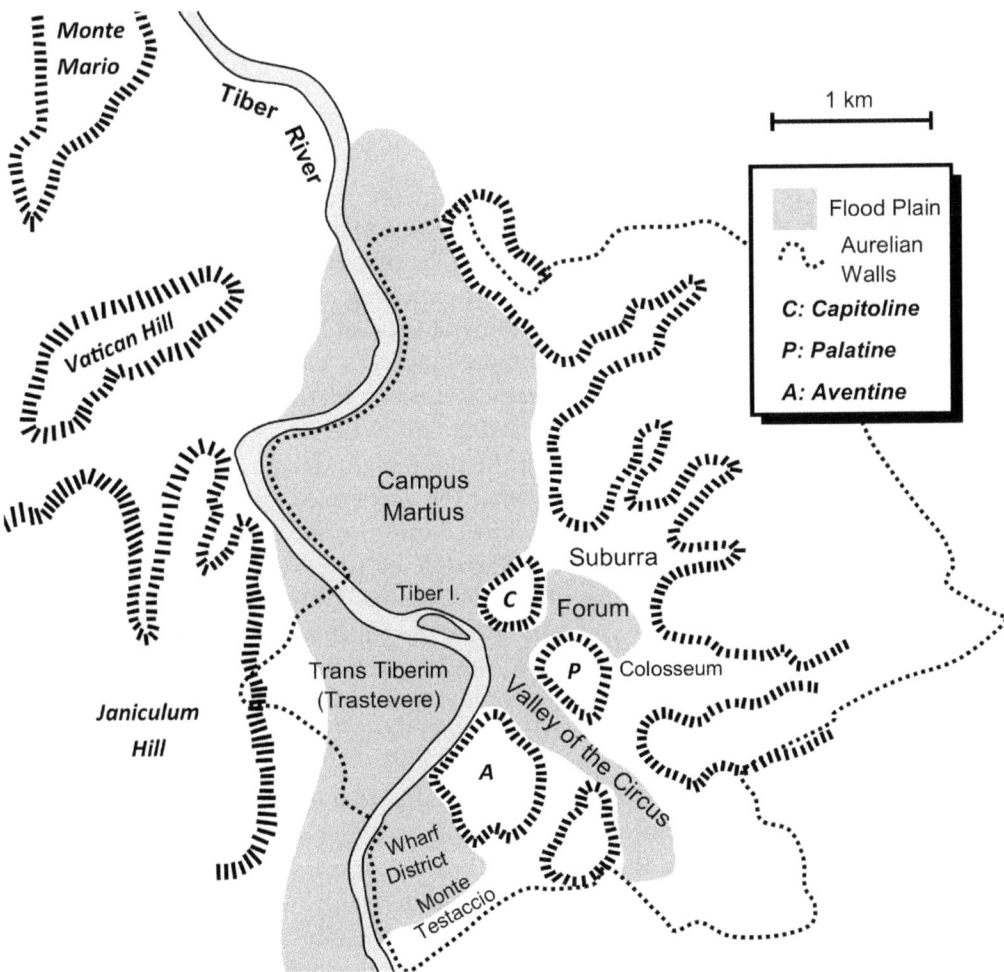

Rome, Hills and Floodplains. Sources: Joël Le Gall, *Le Tibre: Fleuve de Rome dans l'Antiquité* [Paris: Presses Universitaires de France, 1953], p. 34; Penelope J. E. Davies, "Pollution, Propriety, and Urbanism in Republican Rome," in Mark Bradley ed., *Rome, Pollution, and Propriety* [New York: Cambridge University Press, 2012], pp. 67–80.

Flavian amphitheater, an enormous structure better known to tourists today as the Colosseum. Built atop a filled lakebed in 85 CE, the Colosseum could seat an audience of up to 80,000, nearly a tenth of Rome's peak population. The narrow valley between the Palatine and Aventine was drafted into public service as well, becoming the site of religious ceremonies and gladiator games. It also featured chariot races, which gave this place its name: the *Circus Maximus*, so-called because of the circular path of its chariot track.

As housing on the heights became scarce, however, the lowlands were increasingly used for residential space as well. One such neighborhood was the Suburra, a suburb of Rome in a literal sense—it lay beneath (in Latin, *sub*) the urban core of the hilltop city. Nestled between the surrounding hills, the Suburra was warren of tall *insulae* buildings connected by narrow alleys, notorious for its whores, its crime, and its multi-ethnic population, since its cheap housing was favored by foreign migrants to the imperial capital.[12] Rome's population also began to expand into the Campus Martius, a flat plain north of the Capitoline hill traditionally used as a muster-ground for Roman armies preparing for war. By the Imperial age, however, the Campus Martius was increasingly given over to temples, theaters, and residential buildings.

Roman Fever

Unfortunately for the Romans, as the lowlands began to fill, the Tiber turned against the city it had long sustained. The same hills that facilitated bridge-building also bottlenecked descending floodwaters of the Tiber, threatening much of lowland Rome with catastrophic and persistent flooding.[13] The Roman historian Livy reported that in 241 BCE the "nearly all the city in the plain" was submerged under a Tiber flood, which "knocked down" some buildings by the "force of what was nearly a torrent" while other buildings collapsed after being "soaked in the long-lasting floodwaters."[14] As more and more residential buildings were constructed within the flood plain during the Imperial age, the problem grew still worse. In 15 CE, shortly after the death of Augustus, Tacitus reported that "the Tiber, swollen by constant rains, flowed into the flat area of the city" causing "destruction of buildings and loss of life."[15] Plutarch left us a vivid account of a particularly catastrophic 69 CE flood, during which floodwaters "swollen to an enormous size" toppled a wooden bridge over the river, and since the collapsed bridge acted as a makeshift dam, the backed-up Tiber overflowed "not only the flat parts of the city, but also parts usually free of such calamities." Unemployment and food shortages ravaged the poor of the city and apartment buildings throughout Rome collapsed because their foundations were "undermined by the stagnant water."[16]

Making matters worse, the same "stagnant waters" that destroyed human dwellings were themselves ideal habitat for an uninvited guest, *Anopheles* mosquitoes. Even in a normal year the lowland areas of Rome were favorable to mosquito breeding since the land between the hills and along the Tiber was riddled with swamps, depressions, and small lakes.[17] While the ancient Romans never made the connection between malaria and mosquitoes, they did associate marshes and waterlogged land with heavy, miasmic air, which they believed could produce deadly illness especially during the heats of late summer and early autumn—the habitual season of *P. falciparum* infection.[18] Certain low-lying areas in Rome, such as the banks of the Tiber and the valley of the Forum, had a particularly evil reputation for their bad air and fevers.[19] To combat this problem, ancient

Romans built a network of drains to wick away excess water, including the famous *Cloaca Maxima*, a "sacred sewer" that followed the meanders of a holy stream that once passed through the Forum.[20] Similar sewers were built to drain the Valley of the Circus and the Campus Martius, but during flood years these sewers were often overwhelmed and may even have worked in reverse, pumping floodwaters into the very depressions that the sewers were supposed to drain.[21] As a result, each major Tiber flood during the warm months of the year probably triggered a spike in malarial fevers.

Human-induced changes to the Tiber River over time further aggravated Rome's malaria problem. In an effort to satisfy the endless appetite of Rome's burgeoning population, farmers of the Roman *campagna* and the hill country of Latium practiced intensive agriculture, but this in turn triggered large-scale erosion, the rate of which rose by a factor of ten between the 2nd and 1st century BCE.[22] The problem of erosion was probably worsened by Rome's victorious wars, which drained the countryside of freemen and replaced them with agricultural slaves who, unlike freemen, did not own the land they worked and thus had no incentive to retain its soil for future generations.[23] Rome also required timber as well for construction and cooking fuel and the resulting deforestation of the hill country near Rome further compounded the erosion crisis.[24] By the early imperial era, the Tiber's waters were stained with so much erosion sediment that the poet Horace dubbed it the *flavius tiberius*, or the "Yellow Tiber."[25] Most of this dislodged soil settled down in the Tiber Delta, forming vast brackish swamps that were hotbeds for malaria infection.[26]

Farther upstream, deforestation led to a feverish cascade of environmental degradation in the Tiber Valley proper. Lack of tree cover led to increased run-off, while deposition of silt in the river bed reduced the carrying capacity of the river bed. Taken together, these twin processes increased the frequency and duration of the Tiber's floods. Worse yet, the water table level in the *campagna* became increasingly high, leading to further marshification of the soil and resulting pockets of "bad air." As a result the *campagna* surrounding Rome, which had previously supported large villas and substantial agricultural populations, became increasingly unhealthy.[27] Rural Romans would gradually adapt to this by relocating their permanent population to the healthier hills and exploiting the lowland plains mainly for winter-season cattle pasture. In the process, the *campagna* began to adopt the sterile and uncultivated appearance that greeted Charles de Brosses upon his approach to the Eternal City.[28]

Nor was the Eternal City itself immune from fever, despite the partial protection offered by its component hills. Ancient Rome was dotted with temples dedicated to the goddess of fever, *Dea Febris*, who was sometimes worshipped alongside with her sister goddesses *Dea Tertiana* and *Dea Quartiana*. Some of these fever temples, which were most commonly built in quarters of Rome notorious for their bad air, managed to survive into the Christian era, with pagan fever goddess replaced by miracle-working saints.[29] Case in point was the Roman Church of Maria Santissima delle Febbri, or "Most Holy Mary of the Fevers," a sanctuary for malaria-stricken Romans until its destruction in the late 18th century. Nor did ancient Romans rely on supernatural protection alone. Like their rural compatriots, urban Romans who could afford to fled the city's summer heat, waiting out the dangerous fever season in the Apennine foothill town of Tivoli or atop the windy heights of the Alban hills.[30] Despite such prophylactic measures, ancient Roman literature is replete with references to quartan and tertian fevers.[31]

Did the spread of malarial fevers during the Imperial Age help to trigger the fall of Rome? At least one scholar has argued just that. In an influential 1907 essay and subsequent publications, classicist W.H.S. Jones argued that malaria was probably introduced to Italy by the Carthaginians during the Punic Wars and once infected, Rome fell into a downward cycle of annual epidemics and population decline. Most historians of Rome, however, have rejected Jones' thesis. Although interdisciplinary work between history and biology has become more fashionable in recent decades, many historians still recoil at the prospect of combining the two, citing the eugenics movement and the scientific racism of the 20th century as cautionary examples. What is more, scholars have frowned upon Jones' tendency to link malaria to morality: Jones made the argument that malaria corrupted the national character of the Greeks, transforming them over time into weak and inefficient sodomites, while malaria-addled Romans were transformed from civic-minded republicans into "bloodthirsty brute[s]."[32] Still other scholars have attacked Jones on the grounds of biological determinism, despite the fact that Jones himself insisted that malaria was "but one out of many causes" for the decline in Greek civilization, "a single component of a most complex whole."[33]

Most crucially, Robert Sallares has argued convincingly that Jones got the timing of malaria wrong. Jones believed that malaria was not common in Greece until the 5th century and Italy until the Imperial era, but is its now widely accepted that *vivax* malaria was already present in Italy long before the Republic was founded and even *P. falciparum* had fairly deep roots in the southern Italian peninsula.[34] Thus, Romans of both the Republic and the Imperial period would have encountered malaria not as an epidemic disease attacking old and young indiscriminately but as an endemic disease constantly smoldering at a low rate within the population and killing mainly pregnant women and (most commonly) the very young. In the words of the 20th-century doctor and malaria control specialist L.W. Hackett, who knew his opponent well, humans living in the midst of endemic malaria usually "come to some sort of terms with their inveterate enemy, making an annual sacrifice of youth to obtain for the old a certain tolerable freedom from attack." Indeed, Hackett goes so far as to speculate that the myth of the Minotaur, a monstrous creature who demanded yearly tribute of "youths and maidens" from the citizens of Athens, might have been inspired by ancient Greece's own experience with endemic malaria.[35] Hackett did not live to see the excavations of Lugnano, but I suspect he would have interpreted its infant cemetery as a case-in-point example of just such a tribute to fever.

In fact, it would probably be more accurate to turn Jones' argument completely on its head and argue that malaria, far from undermining Rome, may actually have helped to protect Rome from its enemies. On the balance, Romulus had placed his city well. For Romans, malaria was a burden, but perhaps a bearable one, though the aggrieved mothers of nearby Lugnano might have thought otherwise. However, having never sacrificed their youths to the Minotaur, most transalpine travelers who risked the roads to Rome would have had few defenses against that city's malarial fevers. Consequently, over the course of over two millennia, Rome's endemic malaria could flare into deadly epidemics whenever European soldiers, pilgrims, ecclesiastics, tourists, and other travelers crossed the Alps and the Apennines into the Minotaur's domain.

3

Assessing the Threat

So exactly how dangerous was travel to Rome for non–Italian travelers during the pre-modern era? That question lies at the heart of this book.

Unfortunately, questions of this sort are stubbornly difficult to answer. Calculating the disease threat faced by the indigenous population of a historical location—much less short-term travelers to that location—is tricky business. Our greatest enemy in this endeavor is the lack of clear, systematically-collected sources. Ancient and Medieval Europeans did not have the same understanding of infection and disease than we do today, and the terminology they used to describe fevers is often ambiguous, in part because disease was generally ascribed to an imbalance in bodily humors rather than to an invasion by specific pathogens.[1] What is more, even when clear disease symptoms are given by a source, the fact that many diseases have similar or overlapping symptoms further clouds an already murky picture.

One tactic for resolving these problems, as epitomized by the work of disease historian Timothy P. Newfield, is to set a high bar for historical evidence. In his 2017 survey of malaria in early Medieval Europe, Newfield regarded only two types of evidence as definitive "category I" markers of malaria: (1) unambiguous textual references to intermittent fevers—especially tertian and quartan fevers—and (2) DNA recovered from ancient remains. Other forms of evidence, such as general reference to fevers, mentions of an undefined disease in predictably malarial locations, certain forms of skeletal evidence, and seasonality of illness as recorded by funerary epigraphy, are relegated to category II or III status: illustrative certainly, but not definitive on their own in establishing the existence of malaria in any given historical location. Newfield acknowledges that his methodology may seem excessively "narrow-minded," but argues that we must default to assuming *lack* of malaria unless this high standard is met, since it is possible that malaria may have waxed and waned over the course of European history due to climate change, localized extinctions of the plasmodia, and changes in *Anopheles* vector distribution.[2]

The fatal flaw with Newfield's approach, however, is that it can generate false-negative results, and the city of Rome is a case in point. In Newfield's scheme, malaria can only thrive in an environment inhabited by chroniclers who are sensitive to disease pathology and typology. One such locale was early Medieval central France, where the painstaking work of Gregory of Tours clearly established the existence of endemic malaria. In contrast, Newfield was able to discover very little unambiguous "category I" evidence for malaria in Rome. While he acknowledges that a large number of European travelers made reference to fevers when visiting the Eternal City, Newfield notes that these sources do not meet his high evidentiary standards as they fail to make explicit reference to tertian or quartan fever intervals, perhaps because the symptomatic fever from

Rome's *P. falciparum* malaria is often constant and unremitting. Thus, by a strict application of Newfield's scheme, early Medieval Rome must be classified as malaria-free, despite the fact that (as Newfield admits) "with at least 25,000 inhabitants, a riverside setting, and a suitable climate, Rome had the greatest malarial potential in all of early Medieval Europe."[3] Newfield goes on to speculate that "had Gregory of Tours lived in Rome the record would be well marked by intermittents."[4] Newfield's approach, therefore, tells us more about the thinness of certain types of evidence about malaria in Rome than it does about the actual disease situation in the Medieval *caput mundi*.

So by what standards can we measure Rome's malaria endemicity, or at least its relative morbidity and mortality in comparison to the situation that prevailed north of the Alps? I would argue that relative risks are inferable through a close examination of four distinct types of information: (1) anecdotal accounts of "bad air" and fever in the Eternal City, (2) 19th-century medical evidence, collected before eradication of malaria in Europe, (3) seasonal mortality rates as inferable from late Roman epigraphy, and (4) seasonal mortality rates amongst Catholic cardinals from the period from 400–1850. While none of these sources is sufficient on its own, taken together they provide powerful and compelling evidence about the virulence of Rome's resident malaria species in comparison to transalpine Europe's more benign malaria profile. Since the first of these sources, the anecdotal evidence, will be covered at the appropriate time eras in the narrative second half of this book, I will confine myself in the rest of this chapter to the latter three sources: 19th century medical studies on malaria in Italy, late Roman epigraphic evidence, and lessons we can infer from cardinal demography.

Pre-Eradication Medical Evidence

With one important exception that we will discuss below, our medical evidence on Rome and malaria is confined to the late 19th century, when malaria was already in slow retreat due to new medicines and growing population density. Nonetheless, I would contend that the picture we get about malaria during this late date is at least somewhat representative of malaria's impact on Italy in the pre-modern era.

Not all scholars agree, of course. As mentioned above, Newfield is highly skeptical of just such an approach to the topic, arguing that we cannot presume that early disease environments were identical to those of the recent past. As for myself, I think Newfield's extreme caution is unwarranted. Malaria is an endemic disease deeply rooted in specific landscapes, linked to specific geographical conditions and temperature regimens that change only slowly over time. While malaria does exhibit some predictable year to year variation due to changes in rainfall and temperature, the medical evidence we do have on malaria in Italy suggests considerable continuity in infection rates. What is more, Newfield's belief that climate change may have supercharged or suppressed Italy's malaria rate in the past is not supported by recent research, which argues that historical climate change in Italy seems to have been both localized in scale and moderate in scope.[5] Indeed, as we will see later in this chapter when discussing the evidence derived from church cardinal demography, factors other than climate change offer the best explanation for observed gradual changes in Rome-area malaria rates.

Nor does any particular evidence exist to support Newfield's second concern, that plasmodia and *Anopheles* species in Italy changed dramatically over time. Quite the opposite, in fact: according to Robert Sallares and other authors, abundant textual and some forensic anthropological evidence suggests that *P. falciparum* was already commonplace around Rome by the late imperial period.[6] If anything, the range of malaria seems to have further expanded after the empire's fall, with some previously healthy landscapes, such as the mouth of the Po river, succumbing to endemic malaria due to colonization by new mosquito vectors by the end of the 8th century CE.[7] As for *A. labranchiae*, malaria's main mosquito vector in Rome and its surrounding *campagna*, the available evidence suggests it may have been introduced to the west coast of Italy from North Africa via Sardinia as early as the 7th century BCE, and no extant evidence suggests that *A. labranchiae's* habitat shrank thereafter, at least not until the anti-mosquito campaigns of the 20th century.[8] Thus, the available medical evidence we have of malaria in late 19th-century Italy probably gives us some indication about malaria in the pre-modern period as well, since the preceding centuries were probably characterized by roughly similar rates of pathogen presence, vector availability, and ambient temperatures.

So what picture does 19th-century medical science give us about the last years of malaria in Italy? According to data collected by Italian malariologist Angelo Celli, Roman hospitals tallied a total of 92,992 malaria cases from 1864 to 1896. As is typical of malaria, particular the *P. falciparum* variety, the number of cases spiked over the course of the Roman summer, rising from 2,553 cases in June (2.7 percent of the total cases) to 8,844 in July (9.5 percent of cases) and finally to a high of 17,678 cases in August, which accounted for a full 19 percent of annual malaria cases. Malaria levels in Roman hospitals remained high in September (16.3 percent of all cases), the second-most malarial month, before abating in October and November, which accounted for 13.7 percent and 10.2 percent of all cases respectively. By December, malaria rates in Roman hospitals had dropped off dramatically, and would remain low through June.[9] Other hospitals in 19th-century Italy also reported significant numbers of malaria cases, though cities in cooler Northern Italy

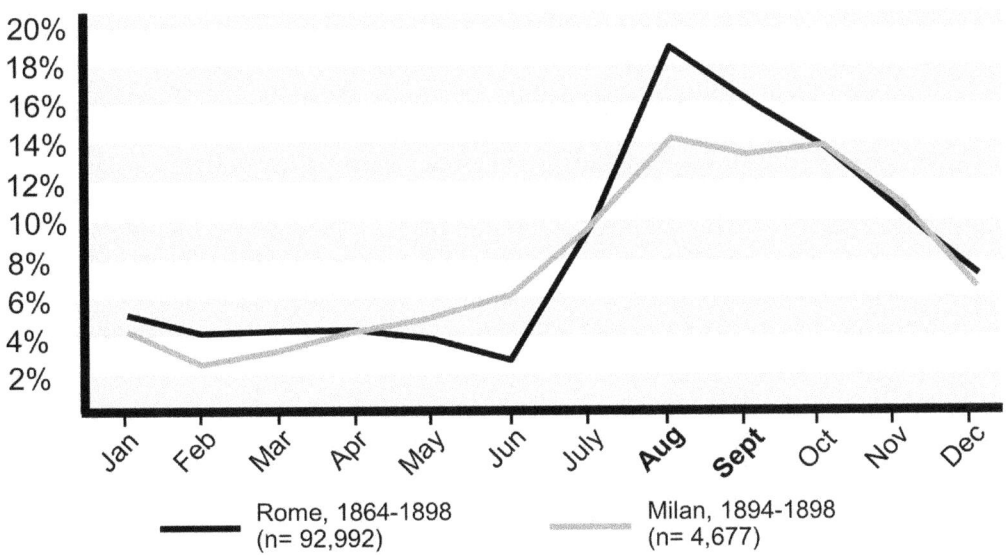

Malaria Cases in Italian Hospitals by Month, Late 19th Century. Source: Angelo Celli, *Malaria, According to the New Researches* (New York: Longmans, Green, 1900), pp. 149, 156).

such as Milan recorded both fewer overall cases and a less pronounced August–September spike, as one might expect in an area where *P. vivax* rather than *P. falciparum* was the predominant plasmodia species.[10]

Other available evidence suggests that Italian malaria rates in the late 19th century were considerably higher, perhaps by an order of magnitude, than in countries north of the Alps. According to statistics collected by malaria researchers Leonard Jan Bruce-Chwatt and Julian de Zulueta, the malaria infection rate in Germany was about 1.23 per 100 per year in 1877. By contrast, Italy still suffered a .75 per 100 *death* rate from malaria ten years later in 1887, which probably corresponds with an infection rate of about 12 per 100—about 10 times the malaria infection rate as Germany.[11] Overall, therefore, 19th century medical records suggest that malaria was a frequent though seasonal affliction in Italy, and that Italy's malaria rate may have been an order of magnitude higher than that of Europe north of the Alps

Military Malaria: Evidence from the French Occupation of Rome, 1849–1850

As we move backwards from 1860, hard evidence about malarial rates becomes far scantier. However, there is one notable exception: French doctor Félix Jacquot's excellent but underutilized medical history of the French occupational army in Rome from 1849 to 1852. The data Jacquot provides are especially useful since they describe malaria infections amongst soldiers, who as we shall see in later chapters were frequent visitors to the Eternal City, especially during the golden age of German Imperial engagement with Rome in the 9th through the 14th centuries. The value of Jacquot's text is further augmented by the fact that he had previous experience with diagnosing and treating malaria infections while serving as a medical officer for the French army in North Africa. Indeed, Jacquot would find that the "miasmic influence" of Rome's *campagna* was equal to that of the "most unhealthy regions of the Algerian coast."[12]

In his medical history of the French occupation of Rome, Jacquot records that 440 French soldiers died in the three largest French hospitals alone during the first seven months of the French occupation. According to official statistics, the greatest single cause of death in those months was typhoid fever, a trendy new disease that had recently been classified and described in mid-century medical literature. In Jacquot's opinion, however, most of the supposed typhoid cases were in reality misdiagnosed malaria, which he believed to be responsible for the vast majority of the casualties.[13] Re-evaluating Jacquot's evidence from the standpoint of modern medical knowledge seems to bear out his diagnosis. Jacquot notes that the number of deaths amongst French troops spiked in August and September before dropping off considerably in the fall, a finding that his highly consistent with malaria infections near Rome, as epitomized by Celli's data. However, Jacquot's data does not match historical evidence about typhoid fever seasonal distribution, which the French official statistics blamed for a majority of the deaths. While typhoid also tends to rise in the summer, it does not exhibit *P. falciparum*'s far more pronounced August–September seasonality.[14] Therefore, Jacquot's claim that malaria, and not typhoid, was chiefly to blame for the illnesses suffered by the French expeditionary force seems to be borne out by the data.

Other evidence collected by Jacquot not only gives further support to his contention

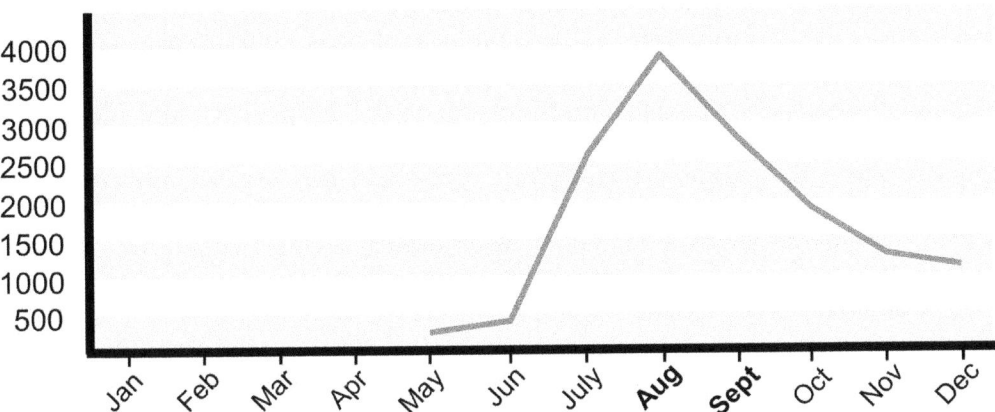

Hospitalizations for Fever in the French Expeditionary Force in Rome, May 1894–1850. Félix Jacquot, *Lettres Médicales sur L'Italie, Comprenant L'Histoire Médicale du Corps d'Occupation des États Romains* [Paris: Librarie de Victor Masson, 1857], p. 74.

that malaria was chiefly to blame for the health woes of the French, it also provides historians with a yardstick for measuring the relative malaria vulnerability of European visitors to Rome vs. local populations previously exposed to plasmodial infection. Jacquot found in 1849 that soldiers who had previously served in highly malarial Algeria—and presumably had gained some measure of acquired immunity to the disease—were less likely to fall sick than troops who had been stationed only in mainland France.[15] What is more, by rotating regiments drawn from different geographic areas into occupied Rome, France effectively carried out an unintentional medical experiment on human subjects concerning relative vulnerability to malaria, and luckily for the modern historian Jacquot was there to collect the data. Case in point was the starkly different fate that awaited Parisian and Corsican troops when they were rotated into the garrison of Rome in 1850. Jacquot notes that the Paris-based regiment sent to Rome withered there during the summer heats to the point that fully 29 percent of the soldiers in that unit were incapacitated by fevers and other ailments during the period from August 26 to September 7. In contrast, only 11 percent of the soldiers who had been previously stationed in Corsica, a notoriously malarial military posting, were on the sick list during the same period.[16] Unacclimated troops from the north, therefore, seem to have been nearly three times as vulnerable to malaria infection as were those with previous exposure to malarial fevers during the peak summer season.

Early Demographic Evidence: Malaria and Epigraphy

A third body of data that is relevant to the question of differential malaria mortality deals with a much earlier period, the Republican and Imperial eras of Roman history. No Roman historian or doctor carried out any systematic study of annual death statistics, malarial or otherwise, in the ancient period. However, we do have the next best thing: tens of thousands of funerary monuments recording the month, and in some cases the day and hour, of a Roman Christian's death. This body of data is of particular utility to those seeking clues about any disease that manifests a highly seasonal pattern of mortality, including *P. falciparum* malaria.

In general, the available epigraphic evidence gives strong support to the 19th century medical data presented above about the seasonal impact of malaria upon Italian demographics. As we might expect, the two highest months of mortality in the late antique city of Rome were August and September, peak *P. falciparum* season.[17] Indeed, as Walter Scheidel has pointed out, the typical *P. Falciparum* seasonal death pattern "corresponds exactly with the mortality pattern as evidenced by the Christian funerary inscriptions."[18] Death rates in Northern Italy were also higher than average during the summer season, though less markedly so than those of Rome, a finding that is again consistent with the 19th century medical evidence discussed earlier in this chapter.[19] This does not mean that Rome's resident malaria plasmodia were directly responsible for all observed summer-season mortality. In many cases, malaria infection may have served as an aggravating factor that increased vulnerability to the real cause of death, such as tuberculosis or food poisoning.[20] Even if this is accepted, however, it is clear that malaria was playing a crucial role in determining demographic patterns in Italy, and most especially in Rome.

Interestingly, the epigraphic materials also suggest that elderly Romans were far less likely to die during the high summer season than younger Romans (ages 20–49), which once again is consistent with the thesis that *P. falciparum* is largely to blame for the elevated August–September death rate. While older Christians were likely to have been long-standing residents of Rome who would have enjoyed some resistance to malaria infection due to previous exposure, younger Christians would have included a number of more recent migrants to Rome who would have lacked acquired resistance to Rome's endemic malarial fevers. The August–September mortality spike amongst this demographic, Walter Scheidel has hypothesized, may therefore represent the high death toll that Rome's resident malaria plasmodia inflicted amongst adults who had recently migrated "from healthier—malaria-free—areas" to the "resource-rich capital."[21] Thus, the sharp differential between the summer-season deaths of the young and the more equally

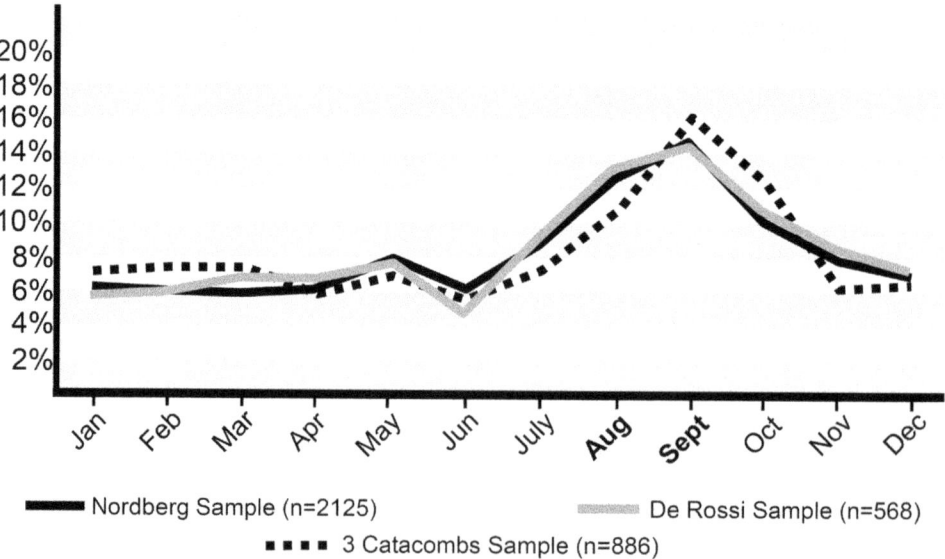

Death in Ancient Rome: Epigraphic Evidence. Walter Scheidel, "Libitina's Bitter Gains: Seasonal Mortality and Endemic Disease in the Ancient City of Rome," *Ancient Society*, Vol. 25 [1994], pp. 167–168.

distributed deaths of the elderly gives further support to the thesis that migrants to Rome with little exposure to malaria, a category that would eventually grow by the early Medieval era to include visiting transalpine Europeans, would have suffered disproportionally from malaria infection during Rome's feverish summer season.

Malaria by the Cardinal Numbers

What about malaria rates during the millennium and a half that separates the late Imperial era epigraphic data from the 19th-century French military expeditions? Do any available data speak to malaria rates in those centuries? While we have plenty of anecdotal evidence that suggests Rome was an unhealthy place throughout this era, especially for unacclimated transalpine visitors, hard numbers are in short supply for the Medieval era. In a perfect world, a researcher would gauge malaria morbidity through a systematic approach: examining demographic data for Roman citizens, identifying the percentage of malarial deaths, and then comparing this death rate to that of non–Italian visitors to the city to determine differential malaria mortality rates. But the data for such a study simply don't exist.

Or so I thought. In 2017, however, I discovered an archive that provides us with fairly robust demographic data for native Romans and European transplants to Rome during the Middle Ages, namely Salvador Miranda's on-line database *Cardinals of the Holy Roman Church*.[22] This digital resource provides biographical data for over 4,000 cardinals for a 16 century period, including their death dates and the causes of death. I initially hoped that it would be possible to search the archive for references to malaria. However, I came to realize that the data that Miranda provides on the causes of death was not very useful, as most deaths recorded in the database are described using antiquated medical terminology and concepts. "Plague," for example, is one of the most common causes of death in Miranda's database, but chroniclers clearly used the term as a catch-all for any serious and widespread disease affliction rather as a designation of a specific pathology caused by a specific pathogen.[23] "Fever" is another frequently mentioned cause of death, but usually without the additional details that would allow us to distinguish malaria's intermittent fever from the fevers caused by typhoid, typhus, influenza, or other diseases. Other cardinals died of the flux, meaning diarrhea, or dropsy, which doctors now call edema. Malaria can cause both of these symptoms, but so can a host of other infections.

While malaria can be a hard poker player to read, it does have a tell: as we have seen throughout this chapter, deaths from malaria tend to follow a very distinct annual pattern of seasonality. Before the advent of the modern era, malaria cases in Rome typically rose sharply in July with the coming of summer heat, reached a crescendo in August and early September, and then declined with the temperature by late September and October, in large part because *P. falciparum* develops far more quickly in the mosquito vector when temperatures rise above 30°C. While other diseases have hot-season spikes as well, including bubonic plague and typhoid, those diseases tend not to display the same narrow August–September mortality maximum. What is more, plague and typhoid were pan–European diseases, striking Italian and non–Italian alike. It occurred to me, therefore, that August–September deaths recorded in Miranda's cardinal database could serve as a useful proxy measurement for the differential malaria death rates of Italians and non-Italians in the city of Rome. Of course, not everyone who died in August and September died of malaria. Nonetheless, I hypothesized that cardinals who came to Rome from transalpine Europe would be much more likely to die during those months than would their Italian counterparts, since French, English, German, and other northern-born cardinals would have lacked the locals' intrinsic and acquired immunity to Rome's endemic malarial fevers.

And indeed, upon crunching the numbers, I found that the data strongly supported my hypothesis. After excluding cardinals from Miranda's catalogue who died outside of the vicinity of Rome or who died by violence or physical trauma, I was left with 1,054 cardinals, of whom 499 died before 1600. As is clear from the adjoining diagram, the 128 non–Italian cardinals of this time period exhibited a distinctly different mortality pattern from the Italian cardinals. While both groups died disproportionally in the August and September months, the spike in deaths during those months was much higher for non–Italian cardinals (36.4 percent) than it was for Italians (22.9 percent). If you subtract away the 8.33 baseline mortality rate that we would expect in any month if deaths were randomly distributed, the difference between the two groups is even more striking. While Italian cardinals experienced 6.23 percent excess mortality in the two summer months, the Northern European and Iberian cardinals suffered 19.73 percent additional mortality.[24] Thus non–Italian cardinals therefore seem to have been about three times as vulnerable to malaria as their Italian counterparts, a finding that perfectly matches Jacquot's observation that Parisian soldiers suffered nearly triple the summer-season morbidity rates as their Corsican compatriots.

The data provided by the Miranda's catalogue of cardinals also has a further benefit: since it is robust and spans a long period of time, it allows us to test Newfield's theory that

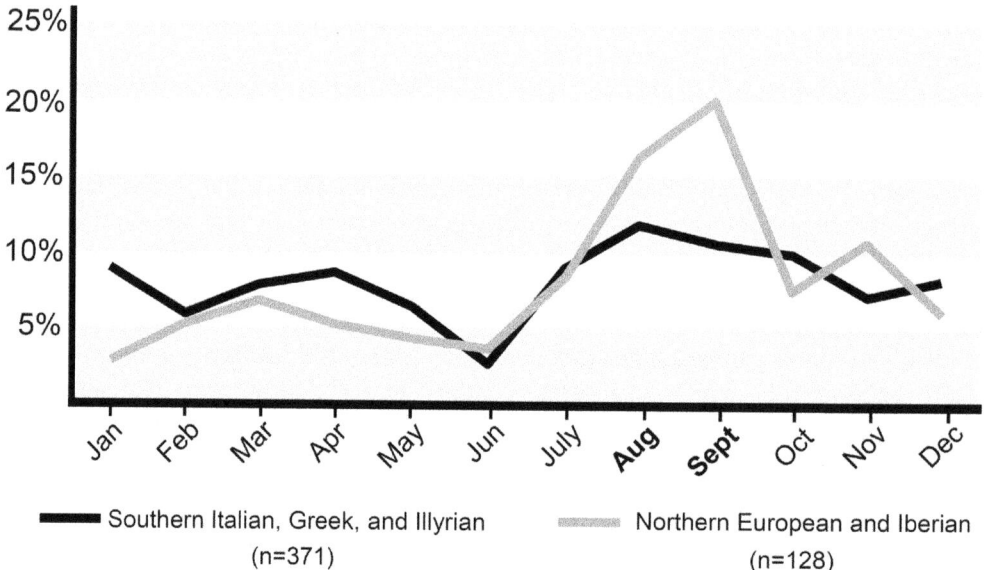

Deaths of Cardinals by Month and by Geographical Origin, 400–1600. Adapted from Benjamin James Reilly, "Cardinal Numbers: Changing Patterns of Malaria and Mortality in Rome, 494–1850," *Journal of Interdisciplinary History*, Vol. 49, no. 3 [2019], p. 415, © Massachusetts Institute of Technology and Journal of Interdisciplinary History, Inc.

periodic climate change might have modulated malaria rates, rendering generalizations from any particular era meaningless. If Newfield is correct, we should expect that summer season excess mortality amongst Catholic cardinals would be negatively correlated with the period of the Little Ice Age, a sustained drop in global temperature that was most pronounced between 1600 and 1850. However, this does not seem to be the case: the data suggest that the Little Ice Age had little impact on August–September death rates.[25] Rather, the gradual decline in August–September death rate amongst the cardinals tracks much more closely with the rise of Rome's population and population density, a theme we will return to in Chapter 15.

Taken together, the evidence is clear and consistent. During the years between the late Imperial Era and early modernity, Rome was a highly malarial location. What is more, the burden of that malaria fell particularly heavily upon transalpine visitors to the city, whose lack of previous expose to malaria (particularly *P. falciparum*) rendered them approximately three times as vulnerable to infection as their Italian during the late summer-early autumn malaria season. Had Rome been an obscure and little-frequented location, this differential mortality danger would have mattered little to European history. But the opposite was true: despite its fall and its fevers, Rome remained the *caput mundi*, and even in ruins Rome was capable of drawing to it an uncountable stream of soldiers, ecclesiastics, pilgrims, and other travelers over the course of a millennium and a half. As we will see over the course of the next section of the book, which re-tells the story of Europe's relations with Rome through the lens of malaria, the interplay between Rome's many attractions and its summer-season dangers would leave an important but under-appreciated mark upon European history.

Part II:
Transalpine Europe
and the *Caput Mundi*

4

GRAVE OF NATIONS

In the fateful year of 475 CE, at around the same time that weeping mothers began to bury their babes in the villa ruins at Lugnano, a teenage boy named Flavius Romulus Augustus became the 87th emperor of Rome. His name probably inspired confidence in his contemporaries, combining as it did the title of Augustus, heir to Caesar, with the name of Romulus, Rome's mythic founder. However, poor Romulus Augustus did not live up to the grandeur of his moniker. After serving as emperor for less than a year, Romulus Augustus was dethroned by military revolt and bundled off into an obscure retirement, vanishing entirely from the historical record.

What happened next was a landmark moment in the history of Europe. While there was nothing new about deposing a Roman emperor—in the extraordinary year of 69 CE no fewer than four self-declared emperors had fallen in quick succession—new candidates had always arisen to claim the vacant imperial office. Not so in 476. Rather, the coup leader Odoacer decided to retain power himself, not as *imperator*, but as King of Italy and as *patrician* (first citizen) of the city of Rome. For the first time in half a millennium, Rome was without an emperor.

Although the roots of this crisis are complex, the fall of empire in the Roman west was both the cause and the consequence of repeated invasions of Italy by "barbarians" from the north. In the 100 years which followed Romulus Augustus's short and sad reign, Rome had already suffered four Germanic sieges and two sacks, leading to a population decline of urban and rural Rome, political chaos, and ultimately the coup by Odoacer, who was himself a Romanized barbarian. The fall of the Western Empire, in turn, opened the door for still more northern invaders: the Ostrogoths and the Lombards. A new and destructive age of transalpine European engagement with the city of Rome had begun.

Threat from the North

Before we delve into the repeated barbarian invasions of the Roman empire, an important caveat is in order: the Roman collapse of the 5th century was only partial. While 476 marked the end of imperial rule in Rome, it did not signal the fall of empire itself, since a Greek-speaking Roman Empire based in Constantinople still held sway in the east. By the time of Romulus Augustus in fact there were in fact two separate "Roman" empires ruled by co-equal courts. This division was born in the Imperial Crisis, a prolonged 50-year period of epidemic disease, civil war, and foreign invasions that nearly destroyed Imperial Rome. Emperor Diocletian (284–305 CE), who reigned immediately after the crisis, had a simple diagnosis for the empire's illness. The body of the empire, he believed, had grown too large to be ruled effectively by a single head. Diocletian's treatment was radical surgery. To shore up the teetering Roman polity, he bisected the state and assigned each half to a separate imperial sovereign.

Diocletian reserved the eastern half for himself, which was a sign of the times. By Diocletian's reign, the center of balance in the empire had shifted decisively to the East, which still boasted large, taxable urban centers with rich foreign trade. Constantinople also enjoyed easy access to the lower basin of the Danube, whose hardened frontier inhabitants increasingly became the backbone of later imperial armies.[1] What is more, basic geography favored the eastern half of the empire. While the Eastern Empire did border on Persia, Rome's great power nemesis, the northern frontier of the Eastern Roman state was fairly secure thanks to the Bosporus straits, the Black Sea, and the Caucasus Mountains, which together offer considerable protection from attack from the various barbarian peoples of the north.

However, no such barriers existed in the Roman west, which had long been vulnerable to attack along its ill-defined northern frontier. As early as 393 BCE, for example, a huge horde of Gallic tribesmen overran a Roman army and seized almost the entire city of Rome. The only part of the city to not to succumb to the Gallic assault was the heights of the Capitoline, where Roman die-hards staged a successful last-ditch stand. Unable to take the Capitoline by force, the Gauls surrounded the hill and dug in for a siege, but were soon besieged themselves by famine and disease. In the words of Roman historian Livy, the Gauls, who were "accustomed as a nation to wet and cold," suffered horribly in the "heat and suffocation" of summer, and since the lowlands around the hill were "full of malaria" the Gauls "died off like sheep." So many perished that the Gauls "soon grew weary of burying their dead singly" and instead "piled the bodies into heaps and burned them indiscriminately."[2] Depleted by fever and famine, the Gauls eventually accepted a cash payment from the Romans in return for peace and withdrew back to the cooler north. As we will see throughout this book, the 393 BCE Gallic invasion would be just the first of a series of a long series of military campaigns by transalpine Europeans that would sputter out in the heat and malaria of the Roman summer.

In the years that followed the 393 BCE Gaulish attack, northern invasion temporarily receded as a threat to Rome. By the time of Caesar, in fact, Rome had flipped the script and invaded the Gauls in turn, eventually bringing all of France and much of Gallic Britain under the wings of the imperial eagle. By Caesar's day, however, the Gauls were no longer the most pressing problem that the Romans faced along their northern frontier. Back in 105 BCE, Rome had suffered its worst defeat since Hannibal's victory at Cannae when Germans of the Cimbri tribe unexpectedly massacred a huge Roman force at Arausio in Southern France. Had the Germans turned south after Arausio and marched directly on Rome, the Roman history section of modern textbooks might be much shorter today. To the baffled surprise of the Romans, however, the Germans loitered for several years in Spain and France, giving Rome enough time to rebuild their forces and revenge themselves against the Germans at the battle of Vercellae. After this defeat, the Germans disappeared from view for over a generation before re-emerging as sideshow players in Caesar's Gallic campaigns. Caesar, who knew the Germans from close experience, described them as a warlike people inured to hardship, whose food was milk and meat and whose glory was valor in war.[3] Consequently, he recruited some German tribesmen into his cavalry and with their help defeated a force of invading Suebi Germans at the Battle of Vosges in 58 BCE.

Caesar's victory stemmed the German threat for another generation, but over the next several centuries the Germans would emerge repeatedly to terrify the empire. These Germans, in the words of Roman historian Tacitus, were "an extraordinarily numerous" people with "fierce blue eyes, red hair, and large frames." Tacitus appreciated their military prowess, though he believed that they were better suited to charges and ambushes than to sustained field combat, lacking as they did the stamina and training of Roman troops. What is more, since the land of the Germans was frigid and full of "tangled forests and dismal swamps" Tacitus claimed that Germans were inured to "hunger and cold" but were unable to endure heat.[4]

What Tacitus did not understand, however, is that the Germans were being pushed towards the heat of southern Europe by demographic and geographic forces. In terms of rainfall and fertility, the Central Asian steppe has a clear east-west fertility gradient, becoming lusher in the direction of Europe. What is more, at least up until the age of gunpowder, the pastoralist nations of the steppe tended to face stronger threats from their east, which was occupied by other horse nomads competing over limited pasture, than from the sedentary agriculturalist societies of Europe to the west. As a result, movement along the steppe corridor generally passed from east-to-west from late antiquity until the pre-modern era. Germans had already pushed the Celtic Gauls before them into conflict with Rome, and by the imperial era Gothic Germans originally based in the grasslands of the Ukraine were now being nudged towards Roman swords in turn, this time by the Huns to their own rear.

In order to counter population pressure from the steppe belt the Romans built a belt of their own, the *Limes Germanicus*, a network of forts and watchtowers strung along their northern frontier. These fortifications were designed to supplement Europe's natural defensive barriers against northern invasion, namely the Alps, the Rhine, and the Danube, which taken together served as a 4,000 kilometer wall and moat. For the first two imperial centuries, the Romans managed to hold the line and even created a province north of the Danube, Dacia, which became the seed of the modern country of Romania. Dacia was abandoned in the late 3rd century to the invading German Goths, but the *Limes Germanicus* held, and the Romans even recruited the increasingly Romanized Goths as imperial soldiers. For another several generations, Germans and Romans enjoyed an uneasy truce along the northern frontier.

In the late 4th century CE, however, the *Limes Germanicus* collapsed. The triggering event, according to historian of Rome Kyle Harper, was a multidecadal drought which withered the grasslands of Central Asia, turning the homeland of the Huns into a veritable dust bowl. This drought transformed the Huns into "armed climate refugees on horseback" whose desperate search for pasture put them at odds with the Gothic Germans to their west.[5] By 376 CE, a group of these Goths became so wearied by their conflict with the Huns that they petitioned Rome for permission to cross the Danube and settle as allies within Roman territory. The Eastern Roman Emperor Valens acquiesced, but the immigrant tribesmen soon rose in revolt against Rome due to hunger and poor treatment by Roman provisional governors. After two years of indecisive conflicts Valens decided to solve the problem himself, personally leading an army of roughly 30,000 troops to quell Gothic resistance.

The result was an unmitigated disaster, the 9/11 of the ancient age. When the two forces met near the Roman city of Adrianople, the numerically inferior Gothic army retreated behind its circle of wagons and managed to hold off the Romans until the

Gothic cavalry, which had been out foraging for food, returned to camp and fell upon the Roman force's rear. Caught between the cavalry and the wagons and unable to maneuver, the Romans were routed, and two-thirds of the Romans fell in the melee, including Valens himself.

Ironically, although the Battle of Adrianople killed an emperor of the east, the Western Roman Empire would suffer the brunt of its consequences. Since the Romans were unable to dislodge the Goths from its Danube provinces after Adrianople, they survived like a cancer within the tissue of Roman territory, sometimes allied to and sometimes at odds with the emperors to their west and east. Like other partially assimilated Germans, these Goths were probably somewhat in awe of the Roman culture. In the words of historian Thomas Hodgkin, Goths had long looked with admiration on the "great roads, the cities, the mines, the baths, the camps, the temples" that Rome had left behind in Dacia, and Gothic mothers entertained their children with stories of Rome's "vast treasure-hoards, guarded by dwarfs or by serpents."[6]

Inspired by these tales and encouraged by Rome's growing weakness, the Goths under King Alaric stormed into Italy in 401 only to be defeated and driven back by the Western *magister militum* Stilicho, a competent commander of half–German ancestry. Stilicho fell prey to palace politics in 408, however, and the Goths roared back, this time overrunning the defenses of northern Italy and descending on Rome. Alaric besieged Rome three times, and while he allowed himself to be paid off twice, he pursued the third siege to the bitter end and finally seized the starving city in August of 410.

The Goths were generous in victory, and although they did ransack the town for three days, there was little bloodshed. Still, the psychological shock of the successful Gothic sack of Rome was immense. "Who would believe," wrote Saint Jerome, "that Rome, built up by conquest of the whole world, has collapsed, that the mother of nations had become also their tomb." This sense of apocalyptic disaster was accentuated by the miserable plight of the thousands of refugees who fled to the eastern half of the empire, "men and women who were once noble and abounding in every kind of wealth but are now reduced to poverty." "There is not a single hour," St. Jerome wrote from his monastery in the east, "in which we are not relieving crowds of brethren" displaced from Rome, and the monkish Jerome complained that "the quiet of the monastery has been changed into the bustle of the guest house."[7]

Alaric himself paid a terrible price for his victory against Rome. Immediately after the sack the Gothic King marched to the toe-tip of the Italian peninsula, probably in hopes of conquering grain-rich Sicily. The first fleet he gathered for the crossing was shattered by a storm, however, and while Alaric was collecting a second one, he died suddenly. While his exact cause of death is unknown, some historians have speculated that malaria was Alaric's undoing. As was often the case with northern invaders of Italy, Thomas Hodgkin wrote, "climate proved itself mightier than armies, and ... fever was the great avenger."[8] If so, Alaric would be in good company. As we shall see repeatedly throughout the coming chapters, transalpine ambitions in the Italian south would routinely be foiled by the region's endemic malarial fevers.

Despite the protection that malaria afforded Rome against foreign invasion, the Visigothic sack proved to be just the first of a series of disasters for the Eternal City. Second on the scene were the Vandals, a Germanic tribe that first popped into view in Poland but which was pushed across the frozen Rhine River into Roman territory in the winter of 406 by rearward pressure from the oncoming Huns. Interestingly, the main military resistance to the Vandal advance came not from the Romans, who had been badly weakened by the Gothic invasion the generation before, but by the Franks, a Romanized Germanic confederation located along the Rhine River. Once in Roman territory, the Vandals migrated down to an area in Southern Spain that still bears their name—Andalusia—though this etymology is contested. A generation later, the Vandals crossed the Mediterranean into North Africa and in 455 CE they took advantage of western imperial weakness to seize the nearly undefended city of Rome in a surprise attack. This time, Rome was looted for 14 days and so thoroughly despoiled of its riches that the name "Vandal" is even today given to a ruthless destroyer of property. Once again, there was little loss of life during the sack, but this is less a tribute to Vandal mercy than to the Vandal's practice of carrying captured Romans back to North Africa as hostages or slaves. A living Roman, the Vandals may have calculated, was worth more than a dead one.

Soon afterwards, Attila the Hun himself invaded Northern Italy, obliterating the ancient port city of Aquileia on the Adriatic coast in the process. The Huns never crossed the Apennines into Rome, however. This may be because they were smarting from a recent defeat at the hands of the Visigoths, though Hodgkin speculated that the "strange awe" which Italy inspired in the hearts of would-be northern conquerors fueled Attila's reluctance to march south.[9] However, fear of fever provides us with the most compelling explanation for Attila's reluctance to march on Rome. Mindful of the death of the Gothic King Alaric in Southern Italy a generation earlier, Attila and his nobles may have reasoned that there was no point seizing Rome if you did not live long afterwards to enjoy the fruits of victory.[10] As a result, Attila "put aside his usual fury" and returned to the grasslands north of the Danube, sparing Rome from what would probably have been a bloody sack.[11] Ironically, Attila would suffer an early death in 453; according to legend, he died of a nosebleed following a night of drunken post-wedding debauchery.

Although safe for the moment, Rome was threatened once again from foreign invasion in 488, this time by King Theodoric of the Eastern Goths, or Ostrogoths. After defeating the last of the Huns after Attila's death, the Ostrogoths allied themselves with the Eastern Roman Empire in exchange for an annual gold subsidy. In 488, Eastern Emperor Zeno gave these Romanized Goths the green light to invade Italy, which at the time was still under the rule of the Odoacer, the Germanic or perhaps a Hunnish mercenary commander who had deposed poor Romulus Augustus 13 years before. It was a testament to the declining stature of Rome in this period that the main wartime objective of the Ostrogoths was not Rome, but Ravenna, a fortress-city located amidst a swamp on the Adriatic that had become the main seat of political power in the Italian peninsula. Once Ravenna fell to the Ostrogoths in 493, Rome acquiesced to Theodoric's rule without a struggle, sparing the city from a further sack.

Theodoric's relationship with Rome was reverential but distant. Like many other Goths, he was probably in awe of the ancient city and during his reign tried to restore some of its fading luster by re-constructing walls, re-building monuments, and staging games in the Circus and the Colosseum. In gratitude, the Senate of Rome erected a gilded statue in his likeness. Nonetheless, Theodoric did not actually visit Rome for the first seven years of his reign, and when he did visit in the year 500 CE he stayed for only six months—presumably in the winter season—before returning to his capital at Ravenna. To some degree Theodoric's decision to set up his throne in Ravenna rather than Rome was a reflection of the political realities of the age: Ravenna enjoyed quick communications with the still-strong eastern half of the empire and was a better base of operations against further incursions from the Germanic north. However, it may also reflect Theodoric's regard for his own health. Ravenna is outside the usual range of *P. falciparum* malaria and did not yet host the *A. sacherovi* mosquitoes which would later become the main vector for malarial infections along the Italian east coast.[12] The fact that Theodoric sponsored drainage works of the Pontine Marshes south of Rome, an area long associated with "bad air" and deadly infections, further supports the notion that Theodoric was factoring malaria into his political and geographic calculations.

While Theodoric basked in the accolades of the remnant Romans of Italy, anti–Gothic conspiracies were beginning to stir in the east. During Theodoric's reign the Eastern emperors, who are usually called the "Byzantines" in the historical sources, had been too weak to interfere directly in the west. As a result, Byzantium contented itself with the legal fiction that the king of the Goths was merely a *magister militium* and therefore an officer of the empire. In 532, however, Emperor Justinian I secured an "Eternal Peace" with his Persian rivals to the east, freeing Byzantium's hand to meddle in western affairs. After first reconquering North Africa from the Vandals, Justinian set his sights on Italy, dreaming of restoring true Roman sovereignty over the lost provinces of the West. In the process, thousands of unacclimated troops from across the Alps would once again be put in mortal danger as they campaigned in the malarial vicinity of the Eternal City.

Rome and Disease in the Age of Belisarius

The Byzantine campaign against the Goths opened with a bang. After first restoring Roman control over Sicily and Naples, Byzantine general Belisarius marched quickly on Rome, which the Goths, rendered leaderless by Theodoric's recent death, were unable to defend. Shocked by this setback, the Ostrogoths raised a new king and new army, marched on Rome, broke the aqueducts that supplied Rome with water, and settled down for a siege. By spring Rome was suffering from famine, but like the Gaulish invaders of Rome in the 4th century BCE, the Goths soon began to suffer horribly from disease. Because of run-off from the severed aqueducts, the *campagna* of Rome turned into a swampy mess, and "pestilence" (possibly malaria) began to ravage the Gothic force. Worse yet, Belisarius managed to seize some towns to the rear of the Goths, threatening their food supply. Complaining that "we are as much the besieged as the besiegers," the Goths withdrew to Ravenna in early 538.[13]

At this point the Goths got some unexpected help: a large Frankish force, led by King Theudebert of the Merovingian dynasty, took advantage of the wartime chaos and invaded the Italian north. While these Franks had formally entered the war as allies of the Byzantines, in practice they were more interested in plunder than in assisting the imperial cause and actually fought several successful engagements against Byzantine troops. What eventually drove the Franks from Italy was not Byzantine military might, but the unhealthy Italian climate. According to contemporary chronicler Gregory of Tours, our main source of the period, the unacclimated Frankish army was "attacked by various fevers" while in Italy, a land notoriously "full of diseases." With the death toll mounting, Theudebert withdrew with his surviving men and his plunder back across the Alps.[14] Shortly after, the Ostrogoths had no choice but to surrender Ravenna to Belisarius' forces.

At this crucial juncture, however, Emperor Justinian snatched defeat from the jaws of victory. Fearing the high-flying Belisarius was about to claim the imperial throne for himself, Justinian recalled him to Constantinople. Soon after, the Goths were driven from the news cycle by two new disasters. The first to strike was the so-called "Plague of Justinian," an outbreak of plague [*Y. pestis*] that slew millions throughout the Mediterranean Basin and the surrounding territories.[15] Secondly, the Persians chose this moment to tear up their "Eternal Peace" with Rome and invade the Byzantine Empire's eastern frontier. Given reprieve by these distractions, the Ostrogoths were able to regroup. Under the leadership of King Totila, the Goths defeated the leaderless Roman armies in Northern Italy and successfully snatched Rome from Byzantine hands, compelling its surrender through siege and hunger.[16]

In desperation, Justinian recalled Belisarius to military service. However, Belisarius was unable to break the siege of Rome. In fact, the siege nearly broke Belisarius. While campaigning near the swampy mouth of the Tiber south of Rome, Belisarius was afflicted by a persistent fever, probably malaria, "which by its long continuance harassed him sorely and brought him into danger of death."[17] In the end, some of Belisarius' own hungry men betrayed Rome to Totila, who considered tearing down the city brick by brick converting the site into sheep pasture much as it had been in the time of Romulus. He was only dissuaded from doing so by Belisarius, who supposedly wrote to Totila that "among all the cities under the sun Rome is agreed to be the greatest and most noteworthy" so to raze Rome would be "considered a great crime against the men of all time." The Gothic King, who like most of his compatriots probably regarded Rome with a certain superstitious fascination, acquiesced to Belisarius' request and contented himself with demolishing some of the city's circuit walls.

He soon regretted this choice—within four months Belisarius craftily re-took the city, forcing the Goths to besiege Rome once again in 549. By the time that the Goths were finally defeated once and for all by the Roman General Narses in 554, therefore, Rome had suffered three major sieges and sacks in less than twenty years. As for the Ostrogoths themselves, they were all but exterminated by these two decades of constant warfare. According to Hodgkin, the few surviving Goths who fled Italy at the end of the wars left the bones of more than "one hundred and fifty thousand warriors ... under the grass of the campagna."[18] This is probably an exaggeration, but one built upon on a kernel of truth.

Nor did Narses' victory mean the end of the German threat to Rome—far from it. During the long Gothic wars, the Byzantines had employed troops of the German Lombard ("Long Beard") tribe as soldiers in Italy. Apparently the Lombards got a taste for Italian life while campaigning in the empire's service, since they swept into Italy *en masse* in 568, taking advantage of the power vacuum left behind in Italy by the extermination of the Ostrogoths. The Lombards, however, had learned from the lessons of previous Germanic invaders and chose their settlements in Italy with the malaria threat in mind. Unlike their predecessors, the Lombards initially left Rome and its *campagna* alone, settling instead in Tuscany, the Apennine highlands of Italy, and the North Italian plain. Their most important capital was Pavia, which lies in the province still called "Lombardy" today. By and large the Lombards avoided settling in warm and flat territory, such as the offshore Italian islands, the mouth of the Po river, and the heel and toe of Italy, and above all the Roman *campagna*, the grave of the Ostrogoths.[19]

For the most part, the Lombards ruled Italy from their healthy hilltop seats, including Spoleto in central Italy and Benevento in the Apennines of the south. The name of the latter town recalls the trait what drew the Lombards to the site—in Latin, Benevento literally means "good wind." This is not to say that the Lombards entirely evaded Italy's resident malaria. In the late 600s, the Lombards of Northern Italy were afflicted by a horrific epidemic which killed so suddenly and liberally that in its aftermath "two were often laid in one grave."[20] This could have been a recurrence of Justinian's plague. However, the fact that that this infection raged from July through September, and the fact that the Lombards tried to flee it by abandoning the Po river valley for the nearby mountaintops, is suggestive of a short-term epidemic of *P. falciparum* in territories that are not normally within its range.

With the coming of the Lombards to Italy, Byzantium's schemes to regain control over the west unraveled and the basic map of Medieval Western Europe began to take shape. Although the Eastern Empire retained a precarious grip on Italy's islands and coasts, most of inland Italy was occupied by the increasingly Romanized Lombards. Visigoth Germans held Spain and the Romanized Frankish Germans ruled France, which still bears their name today. To the east of the Franks, in the area that we now call Germany, lay a tangle of unassimilated Germanic peoples, including Thuringians, Bavarians, Alemannis, and Swabians. Northeast of the Franks were the Angles and Saxons, closely-related Germanic tribes who started migrating across the English Channel in the early 5th century. These Anglo-Saxons eventually carved out a number of small kingdoms in the fertile lowlands of the island of Great Britain, relegating the remnant Celtic population to mountainous margins of Scotland and Wales in the process. Still further to the north were the Vikings, Germanic tribes who occupied the *vík*, or inlets, of the Scandinavian peninsula. Finally, to the east of the Germans lay various Slavic peoples who were migrating along with the Huns along the Asian steppe corridor. The nations that would look in fascination to Rome over the next millennium and a half, therefore, were beginning to emerge into history.

At the same time these new peoples were taking the spotlight, it must have appeared to observers that Rome, once the *caput mundi* and the beacon of the west, was falling into darkness. In the year 400, Rome still boasted a population of about three-quarters of a million souls. In the aftermath of the Visigothic sack of 410, however, thousands of Romans fled the city to the safety of the Byzantine Empire. Following the Visigoths' migration to Spain, the city had the opportunity to recover, but this chance was spoiled by the Vandal invasion of North Africa, which cut the city off from the rich North African grain fields upon which the city depended for its food supply. When the Vandals sacked Rome in 455, therefore, they probably just accelerated a decline that was already well underway.[21] By the start of the Ostrogothic wars, Rome's population was probably down to just 100,000 and during the sieges it declined further still. The last Gothic siege was waged against a city reduced to only 30,000 inhabitants and so much empty land within the city was given over to farmland that Totila found it much more difficult to starve Rome into surrender the third time around.[22]

As for the urban structures of Rome, they fared little better than Rome's people during the Gothic wars. According to Christopher Hibbert, by the time of the Lombard invasion of Italy "buildings were crumbling into ruins; aqueducts and sewers were in

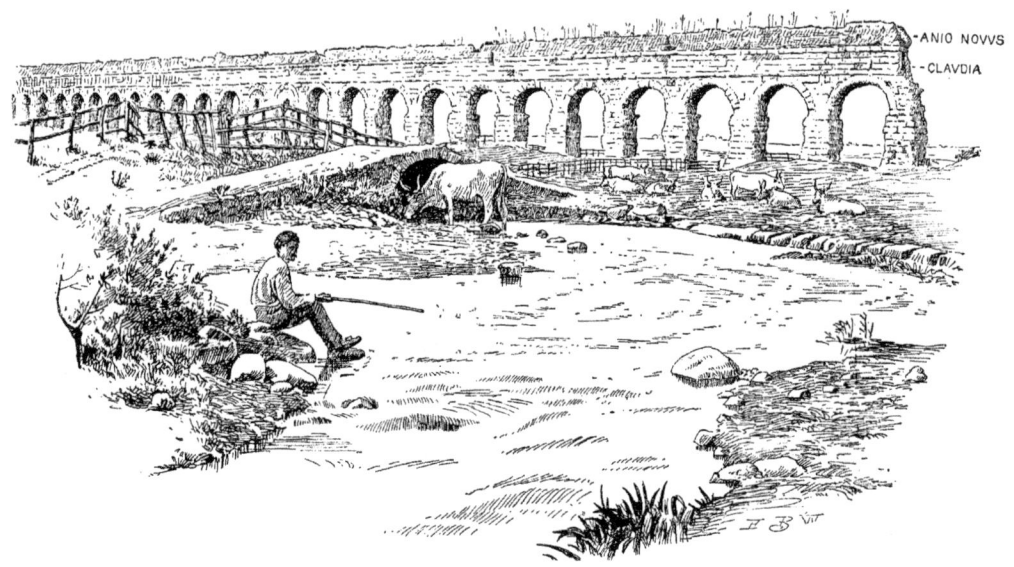

An early 19th-century view of the *Campagna* of Rome, with ruined aqueducts in the background. Hartmann Grisar, *History of Rome and the Popes in the Middle Ages*, Vol. 1 (London: Kegan Paul, Trench, Trübner, 1911), facing p. 178.

urgent need of repair; public granaries had long since collapsed; people were dying of starvation in hundreds." Worse yet, due to wartime neglect and the ruin of the aqueducts, the depopulated outskirts of Rome "degenerated into swamps, and mosquitoes infested the plain of the Campagna."[23] Malaria, always a problem in Rome, was now firmly established as an endemic disease of the remnant population of the half-deserted capital of the world.

At this point, Rome might have joined other fallen capitals such as Carthage, Persepolis, and Ctesiphon on the ash heap of history. But this didn't happen. Instead, Rome's legacy of supremacy was kept alive by one man, who despite the ruins around him maintained Rome's claim to universal spiritual and political dominion over all Western Europe. It is to the Bishop of Rome that we now turn.

5

To Roam/Rome

In his magnificent 1954 book *The English Traveler to Italy*, George Parks of Queens College set himself an ambitious task: to chart the tide of English travel to the Italian peninsula from the age of Caesar to the Renaissance. As Parks was the first to admit, however, the fragmentary and incomplete nature of the available sources means that a full accounting of all English travelers to the Italian south will never be possible. The best we can do, according to Parks, is to treat the few stories that have survived as "stray sparks showing the direction of the wind."[1]

Three of the brightest sparks known to us for the early Medieval period are those of Richard and his sons Willibald and Winnebald, who set out to follow the pilgrim roads to "far ends of the earth" in the summer of 721. Misfortune beset these pious men from the start. Soon after entering Italy, Richard was struck down by sudden illness and was buried in Lucca beneath the flagstones of the Church of Saint Frediano. As for the bereaved brothers, they crossed the snow-topped Apennines, avoided marauding bands of soldiers, and eventually arrived safely before the doors of the "illustrious Basilica of St. Peter," the crown jewel of Christian Rome. This was no mean feat: by reaching Rome, Willibald and Winnebald joined a very small list of known English visitors to Rome and became the first to leave behind a detailed narrative of their travels.

As their account makes clear, however, the hardships of the road paled before the mortal danger that awaited them in the Eternal City itself. In the early summer of their second year in Rome, as the weather turned torrid, both brothers were "seized with great bodily affliction, with heavy breathing and fits of fever, now freezing with cold and now burning with heat, as the fierce disease spread through their limbs." So "ensnared and bowed down" were the brothers that their "vital spirits barely fluttered in their weary bodies" and both were in "great danger of death."[2]

What misfortune had befallen these pious pilgrims in Rome? Some later authors have ascribed their ailments to the bubonic plague, though I know of no other references to plague in Italy that year.[3] In any case, as historians John Theilmann and Frances Cate have pointed out, the term "plague" was used indiscriminately in the Middle Ages for any "disease of great proportions with a high mortality rate."[4] Given the timing of the illness and the symptoms described, it is far more likely that Willibald and Winnebald were amongst the first Christian travelers from north of the Alps to fell prey to malaria, most likely *P. falciparum*, during the swelter of the Roman summer.

Rise of the Papacy

While Willibald and Winnebald's story epitomizes the disease problems suffered by unacclimated Europeans visitors to the Eternal City, it illustrates another truth as well: the irresistible pull that the city of Rome exerted upon the new Christians of Northern Europe. In order to explain why such travelers risked the roads to Rome, however, we should first step backwards and discuss the papacy, the institution that would become synonymous with Rome over the course of late antiquity and the Middle Ages. It is outside of the scope of this book to fully describe how the bishop of Rome rose to a position of prominence over the entire Western Church, but one crucial figure in this story was the miracle-working apostle Peter, who (according to the Romans) was the original founder of the Roman Christian congregation. Peter was not just any apostle, but their leader and spokesman. What is more, Jesus had declared that "you are Peter, and on this rock I will build My church ... and I will give you the keys to the kingdom of heaven."[5] Since the bishop of Rome was Peter's successor, these spiritual keys now fell to the Roman popes, giving the Church of Rome a primacy of place over all other Christian congregations.

In making this argument, supporters of the papacy were indulging in a certain amount of wishful thinking. While tradition holds Peter died in Rome, there is no real evidence he served as bishop there, or even that the Christian community in Rome was in any way united under one head at the time of Peter's death. Modern scholars now argue that the large and fractured Christian community in Rome probably did not have a single leader until at least the time of Anicetus, who served as bishop of Rome from 155 to 166 CE. Even afterwards, not all of Rome's Christian communities accepted that bishop's authority. For a while in the early 3rd century Rome had two dueling bishops, Pontianus and Hippolytus, both of whom were exiled from the city in 235 CE when their partisans began to brawl in the streets. As a result, some scholars claim that Rome was not fully unified under one bishop until as late as the mid–3rd century CE.[6] Like all bishops of the age, the bishop of Rome was informally termed the "pope," or father, of his congregation. The tradition of reserving this title for the bishop of Rome alone was a later innovation.

Our knowledge of the early days of the Roman church is complicated by the fact that the early church had to keep a low profile since Christians were subject at the time to periodic waves of pagan persecution. One of the worst such incidents occurred during the reign of Emperor Valerian (253–260 CE), who ordered the arrest and execution of all high-ranking Church officials throughout the empire. However, persecution under Valerian was cut short when Valerian was defeated in battle and taken prisoner by the Sasanian Persians. Much to the delight of the empire's Christians, the humiliated Valerian lived out his last days as human furniture for the Persian Shah, who reportedly employed the former emperor as a stepstool when mounting his horse. It was during this period of persecution that Christians began to be associated with the catacombs, the warren of underground burial chambers cut into the volcanic tufa rock outside the boundaries of the city. In these dangerous times Christians increasingly began to meet and even conduct worship in these catacombs, knowing that their pagan tormentors associated dead bodies with spiritual corruption and thus were reluctant to venture into the impure darkness of these subterranean boneyards.[7]

Persecution of Christians would continue sporadically for a few decades after Valerian's death, but the tables were about to turn. In 312 CE, during one of the many succession disputes that continued to plague the empire even after Diocletian's decision to divide east from west, Emperor Constantine faced off against a usurper named Maxentius near the Milvian Bridge over the Tiber. Just before the battle was joined, Christian sources tell us, Constantine saw a cross superimposed over the English letter P emblazoned across the sky as well as holy words promising "through this sign you will conquer."[8] While Constantine himself may not have recognized this sign, the denizens of Rome's catacombs certainly would have: this symbol, which combined the Greek letters χ (*chi*) and ρ (*rho*), was an anagram for Christ. Constantine told his men to decorate his shields with this emblem, and as his vision had promised he won the battle and with it the western half of the empire.

Shortly after his victory Constantine and the Eastern Emperor Licinius agreed to promulgate the Edict of Milan, officially legalizing Christian worship throughout the empire. Surprisingly, Constantine himself did not convert to Christianity in the battle's aftermath. Rather, Constantine seems to have hedged his spiritual bets throughout his lifetime and may have combined sympathy for Christianity with continued devotion to the Sol Invictus, or "unconquered sun," a popular Roman soldier's cult. During his reign, in fact, Constantine not only issued coins decorated with symbols of the sun god, he even declared that one day of the week of would henceforth be named *dies Solis*, or "sun day," and celebrated as a day of rest.

Rome and Ruination

Supporters of the pope may have hoped that Constantine's sympathy for the Christian faith would catapult the bishop of Rome to a position of religious prominence in the developing Christian community, but in actuality the opposite occurred. True, Constantine was generous to the Church of Rome. Despite his lingering solar sympathies, Constantine ordered the construction of magnificent new basilica built on Vatican Hill atop the supposed gravesite of Saint Peter. In the long run, however, Constantine's reign created problems for Peter's heir. In 324, Constantine defeated the Eastern Emperor Licinius at the Battle of Chrysopolis and, once in command of the entire Roman Empire, he followed Diocletian's example and decided to base his power in the Roman east. He sought out a new capital accordingly, eventually deciding upon the old Greek city of Byzantium, re-founded by the emperor as the *Nova Roma Constantinopolitana* or "New Rome of Constantinople." As a result, old Rome went from being the *caput mundi* to a political backwater and the influence of the Roman pope declined correspondingly.

The position of the Roman church deteriorated still further by the mid–6th century with the collapse of imperial authority in the west and the depopulation of the Rome in the age of Germanic invasions. Pope Gregory I lamented that, with the coming of the Lombards,

> The population of Italy ... was cut down to wither away. Cities were sacked, fortifications overthrown, churches burned, monasteries and cloisters destroyed. Farms were abandoned, and the countryside, uncultivated, became a wilderness ... wild beasts roamed the fields where so many people had once made their homes.[9]

The city of Rome itself was no better off. "Where is the Senate? Where are the people? The bones are dissolved," Gregory complained, "the flesh consumed. All the glory of earthly dignity has expired within the city. All her greatness has vanished, and yet the few of us that remain are daily oppressed by the sword and afflictions innumerable. ... I do not know what is happening elsewhere," Gregory concluded, "but in this land of ours the world is not merely announcing its end, it is pointing directly to it."[10] In Rome, at least, the Dark Ages had begun.

Gregory did not just chronicle the ills of the age, however: he set about to cure them. Recognizing that the shriveling of imperial power of Italy had left a vacuum, Gregory moved to fill it, and during his reign the papacy became the effective governing body of central Italy. Gregory greatly expanded the size of the papal bureaucracy, appointing (in the words of John Julius Norwich) both high officials and "sub-deacons, notaries, treasurers, and senior executive officers," thus creating a "civil service unparalleled in Europe outside Constantinople itself."[11] Together, these officials assumed responsibility for feeding the hungry, housing displaced refugees, shoring up the faltering economy, defending the city from Lombard attack, and even negotiating treaties with the German tribal kings who now dominated Western Europe. The papacy was able to achieve all of these disparate goals thanks in part to the growing economic resources of the papacy, which during this age of crisis had received huge grants of land from Christian benefactors. The papacy's success was also a tribute to the organizational genius of Gregory himself, who has gone down in history as the founder of the Medieval papacy.

Nor did Gregory confine his ministry to Roman souls alone. As Gregory knew all too well, the Christianization of Europe north of the Alps was still far from complete in the late 6th century. While much of France had been brought into the Christian fold, many Germans were still no more than half-Christianized or remained unrepentant pagans. In response, Gregory inaugurated a papal program of missionary activity to the north, sending forty missionaries to Anglo-Saxon Britain under the leadership of Augustine. These efforts were crowned with success. Within a few months, English King Ethelbert and most of his subjects converted to Christianity, and Augustine established a monastery at Canterbury dedicated to the saints Peter and Paul, thus planting the seeds of what would later become the Church of England. Later popes would send out still more missionaries, forging further ties between Rome and the cold pagan north. In the process, Gregory and his successors laid the foundations of Roman dominance within the wider western church.

One problem that Gregory was unable to solve, however, was the steadily worsening malaria situation both in and around the city of Rome. Following the ruin of Rome's aqueducts, the Roman *campagna* became waterlogged and marshy, a problem exacerbated by the flight of farmers from the area during the frequent sieges of Rome and the consequent ruin of the region's irrigation and drainage canals. The resulting pools of standing water were an ideal habitat for *A. labranchiae* mosquitoes, which probably expanded their habitat range dramatically during the calamities of the 5th and 6th centuries.[12]

As for Rome itself, the destruction of the aqueducts during the Lombard wars left the remnant urban population high and dry, and in this case, it was the *loss* of water rather than its excess that contributed to endemic malaria. Deprived of the aqueduct water the remnant Roman population was forced to abandon the dry hills for the moister flood plains below, where water was still available from wells or the Yellow Tiber. As a result, by the early Middle Ages urban Rome's center of gravity had shifted northward, from the windy heights of Rome's seven hills to the low-lying Campus Martius plain. Spiritually, this made sense: seem from above, it must have looked like the city itself was crawling reverently towards the holy grave of Peter on Vatican Hill. From the standpoint of epidemiology, however, this move was unfortunate, as Rome's shifted population was now living cheek by jowl with *A. labranchiae* and malaria plasmodia. What is more, the sewers that ancient Romans had constructed to drain these lowlands were increasingly inoperative, buried beneath centuries of accumulated urban debris and no longer washed clean by flowing water from the aqueducts. The *caput mundi* thus become a paradise for plasmodia. Small wonder, then, that Gregory himself, like many members of his Roman congregation, suffered repeatedly from bouts of intermittent fever.[13]

Making matters still worse, the depopulation of the city over time probably worsened the malaria threat in a self-strengthening cycle. In general, since high populations mean more people are sharing each other's air and contaminating each other's water, the frequency of disease rises with population density. Not so with malaria. While malaria does require a minimum population density to sustain regular chains of transmission, the fact that it is a mosquito-vector disease means that malaria often declines as population increases since urban development deprives *Anopheles* mosquitoes of the orchards, gardens, and other green spaces that mosquitos depend on for their habitat.[14] The same goes in reverse, with abandonment of developed territory to cultivation or wasteland creating new opportunities for *Anopheles* mosquitoes. The urban farmland that helped the Romans to withstand the third Ostrogothic siege, therefore, probably yielded an unexpected harvest of mosquitoes and malaria.

For the inhabitants of Rome, these geographic and demographic changes were bad but supportable, as each generation of Romans paid for their adulthood by sacrificing a tribute of children to the Minotaur. For the many transalpine Europeans who would follow the footsteps of Willibald and Winnebald to the papal court in the coming centuries, however, malaria posed a serious threat.

Following the Roads to Rome

It is impossible now to guess at how many European visitors Rome received during the early Medieval period, but the sources suggest that they were fairly numerous and became more so over time. According to Bede, a chronicler of early English history, by the turn of the 8th century "many Englishmen, nobles, and commons, men and women, rulers and private persons … began the custom of travel to Rome from Britain."[15] Rome even attracted England's regional kings, such as King Cadwalla of the West Saxons, who came to Rome in 688 to be baptized; when he died soon after arrival he was buried in his baptismal garment.[16] Other English kinglets followed close behind, including Coenred of Mercia, Offa of the East Saxons, and Inne of Wessex. Nor did these kings come alone. To the delight of Rome's resident plasmodia species, each of these kings probably descended upon Rome with a large royal retinue with little or no previous exposure to Rome's endemic malaria infections.

Ecclesiastics crossed the Alps and descended upon Rome in even greater numbers than laymen. Technically, the first known such bishop was Mellitus, who left London for Rome in 605 to confer with the pope. Mellitus doesn't really count, however, since he was not a native Englishman. Rather, Mellitus was a Greek or Italian sent by Pope Gregory to convert the Anglo-Saxons, probably because he was a good speaker—"Mellitus" means "honeyed" or "sweet" in Greek, and the word lives on in the scientific name for diabetes, *diabetes mellitus*.[17] However, the sugar-tongued Mellitus was followed by a number of native English bishops including Wighard, an archbishop-elect of Canterbury who went to Rome in 667 to receive the pallium, a thin band of woolen cloth which was the symbol of an archbishop's authority.

Soon after arriving, however, Wighard and almost his entire retinue perished due to "a plague that broke out at the time."[18] Did Wighard and his men die of malaria? It is certainly possible. While bubonic plague cannot be ruled out—occasional after-ripples of infection recurred for years after Justinian's Plague—Bede's account of "plague" in Italy in 667 is not confirmed by any other source.[19] The fact that this disease seems to have afflicted only Englishmen, and went unnoticed in Italian sources, supports the notion that Wighard's "plague" could have been a malaria outbreak confined to unacclimated English visitors to the city. On the other hand, while we do not know what season Wighard travelled to Rome, there is evidence that even at this early date English travelers may have timed their trips to Rome to avoid Rome's summer fevers. British voyagers to Rome tended to leave England in the summer, cross the Alps in fall, and arrive in Rome around November after the dangerous season was over.[20] Alcuin, a Northumbrian cleric who became the chief scholar of Charlemagne's court, warned that the air of "golden Rome" was is "unhealthy for many men, especially those from afar," and he advised visitors to avoid the summer heats.[21] The visiting ecclesiastics who did not follow this advice, such as the fever-stricken Willibald and Winnebald, became the examples that proved the wisdom of the overall rule. In any case, Wighard's death did not discourage archbishops-elect from visiting Rome in the years to come, including Tatwin, Northelm, and Cuthbert in the 8th century and Wulfred and Ethelred in the 9th.

Why did these men risk the long voyage between England and Rome? The lack of sources makes this a difficult question to answer: as Parks makes clear, our understanding of British travel to Rome before the 7th century "remains vague and shadowy."[22] Two brighter sparks however do shine out of the gloom—the well-documented churchmen Biscop and Wilfrid—and their motives for visiting Rome were probably typical of the group. For Biscop, the main motive seems to have been love and admiration for all things Roman. Biscop's heart was "inflamed with holy Love" for Rome as a youth, and as a result he visited the Eternal City in 653 and then five more times later in life, each time returning with "a large number of books on sacred literature" as well as assorted holy relics. Indeed, Biscop's library would eventually grow to several hundred volumes and would play an important role diffusing Roman religious culture throughout the recently-converted kingdoms of England.[23]

While Biscop's story is a simple tale of English attraction to Roman culture, the erratic trajectory of Wilfrid's spark tells a more complex story. Like Biscop, Wilfrid was reportedly drawn to Rome by the "humble fire" of his faith, which upon reaching Rome was "was blown by God to flame." At this point, however, Wilfrid's story diverges sharply from Biscop's. While Wilfrid would return twice more to Rome, he came not as a pilgrim but as a litigant, seeking Roman help in overcoming his ecclesiastic enemies within England. During his second trip to Rome, Wilfrid appealed to the pope to restore portions of the Bishopric in Northumberland that had been taken from him and given to other dioceses. The papacy decided in his favor, but Wilfrid's English enemies ignored the ruling and insisted that Wilfrid content himself with his monastery in Ripon. The underlying issues was probably financial—Wilfrid seems to have been resented for his lavish lifestyle, and contemporaries accused him of travelling with a retinue of soldiers and dressing his household in an extravagant manner more befitting a secular prince than a servant of God.[24] Frustrated, Wilfrid returned to Rome again in 702 to plead his case. However, he made little headway, perhaps because Pope John VI, who had taken office since Wilfrid's last trip, spoke only Greek and was presumably immune to Wilfrid's oratorical blandishments. Disappointed, Wilfrid returned to England but found the wheel of fortune had turned in his favor. The new king of Northumbria was one of Wilfrid's own former pupils and was happy to restore Wilfrid's control over some of the disputed offices. Afterwards, Wilfrid spent the remainder of his life in relative peace and was eventually buried under the floor of the Church of St. Peter in his beloved first monastery of Ripon.[25]

As the nine Roman voyages of Biscop and Wilfrid illustrate, two main motives drew Europeans to the eternal city in this era. Biscop's story exemplifies the *cultural* attraction that Rome exerted over the English and other European from the north, who arrived wide-eyed in the Eternal City and returned home laden with books, relics, and other bric-a-brac mementoes of Rome. One the other hand, while Wilfrid brought back his own share of Roman souvenirs, his tale testifies more to the *political and institutional* power of Rome. As the seat of Europe's greatest apostolic church, Rome had an outsized influence over European religious and ecclesiastical affairs. While their motives were different, however, the outcome was the same: the biographies of both men were punctuated by frequent visits to Rome. For Biscop and Wilfrid, Rome's cultural attractions and political advantages outweighed the expenses and dangers of the voyage.

Other high churchmen also trekked to Rome in the early Medieval period, including Abbot Ceolfrid of Jarrow, who accompanied Biscop on his fifth Roman trip. Coelfrid's motives were a combination of those of Wilfrid and Biscop. Like Biscop, Coelfrid returned from Rome with a great deal of "spiritual merchandise" such as amulets, books, silk vestments, rich fabrics, and holy relics.[26] However, as with Wilfrid, Coelfrid combined relic-shopping with a political agenda—during his trip, he solicited special papal privileges and exceptions for his Abbey of Jarrow.

Towards the end of his life Coelfrid tried to return to Rome, hoping to spend his last days in the holy city. He never got there, dying in France along the way. His death was not in vain, however, since his aborted second trip to Rome gives the modern reader a clue about the scale of these early Medieval journeys to Rome. According to Bede, Coelfrid was accompanied by a train of Englishmen "to the number of eighty," some of whom continued on to Rome without the abbot while others "abandoning their first intentions, returned home [to England] to relate his death and burial."[27] Bright sparks like Coelfrid, therefore, are reminders that hundreds of dimmer cinders were wafting towards Rome in the same period, though they remain mostly hidden in the undocumented dark. Some of these human cinders probably flickered out in Rome, extinguished by the resident malaria species before they could record their own story or accomplish anything worth being recorded by others. This is one of the perennial problems in studying malaria; like all skilled killers, malaria kills its witnesses.

On occasion however malaria did leave a victim behind to tell its tale. One such survivor was Lullus, an English pilgrim who traveled to Rome in 737 CE. After a harrowing journey, Lullus and his travelling companions finally reached the "shrine of the blessed apostles," but soon after their Roman arrival, Lullus and his comrades were prostrated by illness and began to succumb to "the long sleep of peace." Lullus himself avoided death's long sleep, but the experience left him a changed man. "For five long months the heat and cold of panting fever in turn tortured my sick body," he later recalled. "I did not escape the onslaught of the plague with my former health and robust strength of limb ... all the joints of my limbs were shaken and twisted, and I am still weak and outworn." However, these storm clouds had a silver lining: while sick in Rome, Lullus became the confidant of Boniface, an Englishman recently promoted as archbishop of Germany, who would mentor Lullus through his later ecclesiastical career. Lullus would eventually rise to become the bishop of Mainz and then archbishop of the same town before being given a final postmortem promotion to the sainthood.[28]

Despite Lullus' near-fatal fevers in Rome, the chronic threat that malaria posed to visiting churchmen and laymen seems to have done little to discourage travel to Rome in the age of Biscop and Wilfrid. By the late 770s, in fact, so many Englishmen had come to Rome that they had established their own *schola* within the city, the *Schola Saxonum*. While the name suggests a school, the *schola* was in fact an expatriate colony of Englishmen in Rome residing together in a "group of houses, resembling rather a Saxon hamlet."[29] For the most part, these expatriate Anglo-Saxons made their living selling accommodations and other tourist services to English visitors to Rome. The inhabitants of this *schola* called this neighborhood their "burg"—the old Germanic word for town—which in turn gave its name to the modern-day Borgo district at the foot of Vatican hill in Rome where the old *Schola Saxonum* once lay.[30] Nor was the *Schola Saxorum* the only such expatriate colony in Rome. Other *schola* rose along the banks of the Tiber as well, including a Frankish *schola*, a Lombard *schola,* and a *schola* of the Frisians, a newly-converted Germanic people who lived in and above the north Netherlands coast.[31] As for the Irish, they had no formal *schola*, but the Irish monastery of the Holy Trinity in Rome might have served much the same function for the Emerald Isle's numerous pilgrims.[32]

Rome, Relics and Pilgrimage

As is clear from the voyages of Biscop and Wilfrid, one of the most important factors attracting transalpine travelers to Rome was the Eternal City's stock of holy relics. Already in the 6th century, Gregory of Tours noted that metal shavings from the chains supposedly worn by St. Peter in prison were a much sought-after commodity. Early Christians were also eager to purchase objects infused with the holy radiation that was thought to emanate from the bodies of saints. Handkerchiefs hung near the tomb of a martyr were thought to actually gain in weight as they soaked up the saint's "divine virtue." Similarly, oil from lamps that had hung in the martyr-filled catacombs became tourist commodities highly prized for their supposed spiritual merits.[33]

However, the most desired relics were the bones of the saints themselves. While ancient Romans had associated corpses with spiritual pollution and thus forbade the burying of bodies within the city of Rome, Christians venerated their dead, especially the remains of early martyrs. As a result, during the Gothic and Lombard wars, the Christians of Rome hurriedly re-buried many martyrs inside churches within the walls of Rome to keep them safe from despoilment during the ongoing conflict.[34] From the 4th century onwards in fact it became common practice to incorporate the relics of martyrs, preferably apostles, into newly-constructed churches, usually within a special compartment built into the altar.[35] Since Northern Europe had few martyrs of its own, many Northern European churchmen carted some of Rome's surplus relics back north with them in order to found new places of worship.

By the 8th and 9th centuries, this flow of relics was in full swing, and an "unprecedented" flow of relics streamed northwards from Rome.[36] According to historian Ferdinand Gregorovius, these north-bound martyrs were accompanied to their British, French, or German destinations by a "dismal triumphal procession" of laymen and priests "bearing torches and chanting hymns."[37] Even by Medieval standards, these post-mortem reverse pilgrimages of Roman saints to distant provincial parishes must have been a particularly bizarre spectacle. Some contemporaries, including an anonymous 9th century poet, were dismayed by this commodification of sacred remains. "Rome" he wrote, "you killed the saints with the sword; to-day you sell their bodies."[38]

Ironically, despite this outflow of saints from Rome, Rome's store of relics probably increased on the whole in the 6th and early 7th centuries due to imports from the Holy Land. In this early age, the city of Rome was as much a base as a destination for pilgrims: the most prestigious pilgrimage site during these early Christian centuries was not Rome, but Jerusalem, where believers could walk in the very footsteps of Jesus. On the way to Palestine, many pilgrims stopped in Rome to see Rome's own relics, which certainly outshone those of Northern Europe though they were decidedly second-tier in comparison with the relics of the Holy Land. Over time, however, donated relics from pilgrims returning from Jerusalem gradually bolstered Rome's own collection, which eventually included such Old Testament wonders as Ark of the Covenant and New Testament marvels like the "garment of Saint John the Baptist, and the tongs that Saint John the Evangelist was shorn with."[39]

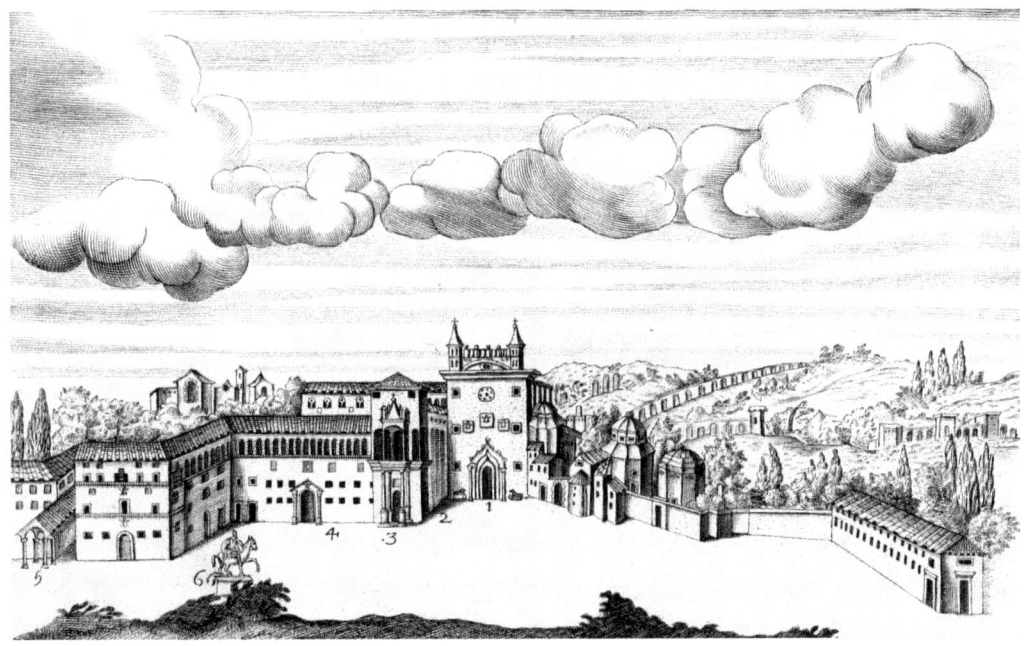

The Lateran Basilica, as it appeared in the Middle Ages. Note the aqueduct ruins in the background. Joannis Ciampini, *De Sacris Aedificiis a Constantino Magno Constructis: Synopsis Historica* (Rome, 1693), p. 17.

During the 7th century, however, Rome's popularity as a pilgrimage center rose dramatically. From 636 onwards, Arab Muslim armies marched from victory to victory in the Eastern Mediterranean and eventually gobbled up nearly half of Byzantium's territories, including North Africa, most of the Levant, and the valuable province of Egypt. Just as Romans had previously fled eastwards in the face of the German invasions, Greeks now fled westwards from the Arab onslaught. These fugitive Greeks were so numerous that they established their own *Schola Graeca* in the area between the Tiber and the Circus Maximus.[40] Some of their descendants later rose to the rank of pope, much to Wilfrid's irritation in 702.

With the Holy Land now in infidel hands, relic-rich Rome rose dramatically in popularity as the destination for pilgrims. Indeed, it used to be said that the English word "to Roam" was derived from the city of Rome, the object of desire of many Medieval European travelers.[41] Modern linguists reject this notion, but the theory itself clearly indicates just how central Rome was to the travel plans to European pilgrims, especially after the fall of the Christian East. Nor were they drawn there for pilgrimage alone. As we shall see in the next chapter, by the start of the Medieval era proper, the legend of Rome had grown to occupy a privileged space in the mindset of Western Christianity.

6

Dragon's Lair

Once upon the time, we are told, a "subtle clerk" was drawn by curiosity to a most peculiar statue standing amidst the ruins of his native city. The statue's arm was raised with a finger extended, and written upon that finger was the mysterious inscription, "strike here." Many of that town had observed this statue before, but none could grasp its meaning. The clever clerk, however, noticed that the statue's silhouette seemed to point towards a particular patch of ground. Taking a spade to the shadow-marked spot, the clerk soon uncovered a mysterious flight of stairs trailing downwards towards a distant light below.

Intrigued, the clerk descended, and there beheld an unearthly spectacle. Before him lay the "hall of a magnificent palace," filled with men wearing costly apparel, but frozen motionless in their places at a great feast table. Nearby lay a bedchamber containing a "multitude of women arrayed in purple garments, but not a sound escaped them" as well as a stable of horses who stood still as statues in their stalls. All of these marvels were illuminated by the light of a single glowing carbuncle, or polished stone, set like a beacon in one corner of the great hall. In the opposite corner stood a motionless archer with arrow aimed directly at the carbuncle, and upon his brow was written the following words: "I am what I am: my shaft is inevitable; nor can yon luminous carbuncle escape its stroke."

Out of fear that no one would believe the story of the wonders he had witnessed, the subtle clerk decided to take mementos of this silent scene back with him back to the sun-lit surface, and in his greed he snatched up a gold cup and golden knife from the feast table. Just as his fingers closed around these treasures, however, the archer in the corner let loose his arrow. It struck the glowing carbuncle, which "shivered … into a thousand atoms," plunging the great hall and the subtle clerk into inky darkness. Unable to find his way back in the dark, the clerk "perished in the greatest misery, amid the mysterious statues of the palace."

As with many Medieval tales, this story was meant to be read allegorically. The statue represented the devil, luring men astray. The subtle clerk was a greedy man, the steps downwards were his passions, the archer was human mortality, and the carbuncle represented the clerk's life. As for the golden knife and cup, they symbolized the fleeting treasures of this world which a good Christian knows to be a distraction from the real treasure that Jesus promised in heaven above.[1]

For our purposes, however, the most significant take-away from this story is where the author chose to set his tale: the subtle clerk lived in Rome. Despite its ruinous state—or perhaps because of it—Rome exerted an enormous pull over the European mind in the early Medieval era. In the words of Italian poet and academic Arturo Graf, "the memory of the formidable power and the boundless empire of Rome excited a particular mood of fantasy in the Middle Ages."[2] Rome's fall into depopulation and disrepair only heightened this sense of awe. Indeed, the ruination of Rome was a commonly employed Medieval metaphor for the transience of all worldly things.[3] Despite the fall of its empire, the city of Rome retained a privileged place in the Medieval psyche.

Rome and the European Mind

Small wonder, then, that fanciful legends about the wonders of Rome circulated widely throughout Medieval Europe. The best-known such tales, including the story of the "subtle clerk" re-told above, were later collected by French, German, or English scribes into a text called the *Gesta Romanorum* or "Deeds of the Romans." Scholars suspect this happened sometime around 1300 CE, though the stories themselves are often much older and derive in part from non–Western sources such as the Greek fables of Aesop and the famous *One Thousand and One Nights* folktales the Islamic Middle East. As if to negate this foreign influence, however, the authors of the *Gesta* are generally careful to ground their tales solidly in Roman history, either by re-setting the stories in Rome or by dating the story by the reign of a real or imagined Roman emperor.[4]

In some cases, the *Gesta Romanorum* not only relocated its stories to Rome but recounted notable incidents from Roman history, albeit with a distinctly Christian spin. Case in point is the story told in the *Gesta* of Caesar's overthrow of the Roman Republic. In the *Gesta* version of the tale, as Caesar crossed the Rubicon he encountered a "phantom of immense stature" who warned Caesar that "if your purpose be the welfare of the state—pass on; but if not, beware how you pass another step." However, since Caesar's love of Rome was pure, he crossed the Rubicon unharmed and went on to defeat his enemies. Once again, this story was meant to be understood metaphorically. Caesar, we are told, represents Adam, who was expelled from the Garden of Eden (Rome) and his crossing of the Rubicon was a re-enactment of the Christian ritual of baptism, allowing Caesar to return to Rome in a state of blessedness.[5] The fact that the real Caesar was a pagan did not matter one whit to the author or his readers; by the Middle Ages, imperial power was commonly associated with Christian virtue, so any good Roman emperor would automatically have been grandfathered into the faith.

This implicit interweaving of Rome, empire, and Christianity in the *Gesta* becomes explicit in a second Medieval text, the 12th-century German *Kaiserchronik* or "Book of Emperors." In the main, the *Kaiserchronik* draws from the same pool of stories used by the authors of the *Gesta*. However, it employs these stories in the service of a quite different objective. While the purpose of the *Gesta* was the moral edification of the reader, the primary goal of the *Kaiserchronik* was to draw an unbroken line of imperial succession from Julius Caesar to the Germanic emperors of the author's own time, thus legitimizing these northern claimants to Roman *imperium*. The common denominator of all these emperors, whether Pagan or Christian, was the seat of their power, the Eternal City of Rome. In addition, the *Kaiserchronik* introduces a second consistent theme not present in the *Gesta*: the central role played by the *German* people in founding and sustaining the empire. Indeed, in the *Kaiserchronik*'s version of the Rubicon crossing so many German cavalrymen rallied to the banners of Caesar that they "invaded the Roman lands like a river in flood." Following Caesar's victory, he paid off his German followers with "gold

6. Dragon's Lair

and silver" from Rome's overflowing treasuries, and as a result "German men have been full of love and praise for Rome ever since."[6]

While many Medieval Europeans learned about Rome through the *Gesta* and *Kaiserchronick*, the most popular available book on the subject was undoubtedly the *Mirabilia Urbis Romae*, or the "Marvels of the City of Rome." Like the *Gesta* and the *Kaiserchronik*, the *Mirabilia* was first compiled in the high Middle Ages, though the stories it contains are much older. And like the other two works, the *Mirabilia* doesn't let the truth get in the way of a good story, especially if that tale could be spun into a lesson about Christian virtues. In the *Mirabilia*, for example, Emperor Augustus is reimagined as a proto–Christian to whom God sends a miraculous vision foretelling that a Virgin would soon give birth to the savior of the world. After this revelation, the *Mirabilia* tells us, Augustus announced to his peers that he was a mortal man like any other and refused the title of "Lord"—an ironic claim, given that the real Augustus was one of the chief architects of the Imperial Cult.[7]

In a similar vein, the author of the *Mirabilia* takes pains to connect the stories of pagan Rome to the people and events of the Christian Bible. According to the *Mirabilia*, Hercules built an early city on the site of Rome somewhere in the shadow of the Capitoline Hill. The hero's descendants later intermarried with new generations of arrivals, including the Trojan refugee Aeneas and his daughter Roma, a distant progenitor of Romulus. Nonetheless, the first founder of Rome was actually Noah, who (the *Mirabilia* tells us) built a city "not far from the place where Rome is now" after he and his sons fled the fall of the Tower of Babel.[8]

Not surprisingly, given the impressive pedigree of Rome's various founders, the city

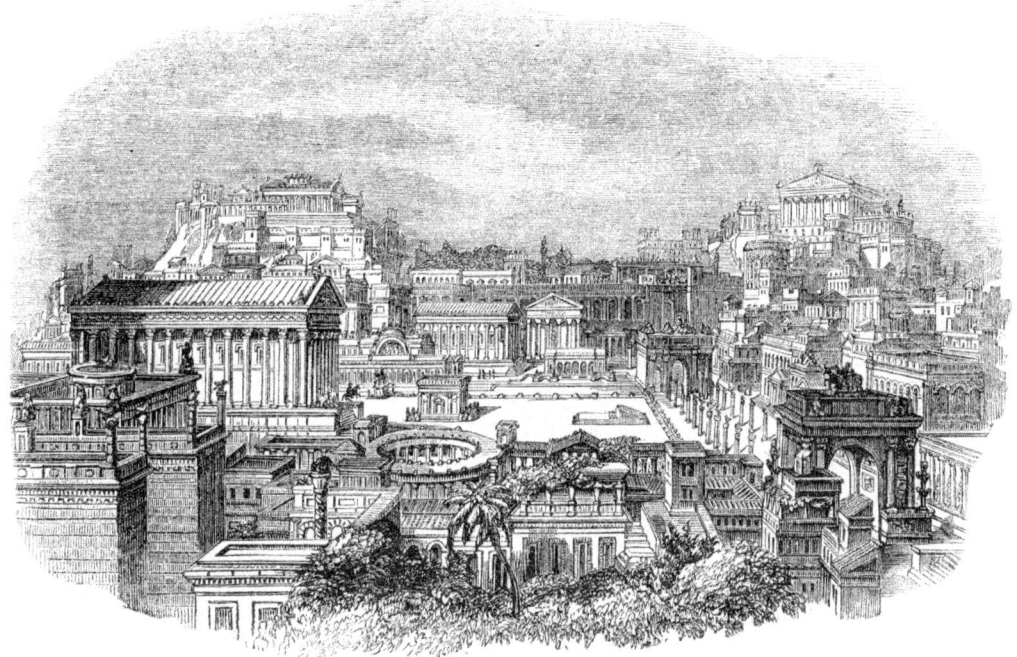

An artist's rendition of the Roman Forum, seen from the Palatine hill, with the Capitoline hill rising in the background. The Temple of Vesta, which supposedly lay atop the lair of the dragon of the Forum, stands in the left foreground (SOTK2011/Alamy Stock Photo).

of Rome itself was replete with marvels. According to the *Mirabilia*, the Colosseum was once a temple of the sun and was originally capped with a dome of gilded brass within which clever Roman engineers manufactured rain, thunder, and lightning for the entertainment of the crowds below. Beneath that dome stood a colossal statue of Phoebus, god of the sun, from which the structure derived its popular name. Another marvel was the Pantheon, a temple-in-the-round decorated with a ring of statues depicting "every kingdom of the world," each outfitted with a bell that rang magically if that country rose up against the authority of Rome. These wonders, however, paled before the opulent structures that once graced nearby Capitol Hill. In ancient times, the *Mirabilia* tells us, the Capitoline was topped by a tremendous palace complex covered "with glass and gold and marvelous carved work" and studded with costly stones; indeed, the combined wealth of the Capitol was said to be worth "one third of the world."[9]

Magic, Monsters and Malaria

The tales contained in the *Gesta Romanorum, Kaiserchronik,* and *Mirabilia*, therefore, illustrate vividly the privileged place that Rome occupied in the minds of Medieval Western Europeans. Some of the stories they tell, however, remind us that Rome could be perilous as well as marvelous. "In the middle of Rome," according to the *Gesta*, "there was once an immense chasm, which no human efforts could fill." According to prophesy this crack could only be sealed by the voluntary self-sacrifice of a man inspired by the good of his country. For a long time, despite earnest entreaties by civil authorities to the people of Rome, no one could be convinced to give himself to the chasm. In the end, Marcus Aurelius—another pagan emperor retrofitted with Christian virtues—took it upon himself to solve the problem. The good emperor mounted his warhorse and galloped into the abyss, which "with a dreadful crash, immediately closed over him." For Medieval Christians, the moral of this story would have been clear: the chasm represented Rome's pagan past, and the good Emperor Marcus Aurelius signified Christ, who sacrificed himself to "ransom the human race."[10]

The story of the chasm in Rome presented in the *Gesta*, however, is a Christian parsing of an older story with a somewhat different moral. During his trip to Rome in the late 1600s, Richard Lassels learned the tale of the "Lacus Curtius" or Lake of Curtius, a "stinking puddle" in the valley of the Forum "which annoi'd the Romans much." Oracles told the Romans that the only way to fill the hole was to throw into it the most precious thing in Rome, so the ladies of the town tossed in their best jewels, but to no avail. Finally, a young nobleman named Curtius realized that Rome's greatest treasure was its young men, so he equipped himself in full war panoply and rode horseback into the lake, thus closing the hole forever.[11]

Lassels gives no moral to this tale, but from the standpoint of geography and epidemiology the meaning is obvious. The Forum lies in a natural depression between hills and was the site of a shallow lake before drainage works were constructed during the Republican era. The story of Curtius' death may have originated in part in a tradition of ancient human sacrifices to that lake, a theory supported by the discovery nearby of the remains of a man, woman, and child who had been ritually drowned.[12] I would argue, however, that most significant detail of the Lacus Curtius story is Curtius' youth. Whatever evil was present in the Forum, it could only be dispelled through a tribute of *young* lives. The

6. Dragon's Lair

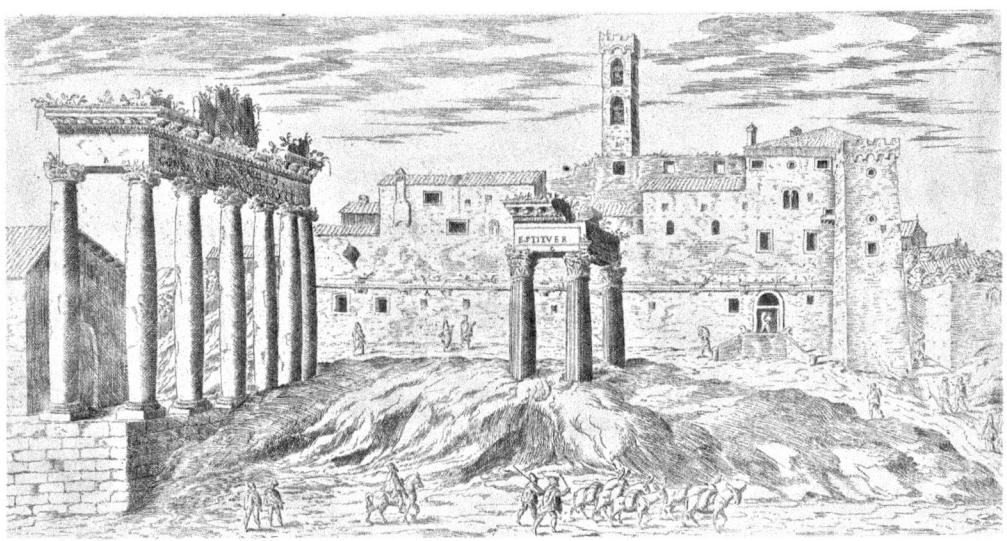

The Forum in the Late Middle Ages. Note that the ruins are still partially buried by built-up debris, washed down from the surrounding hills. Etienne du Perac, *I Vestigi dell'Antichità di Roma: Raccolti et Ritratti in Perspettiva con Ogni Diligentia* (Rome, 1621).

Lacus Curtius tale, then, is arguably a Roman re-telling of the myth of Minotaur: once again, the safety of adults was ensured by the sacrifices of the young.

Other stories reinforce this notion that the chasm story in the *Gesta Romanorum* was inspired by endemic malaria in the lowlands of Rome. The *Kaiserchronik*, for example, records an interesting variant of this tale in which Marcus Aurelius is replaced by a young libertine Roman whose eventual descent into the chasm is presented as punishment for his sexual sins rather than as symbol of redemption for mankind. However, in keeping with Lassal's version, the *Kaiserchronik* variant of the story makes the chasm a threat to Rome's health: in this rendition, the chasm was re-imagined as an "abyss" of "hellfire" which suffocated nearby Romans through the "stench of its flames." Similarly, the *Mirabilia* records that near the Forum was a "place called Hell because in ancient times it burst forth there and brought great mischief upon Rome." In the Mirabilia variant the hole is closed by neither a good emperor nor a sinful pagan but rather a "certain noble knight."[13] Later, a church was built near the site in remembrance of the event: Sancta Maria de Inferno, or "Saint Mary of the Inferno."[14]

While the Forum's gateway to hell was long gone by the time the *Mirabilia* was composed, a second marvel still existed: somewhere underneath the ruins of the Forum lay a dragon, imprisoned there by Pope Sylvester I. The *Mirabilia* only alludes to the story, but a full accounting can be found in the *Golden Legend*, a Medieval collection of stories of holy men compiled in around year 1260, though as usual its component stories are much older. During the reign of Emperor Constantine, the *Golden Legend* tells us, "there was at Rome a dragon in a pit, which every day slew with his breath more than three hundred men." The emperor delegated the dragon to Pope Sylvester, who (as popes are wont to do) prayed to God. As he knelt in prayer, Sylvester received a vision of Saint Peter, who told the pope how to tame the dragon. Following Peter's instructions, Sylvester descended into the liar of the beast, placated the dragon with a prayer, and bound the dragon's mouth with a thread upon which he placed a wax seal stamped with the holy cross. As a result of this miracle, the *Golden Legend* tells us, "the city of Rome was delivered from double death"—not only was the "venom of the dragon" neutralized, but many pagan Romans, impressed by Sylvester's bravery, put aside their false idols in favor of the Christian faith.[15]

As always, variants of the tale exist, and the version told by the *Kaiserchronik* is the most interesting. In the *Kaiserchronik's* telling of the story, a "marauding dragon appeared who brought misery to the Christians. No one dared leave the city of Rome for fear of losing his life on the spot, [and] great lamentations arose through the whole city in Rome." Saint Sylvester prayed to God and was rewarded with a vision from Saint Peter, who reminded Sylvester that as pope he had inherited Peter's power to bind and loose all things in this world and the next. Fortified by this vision, Sylvester took up his key and confronted the dragon, not in the Forum, but on the Mons Gaudii or the "Mountain of Joy," a hill just to the north of Rome now called Monte Mario. There, he punished the dragon by sealing it within a cave until Judgment Day. These changes in location may represent a Germanization of the tale, since Monte Mario was traditionally used as a base of operations by visiting German emperors, and in the *Kaiserchronik's* story the dragon seems to be active mainly in the Roman *campagna*, through which German armies repeatedly marched (and repeatedly suffered illness) during their various coronation trips to Rome.[16] However, most authors agreed with the *Mirabilia* that Sylvester's dragon lay below the Forum, sealed beneath the ruins of the ancient Temple of Vesta.

The dragon of the Roman Forum, it should be noted, was far from the only monster to threaten the health of Europeans in the ancient and early Medieval world. About a century after Sylvester tamed his dragon, another dragon descended on a graveyard in the outskirts of Paris and began to devour a recently-interred corpse, driving the terrified local inhabitants from their homes. In response, Marcellus, the Bishop of Paris, marched forth and challenged the beast, eventually subduing it with three strikes from his hooked bishop's crozier. Defeated, the dragon was driven from Paris and banished by Marcellus to the desert or the sea where it could do no further harm to Marcellus' flock.

According to a fascinating 1992 study by historian Peregrine Horden, Marcellus' dragon was most likely inspired a different sort of beast, malaria. The dragon haunted the wooded outskirts of the city, Horden notes, where it drove people from the homes for fear of infection. What is more, we know from other sources that Paris at the time was subjected to periodic malarial fever outbreaks after Seine River flooding, which happened frequently in that region due to the impervious quality of Paris' heavy clay soils. Indeed, one of the post-mortem miracles later attributed to Marcellus is curing a Bishop of Paris of his "quartan fever," in other words, *P. malariae*.[17]

The idea that the dragon of Marcellus was a monstrous malaria manifestation gets further support from the catalogue of other dragons that ravaged early Medieval Europe, many of which were linked to fever, poison, or malarial terrain. Horden, for example, recounts the story of a dragon which made its den within a mountain spring in the Julian Alps, killing all who approached with its poisonous breath. The Medieval chronicler Gregory of Tours described still another dragon that coiled around an oak tree in a French field, causing "widespread panic and depopulation" throughout the surrounding lands. Eventually the services of the Apostle Andrew were required to slay this beast, which vomited up a river of blood and poison as it died.[18] However, the most well-known Medieval dragon was the infamous dragon of St. George, a lake-dwelling monster near the Libyan city of Sylene which "venomed the people with his breath." Like the Greek

6. Dragon's Lair

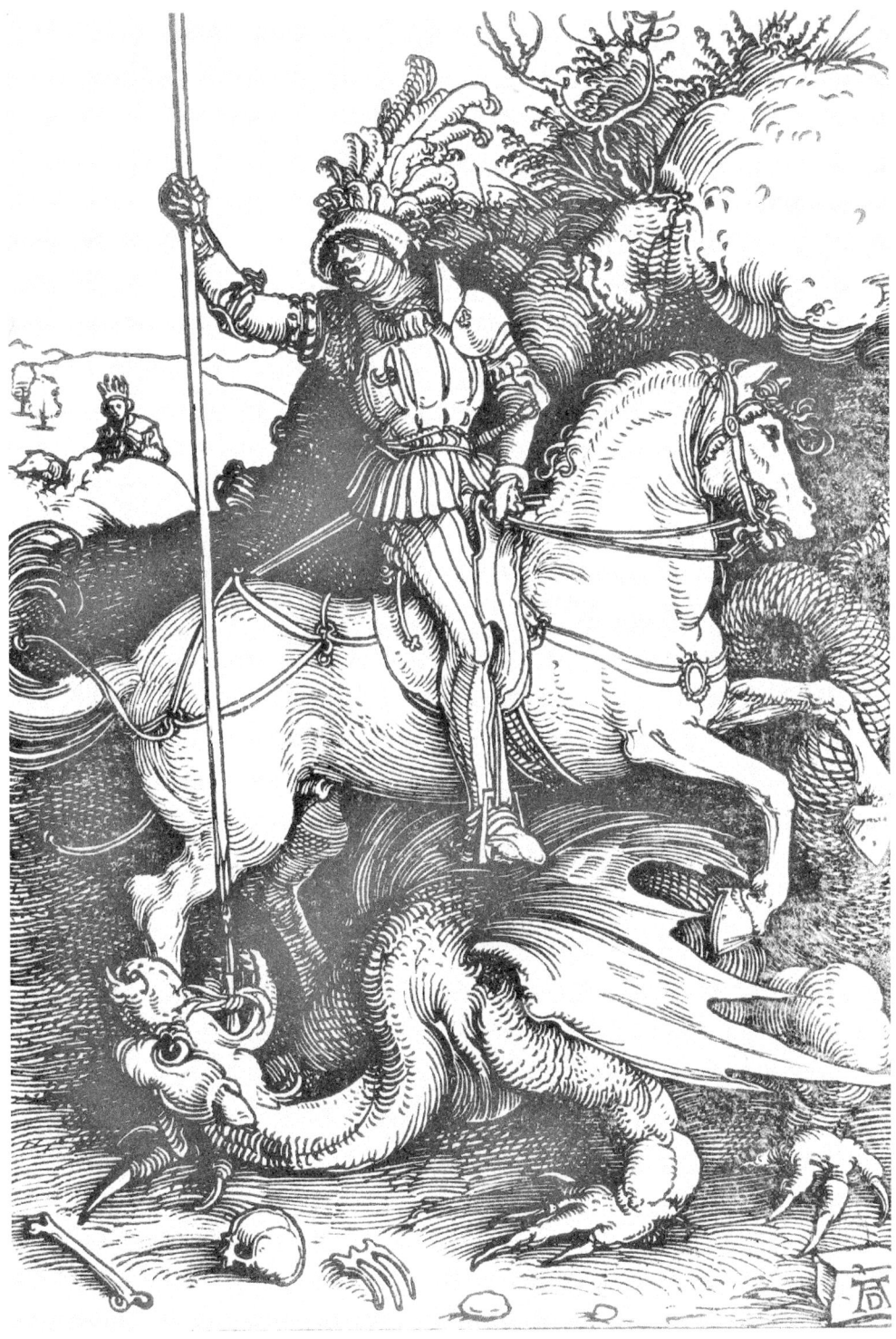

Woodcut by Albrecht Durer of St. George and the dragon, which reportedly inhabited a highly malarial lake near the Lybian city of Sylene. The National Gallery of Art, Washington, Rosenwald Collection.

Minotaur, George's dragon could only be kept at bay through a tribute of "children and young people" who were sacrificed to its endless appetite.[19] Eventually, as is typical of such tales, the local people were liberated from the deadly exhalations of the dragon through the timely intervention of a miracle-working Christian saint.

It is likely that these Christian legends, in turn, owe their inspiration to pre–Christian tales in which divinely-protected heroes defeated monsters associated with malarial landscapes. Case in point is the ancient Greek legend of the hydra, a swamp-dwelling monster with empoisoned breath that only Hercules could defeat.[20] Interestingly enough, the Greeks believed that the hydra's lair, the highly malarial Lernaean swamp, was a gateway to the underworld, a clear parallel to the Roman belief that the forum was both a dragon's lair and a doorway to the inferno. In both Rome and Greece, the fires of fever were likened to the flames of hell.

Dragons of malaria, therefore, built their nests widely throughout Medieval Europe. However, it is important to remember that these dragons were not all created equal. The malaria which likely lay at the root of the Paris, Tours, and Alpine dragon myths was almost certainly of the mild *P. vivax* or even milder *P. malariae* varieties: debilitating diseases certainly, but not typically deadly. The monsters fought by St. George and St. Sylvester on the other hand were more likely manifestations of *P. falciparum*, a far more virulent plasmodia strain. Unlike the dragons of the north, which seemed content merely to drive humans from their vicinity, the dragons of Sylene and Rome were active killers, a horrific annual harvest from the young and unacclimated. Transalpine Europeans who risked a trip to Rome, therefore, were walking into the valley of the shadow of death, the very belly of the beast.

7

The Christmas Crown

In 752, just 15 years after Lullus and his companions shivered with fever in the Eternal City, Pope Zacharias received a remarkable letter from north of the Alps that inaugurated a new set of connections between Rome and Northern Europe. In this letter Pepin, the Mayor of the Palace of the Frankish Kings, reportedly asked the pope "in regards to the Kings of the Franks who no longer possess the royal power: is this state of things proper?" In effect, Pepin was asking papal permission for a palace coup. And Pepin was not disappointed: Zacharias assented to Pepin's request. Green-lighted, Pepin dethroned the last king of the Merovingian line and had himself proclaimed King of the Franks by his assembled nobility.[1] In doing so, he inadvertently began a process that would propel hundreds of thousands of European travelers and soldiers over the Alps to Rome in the centuries to follow.

From Merovingians to Carolingians

So who were these Franks? They were not really a tribe per se, but rather a loose confederation of German speakers whose collective name probably derived from an ancient Germanic word meaning "free" or "fierce." Up until Pepin's coup, the Franks were ruled by the Merovingian dynasty, pagan kings who claimed quasi-divine ancestry through the Quinotaur, a magical five-horned sea-monster who copulated with a Frankish queen. Despite these pagan origins, the Merovingians had adopted the Christian faith in the 5th century and afterwards generally enjoyed good relations with the papacy. By the middle of the 7th century the Merovingians were past their prime. In the words of Carolingian chronicler Einhard, these long-haired and bearded Merovingian monarchs had become non-entities, kings in name only, "content … to sit on [their thrones] and play the ruler."[2] Real power was monopolized by the Frankish "mayors of the palace" who held the reins of government but lacked the formal title of kings, not to mention the otherworldly mystique of belonging to a sanctified royal lineage. The greatest of these mayors of the palace was undoubtedly Charles Martel, or Charles "the hammer," who dominated the Frankish kingdom from 718 to 741. Charles Martel is perhaps best remembered today for his 732 CE victory at the Battle of Tours against the Muslim Arabs, who had had conquered the Visigothic state of Spain during the 710s.

From the standpoint of the Papacy, the main value of these Franks was as a counterweight to the "perfidious and most foully stinking" Lombards, who by then were becoming an increasing threat to the independence of the papacy.[3] The Lombards had marched on Rome in 728, though on this occasion the Lombard King Liutprand was dissuaded from attacking papal territory by an impassioned personal appeal from the pope. In the 740s, however, Liutprand once again sallied southwards from his capital at Pavia and this time managed to secure the submission of the local Lombard dukes in Spoleto and Benevento, long-standing supporters of the autonomy of the papacy. Worse yet, Liutprand seized control over a large swath of territory near Rome previously administered by papal officials.[4] These Lombard attacks on the papacy continued even after the popes had forged an alliance with the Franks. In fact, Lombard interference in Roman affairs reached a new peak in the 670s, when Lombard King Desiderius tried to install his own client pope in Rome following the death of Pope Paul I.

War between the Franks and the Lombards broke out soon afterwards, though it was triggered as much by dynastic disputes as by Liutprand's mistreatment of the papacy. After Pepin's death, authority in the Frankish territories was divided between his two sons, Charles and Carloman. As brothers have done since the age of Romulus and Remus, the two began to quarrel and the Lombards took the opportunity to meddle in Frankish affairs, allying themselves with Carloman against Charles. However, while the brothers were gathering their forces for war, Carloman died unexpectedly. In a bizarre twist, contemporaries attributed Carloman's death a violent nosebleed, the same fate that had befallen Attila the Hun over three hundred years before.

Carloman's demise proved to be a disaster for the Lombards. Immediately after Carloman's death his widow fled to the Lombard court to seek its support in putting Carloman's children upon the Frankish throne. Charles interpreted this as an act of war, invaded Italy, besieged the Lombard capital at Pavia, and forced the unconditional surrender of the Lombard King, who spent his last days as a monk-prisoner in a remote abbey. As for the Lombard Kingdom, Charles decided to formally annex it to the Frankish domain. Gathering up the Lombard lords, Charles staged a coronation ceremony in Pavia in which he claimed the Lombard crown, later known as the Iron Crown since it supposedly contained metal from one of the iron nails hammered into the body of Jesus during his crucifixion. Some Lombard lords refused to kneel to Charles, especially those in the less accessible Italian south, but overall the Lombard threat to Rome had effectively been defanged.

Even after the annexation of the Kingdom of the Lombards, Charles' appetite for territorial gains was far from satisfied. During his long reign Charles waged unremitting military campaigns from his capital at Aachen into the Iberian south and the half-pagan German east, eventually adding the

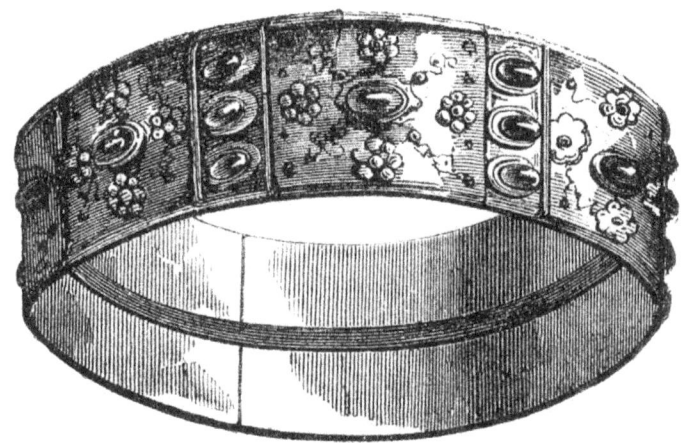

The Iron Crown of the Lombards, depicted in a mid–19th century engraving by Cesare Cantù. *Grande illustrazione del Lombardo-Veneto ossia storia delle città, dei borghi, comuni, castelli, ecc. fino ai tempi moderni* (Milano, Corona e Caimi Editori, 1858).

provinces of Saxony, Bavaria, Carinthia, and the Spanish March to the already sprawling Frankish state. By the time of his death, Charles' domain spanned over 1.1 million square kilometers—over twice the size of modern France—and had an estimated population of 10–20 million people, making it by far the largest state in Europe since the fall of the Roman Empire.

Empire Reborn

The apex of Charles' political career, however, occurred not on the field of battle but within a Church in Rome. To understand what happened in Saint Peter's Basilica in Christmas of the year 800 requires a brief primer in 8th century Roman politics. By the late 700s, the papacy and the papal court had fallen increasingly under the control of Rome's powerful noble families who now fought over clerical offices much as their pagan ancestors had competed for consulships and other political ranks during the time of the Roman Republic.[5] Unfortunately, these squabbles over sacred office could take on a quite profane level of violence. In April 799, supporters of a previous pontiff attacked Pope Leo III in the streets of Rome and tried to blind him and cut out his tongue, thus rendering him unable to continue as pope. Leo survived the attack, but recognizing that his position in Rome was weak he fled to Charles, who was then making war against the German Saxons. Wrapping up his campaign, Charles marched to Rome, re-installed Leo III on the papal throne, and condemned many of Leo's Roman enemies to life imprisonment.[6]

In gratitude for this support, Leo III did something remarkable: he made Charles an emperor. According to an often-repeated story, Charles was attending Christmas mass when Leo III placed a crown on the king's unsuspecting head and, despite Charles' protests, proclaimed the Frankish King the Emperor of the Romans. In actuality, of course, the details of the coronation were almost certainly cooked up between the King and Pope beforehand and Charles' supposed unwillingness to accept the burden of the crown was a piece of political theater designed to illustrate Charles' humility and worthiness for the office.[7] Charles now wore three crowns, the crown of the Franks, the crown of the Lombards, and the Imperial Crown, which made him theoretical sovereign of the whole Christian world. Small wonder, then, that Charles is known to history as Charles the Great—or Charlemagne, in French.

From a political standpoint, Charlemagne's coronation was a watershed moment for the history of the Medieval west. Equally importantly, though less well appreciated, is that his crowning also marked a major change in transalpine Europe's *biological* relationship with the city of Rome. There was nothing new about large-scale German migration into Italy; repeated waves of Germanic invaders had been crossing the Alps for centuries, most recently the Ostrogoths and the Lombards. By and large, however, these Germans came as settlers and later generations born upon Italian soil would have enjoyed some resistance through childhood exposure to Italy's resident malaria plasmodia or intermarriage with local populations that had genetic defenses against malaria such as thalassemias or favism. What is more, while both the Ostrogoths and Lombards occasionally looked to Rome with covetous eyes, neither group seems to have regarded possession of Rome as vital to their political legitimacy.

Charlemagne and his successors however differed from their Germanic forebears in both of these respects. Unlike their predecessors, the Frankish Germans did not migrate

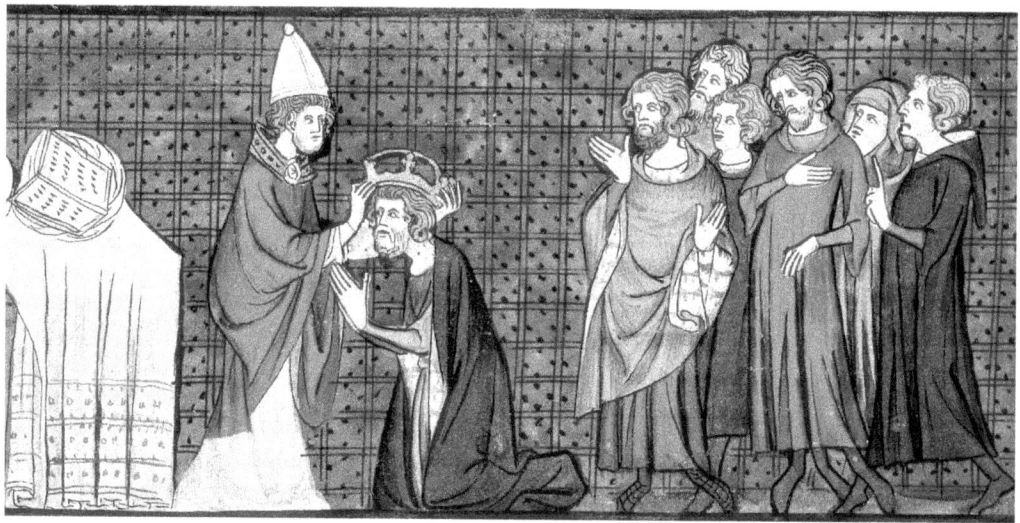

Coronation of Charlemagne by Leo III. *Chroniques de France ou de Saint Denis*, Vol. 1, photograph by Levan Ramishvili, Wikimedia Commons.

en masse to Italy but rather added Italy as the southernmost appendage to a larger empire. As a result, when Frankish armies mustered north of the Alps marched into Italy, their unacclimated armies would routinely fall prey to Italy's resident malarial fevers. What is more, Rome became crucial to the political legitimacy of Frankish and later Germanic emperors, for whom coronation in the Eternal City was tantamount to "possession of a legal diploma, genuine and hallowed by antiquity" validating their claims of imperial rule.[8] The conjunction between these two factors—the imperative need of these emperors to control Rome, combined with the biological vulnerability of European visitors to Rome's malaria plasmodia—would wreak havoc in European history for the next half-millennium.

The peril faced by transalpine troops in Italy is illustrated vividly in the map below, which overlays Charlemagne's domain atop a historical malaria map of Europe. Almost all of Charlemagne's territory, with the exception of the swampy headwaters of the Rhine River just north of the Alps, are within the epidemic zone of malaria. While "epidemic" sounds serious indeed, the term is somewhat deceiving: in actuality, territories classified as hosting "epidemic malaria" suffer only occasional flare-ups of fever, with years going by without any serious outbreaks. Large-scale infections only occurred during particularly warm and/or moist years when malaria might strike the old and young alike. However, this happened too infrequently for the resident populations to develop immunity to the infection. Overall, the death toll due to malaria was fairly low in transalpine Europe, in part due to its rarity, but also due to the fact that the malaria of the Frankish Empire consisted mainly of the relatively mild *P. vivax* and *P. malariae* species.

I should point out that this map somewhat oversimplifies the malaria situation of northern Europe.[9] Pockets of endemic malaria did exist in the north, such as in the Fenlands of Eastern England or the coastal marshes of the Netherlands and Germany.[10] The best known such malarial hotspot of northern Europe was probably the Dutch coast, the site of the famous Walcheren campaign of the Napoleonic Wars. The British forces that disembarked into Walcheren in 1809 expected to encounter French troops, but were

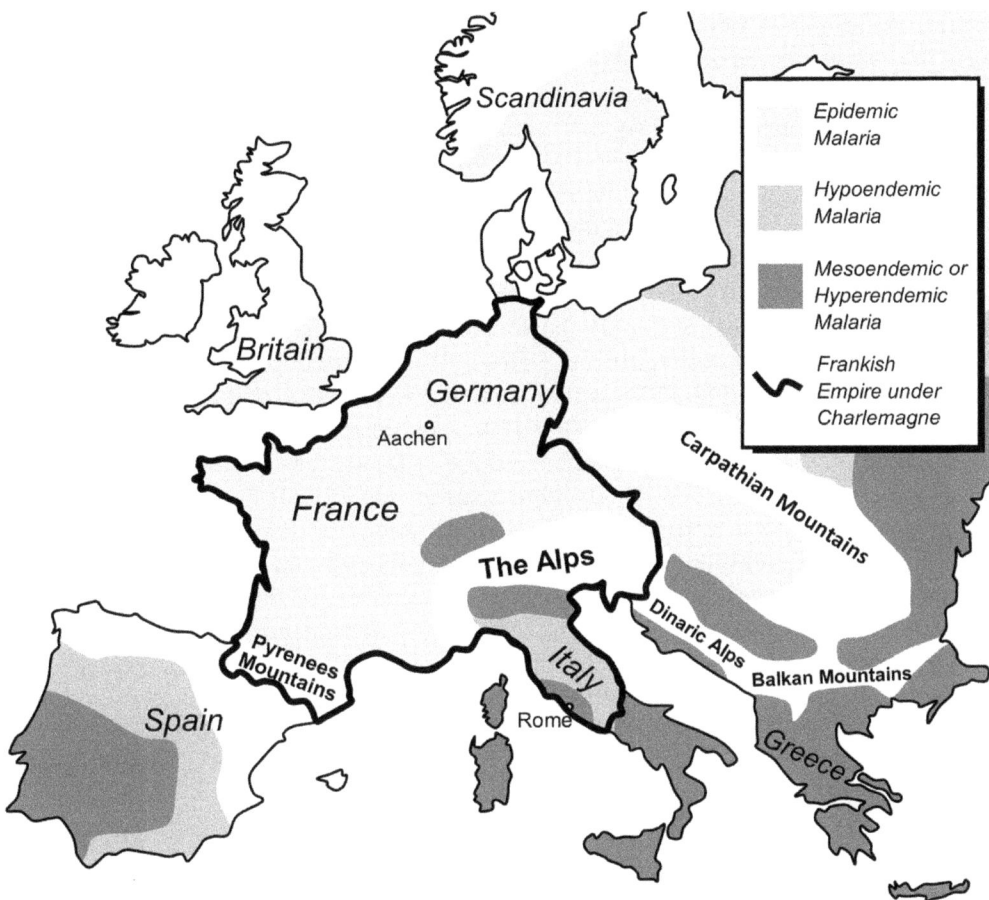

Historical Intensity of Malaria Infection in Europe. Modified from Benjamin James Reilly, "Cardinal Numbers: Changing Patterns of Malaria and Mortality in Rome, 494–1850," *Journal of Interdisciplinary History*, Vol. 49, no. 3 (2019), p. 404, © The Massachusetts Institute of Technology and The Journal of Interdisciplinary History, Inc.

assaulted instead by "unexpected swarms of mosquitoes ... which bit them until their faces swelled." By September 8,000 men were ill, and ultimately the Walcheren campaign cost the British nearly 4,000 men and 60 officers. Such a high death toll probably indicated that diseases other than malaria were involved in the casualties, but malaria certainly played a contributing role in the carnage. Not only did Walcheren Island lie within a known endemic zone for malaria, British army doctors later determined that soldiers from "dry mountainous districts" in England suffered far higher death rates at Walcheren than those from "flat and fenny countries" where malaria was an endemic disease.[11]

In Northern Europe, pockets of endemic malaria such as Walcheren and the Fenlands were the rare exception. Not so in Italy. Once through the Alpine passes, Italian-bound German troops would have first descended into the Po river valley, where they found malaria to be mesoendemic; in other words, at any given time, a significant proportion of the population was suffering from active malarial infections. As German armies continued south the epidemiological situation would have briefly improved, since overall malaria rates were lower in the Apennine interior highlands of Italy than they were in the river towns of the north. By the time the German army reached the lowland plains of the Roman campagna, however, malaria frequency would have risen once more to mesoendemic levels. Not only that, these hypothetical German soldiers would have entered the habitat range of voracious *A. labranchiae* mosquitos and heat-loving *P. falciparum* malaria, the deadliest plasmodia species. South-bound imperial armies, therefore, were obliged to climb a substantial disease gradient, to borrow a term first coined by William McNeill in his seminal *Plagues and Peoples*.[12]

Making matters still worse was the condition of itself Rome in the time of Charlemagne. The final defeat of the Lombards brought peace to Rome but nonetheless the city remained in a ruinous condition. Rome's steady-state population by this time had declined to only about 50,000—less than one-twentieth of the total it had boasted in the imperial era—and these inhabitants lived like squatters amidst and within the ruins of the *caput mundi*. Little work had yet been done to repair the aqueducts, and as a result the healthier but dry hills remained all but abandoned. Still less had been done to repair the sewers or otherwise improve drainage in the lower-lying district of the Campus Martius, where Rome's remnant population was now concentrated. The other two-thirds of the area within the city walls was occupied by orchards, farmsteads, gardens, animal pasture, or marshy wastes, perfect habitat for *Anopheles* mosquitos. As a result of these changes, Peter Llewellyn observed, Medieval Rome had become "a death-trap, especially for unacclimatized visitors from the north."[13]

From the standpoint of biology therefore, Charlemagne's empire was erected upon a shaky foundation. True, it was a political triumph: by accepting the imperial crown, Charlemagne had transformed himself from a Germanic warlord into an heir of the Caesars, and the status of the Germanic peoples in Europe rose accordingly. However, the costs were enormous. Charlemagne's crown ultimately bound together transalpine Europe, where malaria was rare and epidemic in character, with the much more malarial Italian peninsula. In the long run, the Christmas Crown would prove to be a disaster for Italians and Germans alike.

Carolingian Decline

The revival of empire in the West proved to be unfortunate not just for the Germans, but for the papacy as well. Indeed, almost from the start, the Frankish Empire failed to its primary objective: the protection of the papacy against its outside enemies. In 846, a just a generation after Charlemagne's death, Rome was sacked yet again, this time by Arab raiders, who landed in 73 ships near the mouth of the Tiber, defeated a hastily-mobilized Roman defensive force on the outskirts of the city, and ravaged the foreign *scholae* of the Borgo district. What is more, the Arabs despoiled the undefended Basilica of Saint Peter, which had been built atop Peter's grave and thus sat outside the protective embrace of Rome's Aurelian walls. These raiders soon fled in the face of an oncoming relief army from the Duke of Spoleto, but not before the Arabs stripped Saint Peter's bare of gold and jewels. Some of this treasure was later recovered from the bodies of drowned Arabs, since the escaping Arab fleet was ravaged by in a storm off the Italian coast. Nonetheless, the Arab sack of Saint Peter's probably marks the nadir of the fortunes of Rome and the papacy during the early Middle Ages.

Following the 846 sack, the popes bolstered their defenses by constructing the Leonine Walls around Vatican Hill and the Borgo, walls that roughly define the borders of the Vatican City micro-state even today. Nonetheless, the Arab threat was far from over. By the mid–9th century the Arabs had consolidated control over the island of Sicily and used it as a jumping-off point for repeated attacks into the Italian peninsula.[14] "Cities, fortresses, villages have perished with their inhabitants, their bishops are dispersed," Pope John VIII complained in a letter to the Frankish emperor. "The whole Campagna is depopulated, nothing is left to the convents or other places of religion ... the neighborhood of the city has been so utterly devastated, that not a single inhabitant, man or child is to be found."[15] Rome itself was crowded with people displaced by the Arab raids. These impoverished refugees were the lucky ones: as in the days of the Vandals, many Italians were captured and sold off as slaves in North Africa.

So where were the Franks in all of this? When Zacharias gave his blessing to Pepin's coup, he did so in hopes of harnessing the Franks as the papacy's protectors against its enemies, the Lombards included. In the long run, however, the papacy may have been better off with the devil they knew: Pepin's descendants would eventually prove to be a much greater threat to the power and autonomy of the papacy than the Lombards ever were. Even during the age of Charlemagne points of friction were already emerging between popes and Frankish emperors. While Charles dutifully returned the territory that the Lombards had taken from the papacy, he seems to have regarded the pope as his political subordinate—as the Frankish "viceroy in central Italy" in the words of Roger Collins.[16] More ominously for the future, the Franks even challenged the papacy's right to parcel out ecclesiastical appointments even within Italy itself. Much to the dismay of the papacy, for example, the Franks like the Lombard rulers before them asserted the right to confirm the appointment of the archbishop in the strategically important city of Ravenna.

Such interference in papal affairs might have been acceptable if the empire had protected the papacy from attack, but that was far from the case. After Charlemagne's death the empire's attention was distracted from Rome by internal turmoil, largely because Charlemagne's successors did not live up to their forebear's illustrious example. In the words of 19th-century historian Robert Comyn, "the Glory of the Carolingian race, which had been carried to the highest pitch by Charlemagne, expired with that Monarch; and the history of his descendants is little more than a series of errors and misfortunes."[17] Modern historian Roger Collins has made much the same point, though more succinctly: the later Carolingians, he noted, have "something of a 'bargain basement' feel."[18]

Charlemagne's chosen successor was his son Pepin, who ruled as King of Italy during Charlemagne's lifetime. Unfortunately for Pepin, Italy was his undoing; after conducting a long military campaign in the swamps outside of Venice, during which his forces were ravaged by disease, Pepin was "seized by illness and ended his final day" in July of 810.[19] Pepin may very well have been an early transalpine victim of endemic malaria in the Po Delta region, which was becoming increasingly prevalent by the 8th century due to colonization of the Italian east coast by *A. sacherovi* mosquitoes from the nearby Balkans.[20] Whatever his cause of death, Pepin's passing meant that the entirety of Charlemagne's empire was inherited in 814 by his son Louis the Pious, a reasonably competent ruler, but one with several sons too many, and much of his reign was given over to negotiating disputes between them. Largely because of these domestic troubles Louis gave little attention to Italy and never went to Rome for a papal coronation. Rather, Louis hastily crowned himself emperor in Aachen after his father's death, in part to forestall possible dynastic challenges from Pepin's own offspring.

Louis the Pious reigned for 27 years—far too long in the opinion of his sons, who plotted against him and each other even during Louis' own lifetime, triggering three bloody civil wars. Still another war erupted after Louis' death, leading to what a contemporary chronicler called "a massacre whose equal no one could recall ever before witnessing amongst the Franks" during the 841 CE battle of Fontenay.[21] After years of negotiations the brothers Lothair, Louis "the German," and Charles "the Bald" settled matters with the Treaty of Verdun, which partitioned Charlemagne's inheritance into three parts. Charles took the highly Romanized territories of the Frankish west while Louis received newly-conquered Saxony and the Germanic east (hence his nickname). On paper, Lothair did the best in the settlement, receiving the title of emperor, the Kingdom of Italy, and the Kingdom of Burgundy, a strip of territory stretching from Southern France and the Alps all the way to the Dutch coast. In the long run, however, Charles and Louis' kingdoms had the brightest future ahead of them, becoming the core territories of the Medieval French and German states respectively. As for Burgundy, it soon became a kingdom in name only and its territory would be steadily absorbed by its stronger French and German neighbors.[22]

From the standpoint of Rome and the papacy, this sub-division of Charlemagne's empire was far from satisfactory. Since its component parts were individually weaker than the whole and were often at war with each other, the fragments of Charles' old empire could do relatively little to protect Rome from assault, as the 846 Arab raids made painfully clear. Nonetheless, despite their diminished military capacity, Charlemagne's successors continued to insist on their right to approve the results of papal elections. In the long run, this was an unsupportable situation.

From the Frankish point of view, however, their reluctance to come to Rome's defense is understandable given that horrific disease outbreaks regularly assaulted German armies that dared to cross the Apennines into the Italian center and south. The disastrous Italian campaigns of Louis II and Lothair II are a case in point. Louis II, the titular King of Italy, first came to central Italy in 863 not to protect Rome but rather to pressure the papacy into sanctioning his brother Lothar's divorce from his barren wife Teutberga. Soon after arriving, however, Louis II was seized with fever, made peace with the pope, and fled back north. Four more years would pass before Louis finally got around to answering papal calls for a military campaign against the Arabs. When he finally resolved to march on the Arabs in 866, he enlisted the assistance of his brother Lothair II, who had inherited both the imperial title and his father's Burgundian lands. Thanks to this infusion of troops from the north the Frankish forces won several battles against the Arabs, but during the campaign Lothair's troops were afflicted by a "serious pestilence" which killed a "countless multitude," caused by the "unaccustomed heat and the intemperance of the climate.… This is why he did not return to Francia without, as has been said, serious losses amongst his men."[23]

Contemporary chroniclers ascribed Lothair's losses mainly to dysentery (diarrhea), while noting that "many also died of spider bites."[24] However, malaria is a far more reasonable diagnosis given the mention of great heat and the southern Italian location of the campaign—not to mention the fact that Italy hosts no native spider species capable of harming man. It is also suggestive that Lothair's army, recruited north of the Alps, seems to have suffered disproportionally from disease. Louis's army seems to have been less affected, which makes sense: his troops were drawn from the Kingdom of Italy and thus probably included many Italian troops as well as transalpine northerners who had become acclimated to malarial fevers through continuous residence in the Italian peninsula.

Fever struck the unfortunate Lothair II once again in 869. Poor Lothair was desperate to secure the legitimacy of his marriage to a second wife, who unlike Teutberga had borne him a son and potential heir. He had already dispatched several Archbishops and other high ecclesiastical delegates to plead his case in Rome, but to no avail—indeed, most of these delegates were eventually "overcome by illness in Italy and died as exiles and foreigners."[25] Thinking he could accomplish himself what his subordinates could not, Lothair came to Rome to plead his case. According to the chronicler, the pope received Lothair and offered him and his retinue the holy Eucharist but warned Lothair to be faithful to Teutberga, as "anyone who eats and drinks unworthily, eats and drinks judgement on himself." Heedless of the risk, Lothair took the sacrament and proclaimed his innocence of the sin of adultery. Shortly afterwards taking the holy host, however, the emperor was "gripped by an illness" and "he ended his final day on 8 August" in the city of Piacenza. His men shared the same fate. "There were so many casualties among the king's followers," the chronicler tells us, "that it seemed as if an enemy sword rather than a plague had cut down the nobility and manliness of the whole realm."[26] While supporters of the Papacy claimed that the Eucharist had turned to poison in Lothair's lying mouth, malaria is the most plausible explanation for this outbreak of illness. Although no symptoms are given by the chronicler other than death, the demise of so many unacclimated transalpine soldiers during the late summer after visiting Rome and crossing the *campagna* and the marshy Maremma coastal plain in Tuscany is once again consistent with *P. falciparum* infection.

As for rest of the Carolingians, the less said the better: in the disparaging judgment of 19th century historian Robert Comyn, "from the death of Charlemagne to the election of Otho [Otto I] the annals of the empire are little better than a dry and unprofitable enumeration of names."[27] Several of these later Carolingians came to Rome for coronation, including Charles III, "the Fat," an inert and ineffectual figure who seemed more interested in convincing the pope to legitimize his bastard son than he was in the imperial crown. After Charles III's death the empire passed to that bastard, and then to Louis "the Child," but upon the latter's premature death in 911 the Carolingian dynasty in Germany sputtered out entirely. The papacy responded to the resultant power vacuum in Italy by pawning off the imperial title to local Italian notables who could offer some measure of protection for the beleaguered papacy such as the nearby Duke of Spoleto.[28] The popes were in desperate need of military assistance during the 10th century due to repeated invasions of Italy by the Hungarians, the latest group to be pushed into Europe by population pressure from the rear along the steppe nomad belt. Nonetheless, like the Carolingians before him, the Duke of Spoleto proved ultimately to be more interested in meddling in papal affairs than in protecting church territories.

The Ottonians and the Lure of Rome

By the middle of the 10th century, however, Charlemagne's old empire experienced a revival of sorts under a new German-based dynasty. Its founder was Conrad I, Duke of Saxony, who was elected King of East Francia by the other German dukes in order to secure stronger military leadership in this era of Hungarian depredations. Under Conrad's successor, Henry "the Fowler," the dynasty became further consolidated. Henry was followed by Otto I, who marched into Italy early in his reign to be crowned King of Italy and to put an end to Italy's chronic post–Carolingian chaos. While he succeeded in the former he failed in the latter, in part because he has brought insufficient forces with him to force Berengar II, the *de facto* King of Italy, into submission. For the time being Otto could do little, since he faced active opposition to his rule from many German lords including his own son Luidolf.

In 955, however, Otto's hand was strengthened immeasurably by his victory at the Battle of Lechfeld, a stunning triumph that put to an end over 100 years of Hungarian invasions into Western Europe. In the old Roman tradition, Otto was proclaimed *imperator*—emperor—by his triumphant soldiers in the battle's aftermath. With Germany now firmly under his rule, Otto returned his attention to Italy, inaugurating a half-century of sustained engagement between Rome and the German Empire. As an opening move, Otto sent his son Luidolf in 957 to deal with Berengar. Luidolf's forces were initially successful, forcing the troops of Berengar to flee before them. In the end, however, Luidolf suffered the same fate as Charlemagne's son Pepin, dying in Northern Italy of an unexpected fever—perhaps malaria—on September 6.

Despite his own son's death from an Italian illness, Otto remained resolute in his desire to restore order in Italy, in part because he wanted to follow the tradition of Charlemagne and receive the imperial title in the sacred city of Rome. To this end he crossed the Alps in 961 and descended upon the Eternal City with a large force, arriving at the end of January 962. Once there, Otto made it clear he wanted more from Italy than just a crown. Shortly after his coronation, he cajoled Pope John XII into agreeing to the *Diploma Ottonianum*, establishing a framework for future relations between the German empire and the papacy. In this document Otto acknowledged the spiritual authority of the pope, recognized the land grants of Pepin and Charlemagne, and promised to defend both the properties and the independence of the papacy. The pope in turn agreed to the formation of several new archdioceses in Germany, pledged that future papal elections would adhere to established legal forms, and granted the emperor and his representatives the right to confirm the results of those elections. Had both sides faithfully followed the provisions of the *Diploma Ottonianum*, it might have set the tone for mutually beneficial symbiotic relations between the spiritual and secular spheres for centuries to come.

In reality, however, the document was a dead letter almost before the ink had dried. The day after its signing Otto and his army marched north to take on Berengar II, who was still clinging to power in Northern Italy. As soon as Otto's back was turned, the distrustful John XII began to connive against him, seeking to forge a grand anti–German coalition between Berengar, the Hungarians, and the Byzantines, who still harbored their own ambitions in Italy. Unfortunately for the pope, Otto got wind of these back-alley machinations. Furious at the pope's betrayal, the Otto quickly crushed Berengar's forces, forced Rome's surrender with "catapults and hunger," and deposed the fugitive John XII in absentia.[29] Convoking a synod, Otto appointed a supporter, Leo VIII, as pope in Rome.

However, the matter did not end there. By late 963 Otto thought he had Rome firmly under control, so he and his army headed back to Germany. In his absence the Roman populace rose up, deposed Otto's pliant pope, and restored John XII to the papal throne.

Adding insult to injury, upon John's death shortly afterwards the Romans elected Benedict V to replace him without bothering to seek imperial confirmation of their decision as the *Diploma Ottonianum* required. Outraged, Otto recruited a new army, marched on Rome, re-installed Leo VIII as his chosen pope, and sent Benedict V into exile. Rome was once again under secure imperial control, at least for the time being.

Unfortunately for the Germans, Otto's victory over the papacy came at a terrible cost. While campaigning against the pope in 963 Otto had been careful to avoid Rome during the malarial season; Otto had withdrawn "far from the Roman walls" during the "hot season, boiling over with the rays of Phoebus," in the words of contemporary chronicler Liutprand of Cremona.[30] In 964 however the frustrated Otto mistimed his withdrawal from Rome. During July, as the Germans began their return march through the *campagna*, Otto's army was "attacked by so deadly an illness that a healthy man hardly had any hope he would live from morning to evening or from evening to morning." By the time the pestilence had passed, many of Otto's chief supporters had perished, including the Archbishop of Trier, the Abbot of Wissemburgh, the Duke of the Lotharingians, and "a countless multitude of others, noble as well as non-noble."[31] The pestilence only abated with the coming of autumn after Otto's army had reached Liguria in the Italian north. While there is no way to be sure, the timing of the disease, the geographic location, and the scale of the casualties is all highly consistent with *P. falciparum* infection amongst immunologically vulnerable German troops.

After licking his wounds in Germany for a year, Otto returned to Rome to in 966 to restore another imperially-favored pope to the papal throne, and this time he stayed, making Rome his permanent capital. For the next six years Otto endeavored to solidify the empire's position in Italy through frequent military campaigns against the Lombard states of the Italian south, though he was careful in light of the disaster he had suffered in 964 to confine these campaigns to the healthier months of winter and spring.[32] He also opened negotiations with the Byzantines, who were still not reconciled to the unwelcome rebirth of imperial power in Western Europe. In 969, however, Otto made a breakthrough with Byzantium, which had fallen into the hands of the soldier-emperor John I Tzimskes. Since John's position was insecure—he had taken the throne through rebellion and assassination—the emperor of the East was

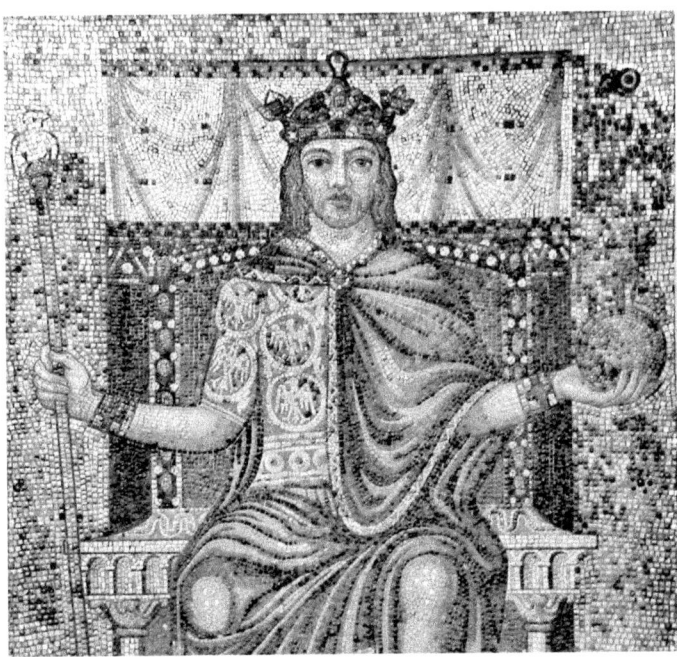

Mosaic of Otto I in the Richard-Wagner-Platz subway station in Berlin. Axel Mauruszat, Wikimedia Commons.

more than willing to make peace with his western counterpart. In addition to recognizing Otto's imperial authority, John agreed to Otto's control over Capua, Benevento, and Salerno in the Italian south, and even gave his niece Theophanu as a bride for Otto's eponymous son. Shortly after, Otto returned to Germany, where he died in May of a sudden fever, as if to remind us that fevers are not restricted to Italy nor are they all malarial in nature.

Otto was succeeded by Otto II, who like his father descended on Italy as soon as he had settled affairs in the Germanic north. His presence was badly needed. In the eight years between Otto I's death and Otto II's arrival, the imperially-appointed pope had been imprisoned and killed and there were two rival claimants to the papacy. What is more, the Lombard principalities of the south were in turmoil, Muslim raids from Sicily had resumed, and relations with Byzantium had reverted to hostility after the assassination of John I Tzimisces, in part because Otto's Byzantine wife Theophanu blamed the new Emperor Basil II for her uncle's murder.

For a while, it appeared that Otto II's reign would be as successful as that of his father. After being anointed King of Italy in Pavia, as was customary, Otto marched on Rome and installed his chosen pope Benedict VII upon the papal throne—there was no need for Otto II to be crowned emperor, since he had been co-crowned with his namesake father years before. Like his father Otto made Rome his official capital and notables from all over Europe flocked to Otto II's court to celebrate Easter of 981, including Hugh Capet of France and King Conrad of Burgundy. However, triumph soon turned to disaster. In 982, Otto invaded the Byzantine state of Apulia on the heel of Italy, seeking to annex it to his empire. The Byzantines responded by allying with the Muslims of Sicily, who duly dispatched an army to Southern Italy to counter Otto's ambitions. The two forces met in South Italy at Stilo, and the result should have been an easy imperial victory: the Arab troops were outnumbered and blockaded from the sea. However, perhaps driven by desperation, the Arabs inflicted a terrible and unexpected defeat on Otto II, who lost as many as 4000 men in the melee.

Otto himself survived the slaughter, but Stilo proved to be the beginning of the end for his reign. News of his defeat crossed the Alps and triggered numerous revolts against Otto's rule. To counter this, Otto called an assembly of his nobility in Verona in Italy to shore up his support and levee new troops. In addition, perhaps worried about his own mortality after the deaths of so many of his men at Stilo, Otto had his son (another Otto) officially elected as King of Germany and heir apparent to the imperial throne. Events would soon prove the wisdom of Otto's decision. Before Otto could march north to deal with pressing matters there, Otto's client pope Benedict VII died, forcing Otto to march to Rome in order to oversee the next papal election. As misfortune would have it, however, Benedict's death occurred in July, so Otto's trip to Rome by necessity coincided with the summer malaria season. As conclave dragged on into September and October, the emperor and many of his followers fell ill with malaria. Otto languished in his Roman palace for months before finally expiring in early December of 983. No doubt many of Otto's soldiers and men of his entourage succumbed to fever as well, but our sources for this time period tend to confine themselves to the affairs of the mighty and do not always deign to comment on the fates of lesser personages.

After Otto's death, the German Empire was thrown into a period of crisis during which Theophanu and other regents tried to manage affairs on Otto III's behalf. German engagement with the Italian south entered a brief lull during this period, though the young king and his mother did visit Rome in 989 to adjudicate some ecclesiastical matters and visit Otto II's grave. When Otto finally came of age in 995, however, he followed his father and grandfather's footsteps on the roads to Rome. Indeed, it soon became clear that Otto intended to exert even more control over Rome than either of his successors, to the point of installing his own cousin, Bruno, as Pope Gregory V. After receiving the imperial crown from his own cousin's hand in late 996, Otto left his kinsman in Rome and returned to Germany to wage war against the Slavs. However, he was forced back to Rome in late 997; as had become customary, the imperially-backed pope had been driven from the city by angry Roman aristocrats during the imperial absence.

Resigned now to the fact that Rome was ungovernable from a distance, Otto settled in for a long stay in a fortified palace atop Rome's Aventine hill, which was reputed to offer protection from Rome's summertime fevers.[33] During this time, in keeping with his imperial motto of *Renovatio imperii Romanorum*, or "Renewal of the Roman Empire," Otto tried to turn the city of the popes back into the city of the emperors.[34] To this end, Otto revived the old imperial system of governance in Rome, promulgated Roman law, established elaborate court ceremonials modeled on Byzantine practices, and even planned to restore the old Senate.[35] What is more, to the dismay of both the papacy and Roman aristocracy—indeed, as we will see in the next chapter, there was little difference between the two during this time period—he also made it clear that he regarded himself as head of the Church and treated the Bishop of Rome as his own chaplain. Upon the death of Gregory V Otto even forced the church to accept his former tutor, the French ecclesiastic Gerbert of Aurillac, as Pope Sylvester II.

Otto returned to Germany briefly in 1000, in part because he was suffering from bouts of illness; as he complained to Pope Sylvester, "the air of Italy is hurtful to my health."[36] But he had by no means turned his back on Rome. Indeed, as part of his plan of Roman imperial restoration Otto traveled to Aachen, the old Carolingian capital, and raided Charlemagne's grave. After breaking down the crypt walls Otto found the great emperor's body seated in a throne "as if alive" and to be almost uncorrupted—a sign, supposedly, of Charlemagne's saintly purity—though one contemporary account reported that Charlemagne's fingernails were poking through his gloves and the tip of his nose had rotted away.[37] Why Otto felt compelled to exhume his predecessor in the imperial office is unclear, but it may be that he wanted to investigate whether Charlemagne was indeed the Last Emperor of legend, prophesized to return and defeat the Antichrist in the endtime of the world before laying down his crown in Holy Jerusalem. Alternatively, Otto may have wanted to establish Charlemagne's holy sanctity, which would be politically useful, or wanted to raid Charlemagne's crypt for holy relics, perhaps seeking to trade them with Duke Boleslaw of Poland for the arm of Saint Adalbert.[38] But these are just speculations—Otto's real motives are unclear.

By the start of the new century, however, the Romans had had enough of Otto's antics. In 1001, the flame of revolt broke out in Rome, sparked by Otto III's lenient treatment of the rival city of Tivoli but fueled by deeper Roman grievances against Otto's imperial ambitions, which were being achieved at the expense of the Roman aristocracy. Otto and his puppet pope were driven from Rome. While waiting for the arrival of the northern reinforcements he needed in order to retake the Eternal City, the deeply religious Otto made a pilgrimage to the monastery of Sant'Apollinaire in Classe amid the swamps outside of Ravenna. There, the emperor fasted, did penance, and probably contracted malaria. By the time his troops arrived and he began his march on Rome, Otto

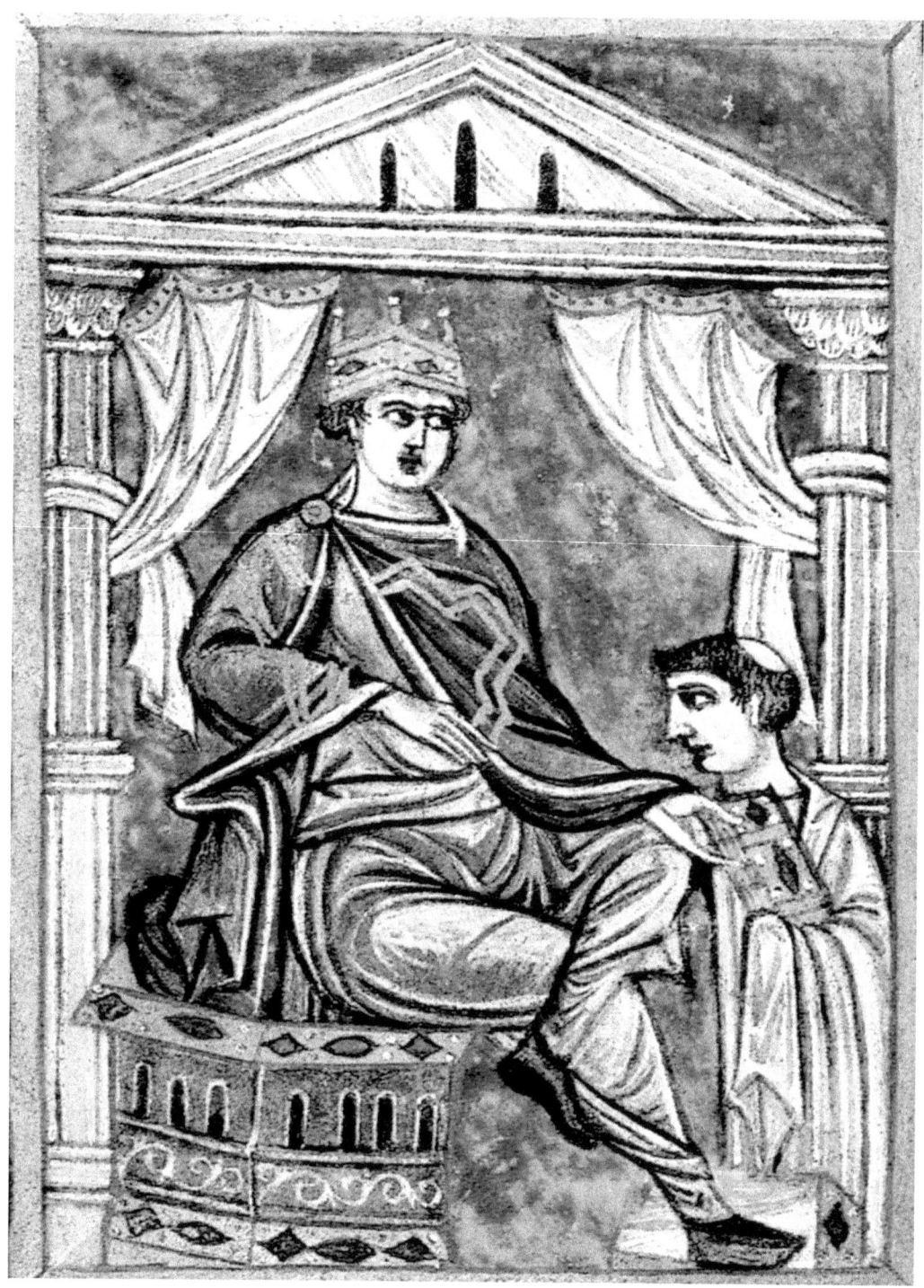

Otto III, depicted in a position of authority over a clergyman, seated on his throne in Rome. *Meister des Gebetsbuchs Ottos III*, fol. 43r.

was already in the grips of *morbus Italicus*, as contemporary sources termed the disease. Shortly after an unsuccessful attempt to retake the Eternal City, Otto followed in the footsteps of his father and succumbed to fever.[39]

In total, historian Eckhard Müller-Mertens points out, Otto III and the other Ottonian emperors spent "sixteen years and ten months in Italy," during which "numerous Italian expeditions…" followed one another in rapid succession, "lengthy courts" were held in Italy, and countless "German princes and their followings—mailed horsemen and other fighting men as well as servants," passed over the Alps into Germany. The sum result of this, Müller-Mertens argues, was the dramatic "lengthening and strengthening of the north-south axis of the Ottonian Reich."[40]

But what was it all for? In later years, German intellectuals and nationalists turned hostile to these impractical Ottonian emperors, especially Otto III, whose magnificent Italian fantasies moved in "magic circles" and were built "upon a foundation of air."[41] In a characteristic passage, German poet August von Platen-Hallermünde puts this lamentation in the mouth of the dead emperor:

> *Oh Rome, where all my blossoms*
> *Have withered into Dust*
> *To guard the Royal coffin*
> *Does not befit your cast!*
> *You have destroyed my honor,*
> *Have broken every limb:*
> *In Aachen with great Charlemagne—*
> *There I will lie by him*[42]

Such complaints about Otto's Italian dreams no doubt made sense to 19th-century German nationalists, whose longing for German statehood outweighed every other consideration. However, they would have rung hollow to the Ottonian emperors themselves, whose sense of identity was linked not to Germany but to God and empire—and both God and empire were tied inextricably to Rome. Even Platen himself was by no means immune to the lure of Italy. After visiting Italy in 1826, the smitten Platen made it his home and like Otto III passed away far from Germany, on Italian soil.

With Otto III's death, Germany's imperial ambitions in Italy ground to a temporary halt. But the imperial struggle with the papacy was far from over—and during these struggles, malaria gave the papacy a consistent home field advantage. As 19th-century historian James Brice observed,

> … not all the efforts of Emperor after Emperor could gain any firm hold on the capital they were so proud of. Visiting it only once or twice in their reigns, they must be supported among a fickle populace by a large army of strangers, which melted away with terrible rapidity under the sun of Italy amid the deadly hollows of the Campagna.[43]

8

Brood of Vipers

The half-century after Otto III's death was marked by a temporary lull in imperial interest in Italy and Rome. While the Ottonians had spent the bulk of their reigns in Italy, Otto III's successor Henry II kept to Germany and delayed his expected Roman coronation until his ninth year. When he finally crossed the Alps, Henry kept his time in Italy to a minimum, arriving in Rome for his public crowning in February of 1013 and then scurrying home via Pavia shortly afterwards. Control over Rome, it appeared, was no longer of crucial importance to the emperors of Germany.

As events would prove, however, 11th-century German disinterest in Rome would only be a temporary state of affairs, the result of Henry's personal ideology and his distraction by events closer to home. Much of Henry's reign was consumed by a brutal 16-year war with the Duke of Poland. However, Henry's disengagement from Italy also reflected a conscious program of refocusing imperial energies north of the Alps. While Otto III had chosen *Renovatio regni Romanorum*, or "restoration of Rome" as his motto, Henry II contented himself with the more modest goal of *Renovatio regni Francorum*, or "restoration of the Frankish state."[1]

As a result of this Frankish focus, Henry would only descend into Italy once during his later reign—and the results of his 1021–1022 military campaign demonstrate the wisdom of his overall disinclination to meddle south of the Alps. Henry's objective in this campaign was to annex the Southern Italian coastal territories of the Byzantines, who were temporarily in ascendency after defeating the Lombard dukes and their Norman mercenaries at the battle of Cannae in 1018. As was typical for unacclimated northern European troops in southern Italy, however, Henry's campaign was spoiled by disease, which "ravaged his army" and forced him to flee from the "ungenial heats of the south" back into German territory.[2]

Henry II's disinterest in Italy was inherited by his successor Conrad II, a somewhat distant descendent of Otto I. True, Conrad's coronation trip was somewhat more protracted than Henry's, in large part because his attempt to be crowned King of Italy in Pavia, the old Lombard capital, was foiled by local aristocratic resistance. Conrad would ultimately have to settle for coronation in Milan instead. Slowed down by this unexpected delay, Conrad wisely held off marching to Rome until early spring of 1027 and then fled Italy before the coming of the feverish summer. Like Henry II, Conrad did not return to Italy for a decade, and when he did finally revisit Italy for a 1036–1038 military expedition, the result was a near-exact replay of Henry's campaign 14 years before. After a short visit to Rome, Henry marched into southern Italy to impose order in the Lombard dukedoms, but as spring turned into summer a "destructive contagion" broke out in his army.[3] Conrad would live to return to Germany, but his stepson and daughter-in-law did not. Like many other members of the unacclimated German force, both had fallen prey to disease, most likely malaria, in the Italian south.

Rome's Saeculum Obscurum

The factor that did the most to re-establish close German imperial relations with the state of Rome after Conrad's reign was the growing corruption in the papal office. Even before the age of Charlemagne, the office of pope had become the plaything of the Roman aristocrats, who fought and killed each other for access to the papacy and the resources it commanded. The century after the death of Charles the Fat was particularly notable for papal misdeeds; church historians have labeled this era that century *saeculum obscurum*—the dark or obscure century.[4] Others call this period the pornocracy, since the popes of this age were dogged by accusations of "murder, black magic, adultery, [and] sexual perversion."[5]

The situation improved somewhat during the reigns of the Ottonian emperors, who pushed aside these aristocratic popes in favor of their own candidates. However, after Otto III's death the papacy once again fell to the control of the Roman aristocracy, whose urban towers, numerous as the spines of a hedgehog, dominated the *Caput Mundi's* skyline.[6] Indeed, with the exception of a few popes appointed by the Ottonian emperors, every pope in the 200 years following 816 was a member of a Roman aristocratic family.[7] The Teofilattos alone managed to seat five of their members upon the papal throne between 816 and 1032.[8] Very few of these popes survived into old age, since assassination had become the new normal. As historian of Rome Ferdinand Gregorovius has quipped, during this era "Saint Peter's chair became the prey of the nobles, and was occupied by a series of popes in such quick succession, that scarcely had they ascended it before they sank into a bloody grave."[9]

While most of the post–Ottonian emperors were willing to turn a blind eye towards the corruption gnawing at the papal office, Conrad's successor Henry III did not have that luxury. Henry III's reign coincided with the papacy of Benedict IX, who outdid the worst excesses of the pornocracy era. A scion of the powerful Theophylactus family, Benedict took power in 1032 as a result of "wholesale bribery on the part of his father." As pope, Benedict was a "shameless debauchee" who "led unchecked the life of a Turkish sultan in the palace of the Lateran."[10] By 1045, the people of Rome rose in rebellion against this dissolute pontiff, leading to the election of Sylvester III. However, Benedict refused to stand down and his powerful family soon drove Sylvester from the city. Making matters worse, after dislodging Sylvester from the Lateran, Benedict sold the papal office to his godfather, who became Pope Gregory VI. But then the fickle Benedict changed his mind and tried to depose Gregory in turn.

When Henry III descended on Rome for his papal coronation in 1046, therefore, Rome had no fewer than *three* popes, each of whom had excommunicated the others. Rather than accept three crowns from three feuding popes, or risk the wrath of two popes by picking the third, the pious Henry III decided to clean house in Rome altogether. Calling together a synod at Sutri in December of 1046, Henry deposed all three papal claimants and installed the German Bishop of Bamberg as Clement II, who then crowned Henry as emperor of the Romans on Christmas day. Clement didn't last very long, dying in Pesaro on the Adriatic coast on October 9, 1047; he may have been poisoned by agents of the still-at-large Benedict IX, though given the date and location malaria may have played a role in the unacclimated German's death. Henry then placed a second German on the papal throne, Damasus II, who survived in the office a mere 23 days. After ordination in Rome, Damasus fled the heat of the city for the relative cool of the nearby hill town of Palestrina, but he probably contracted malaria before leaving the Eternal City. He died on August 9 as he had lived—a virtuous man, but one without any intrinsic or acquired resistance to *P. falciparum* malaria.

Undeterred, Henry appointed yet another German pope in Rome, and this time his appointment stuck. The man who would be called Pope Leo IX was Bruno, a distant relative of Henry III and a committed churchman. During his five-year reign as Pope Leo filled the city of Rome with reformers from north of the Alps who together wrenched control of the papacy—at least for the time being—from the Roman aristocracy.

The Reform Papacy, the Empire and Investiture

Ironically, the reform popes of the 11th and 12th century that the German Empire installed in Rome would ultimately prove to be a far greater threat to the empire than the aristocratic popes that preceded them. Shortly after being established in office, the reform popes passed two major resolutions that challenged the very basis of German imperial power. First, during the synod of 1059, the reform papacy established new rules of papal elections. Henceforth the cardinals of the Church, and *only* the cardinals of the Church, enjoyed the right to elect the pope. In effect, the College of Cardinals became the "spiritual Senate" of Christianity, and the pope its elected emperor.[11] This decree was directed mainly against Rome's aristocracy, which had interfered repeatedly in papal elections using various mechanisms during the *saeculum obscurum*. However, this new arrangement also threatened the empire's long-established right of oversight over papal elections. Given the fact that 12 of the 25 popes to reign between 955 and 1057 had been imperial appointees, the 1059 synod represented a direct challenge to the traditional rights of the German Empire.[12]

Even more troubling for the German Empire, in the long run, was the new papal stance on simony, the buying and selling of spiritual things. The Reform popes considered all holders of ecclesiastical office, from priests to popes, to be God's representatives on earth. By their words, two people joined as one in marriage; by their voice, bread became the body of Christ; by their intervention through confession and penance, a sinful man could escape the fires of hell. Such offices should not be bought and sold like cattle in the marketplace, nor should their possessors be under the thumb of mere secular lords.

Ideals such as this, however, were antithetical to the political constitution of the German Empire, where from the 9th century onward emperors depended heavily on ecclesiastical office-holders to shore up imperial authority. From the time of the Ottonians onwards, the emperors had tapped the military potential of Germany's church lands by relying heavily on the support of high German ecclesiastics whom the emperors personally appointed to their dioceses. Most of these "bishops" were really young aristocrats excluded from inheritance of their father's lands by primogeniture, a system of inheritance where a family's property passed exclusively to the first-born male child. Although these late-born sons were technically clerics once they were appointed to ecclesiastical office, many resembled the decidedly secular Archbishop Christian of Mainz, who "remained a jovial knight until his death, kept a harem of beautiful girls, and, clad in glittering armor, rode a splendid horse, swinging the battle axe with which he shattered the helmet and head of many an enemy."[13] Christian, incidentally, would meet his end not on the battlefield, but from Roman Fever, perishing in August of 1183 during a later German imperial campaign in Rome. The importance of such military-minded bishops and archbishops to imperial power was exemplified by the Italian campaigns of Otto II, in which 15 bishops campaigned in Italy, each with a retinue of 200–400 armed vassals.[14]

During the 1070s, however, the Roman Church under Pope Gregory VII moved to formally outlaw "lay investiture," in other words the right of a king or emperor to endow candidates with ecclesiastical positions and their associated feudal land holdings. In the mind of the reform papacy, churchmen were supposed to be dedicated to the well-being of their congregation and thus it was not proper that they "bear arms or … be zealously engaged in military service."[15] What is more, the papacy considered royal grants of ecclesiastic offices to be simony since their recipients had in effect purchased their sees through their oath of support to the emperor. Therefore, during a series of church councils from 1074 to 1075, lay authorities were expressly forbidden to invest ecclesiastical officials to their offices. In one stroke, the German emperors were (in theory) divested of nearly half their lands.

The result of these decrees was a sustained century of repeated German imperial military campaigns into Italy, this time directed against the popes and their Italian allies. The most important such allies were the Normans, descendants of Vikings who had become Romanized in the province of France which still bears their name today. These Normans came to Italy first as pilgrims, then as mercenaries in the struggles between the papacy, Lombard dukes, Arabs, and Byzantines, and finally as immigrants, leaving their overcrowded home in France for the land of opportunity in south Italy. Following the tradition set by the Ostrogoths and the Lombards before them, the warlike Normans avoided settlement in the malarial coastal plains of south Italy, preferring instead the windy hills of the Apennines, and they timed their frequent military campaigns to the healthier months of winter and spring.[16] In order to legitimize their rule in the Italian south, the Normans hitched their power to the rising star of the reform papacy. In the process, the popes gained powerful military allies against the Roman aristocracy and, if need be, the German Empire.[17]

Confident of Norman support, Pope Gregory took the dramatic step of excommunicating the Emperor Henry for ignoring his decree against lay investiture. Henry tried to depose Gregory in turn, but his words rang hollow, and the outlawed emperor Henry found himself in danger of being deposed himself. Abandoned by many of his allies, the emperor was eventually forced by desperation into a humiliating show of repentance. Indeed, Henry's famous meeting with Pope Gregory in the Apennine mountain town of Canossa, where the emperor stood for three days "in a wretched condition, barefoot and clad in wool" before the pope consented to forgive him, is one of the most famous set pieces of the Middle Ages.[18]

Gregory had won the first round of the papal/imperial conflict, but the newly-forgiven Henry was far from finished. Despite papal declarations that Henry had merely been absolved of his sins at Canossa, not restored to power, Gregory was unable to prevent Henry from returning to Germany and cleaning house of his domestic enemies. Henry then roared back into Italy once again, this time clad in the armor of a conqueror

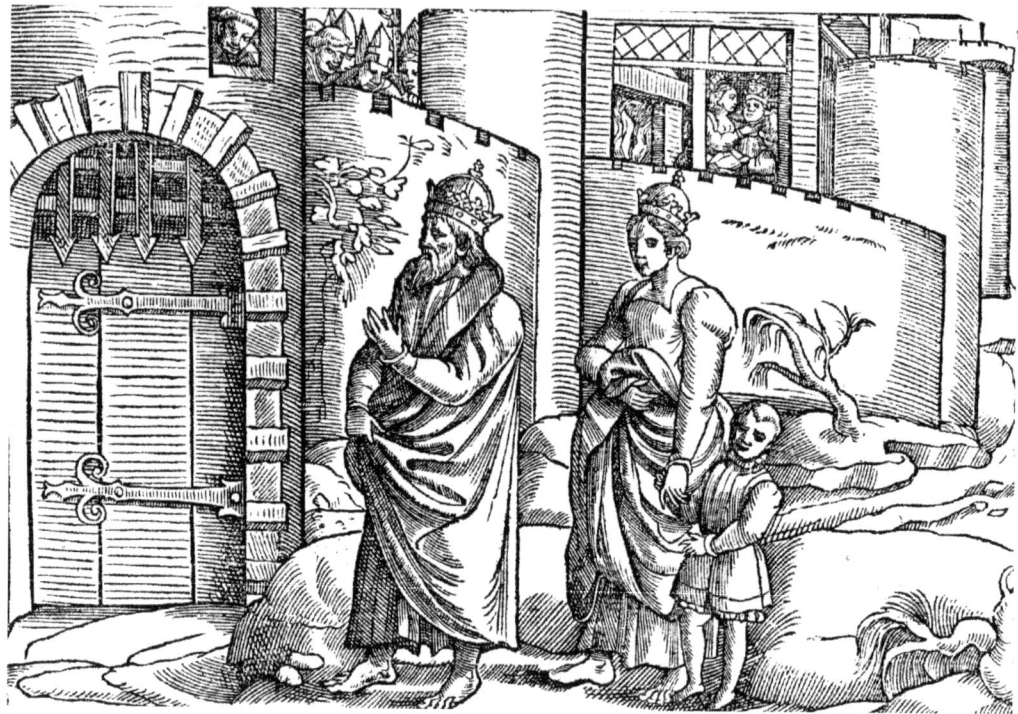

Henry IV and his family barefoot at Canossa, awaiting absolution from Gregory VII. In this anti–Catholic engraving, the pope is depicted in the background cavorting with Mathilda of Tuscany in a manner rather unbefitting of his office. *John Foxe's Acts and Monuments* (London: John Day, 1570), p. 232.

rather than the coarse wool of a penitent. In both 1080 and 1081, Henry's forces tried and failed to breach the walls of Rome, in part because Henry wisely gave up the sieges each summer rather than risk exposing his men to Roman Fever. Finally, in June 1082, Henry's forces broke through the Leonine Walls of Vatican Hill, though they failed to seize Gregory himself, who had retreated to the powerful fortress of St. Angelo in the Borgo district. Since the summer was now nigh, Henry withdrew northwards once more, leaving behind a detachment of about 300–400 knights to defend territory he had seized during the siege. This proved to be a mistake; by the time Henry returned to Rome in Christmas of 1083 "fever had swept away the garrison," forcing him to start the siege of Rome from scratch once more.[19]

By 1084 the people of Rome, who were tired of serving as pawns in this endless chess match, decided to settle matters themselves. Pro-imperial Romans opened the gates to Henry's forces, forcing the pope to flee to the papal fortress of St. Angelo. Henry put the castle to siege but his grudge against the pope was interrupted by the arrival of the papal ally Robert Guiscard, Norman Duke of Sicily, who forced the outnumbered Henry to flee back to the north. Rome now found itself at the mercy of the Normans, who showed their Viking roots by putting the city to a three-day sack and then setting it aflame when the despairing Roman populous finally rose against them. Soon after, Robert Guiscard and his Arab allies left Rome, the latter in the company of hundreds of Roman captives destined for the slave markets of North Africa. It was the Vandal invasion all over again. As for Gregory, he was now *persona non grata* in Rome and was forced to tag along in the trail of the Normans before dying in Salerno a year later.

Although Gregory was dead, the investiture controversy between emperors and popes lingered for another generation. Henry IV's heir, Henry V, tried to settle matters with military force again in 1117, taking advantage of temporary chaos within Rome to seize the city, though the pope himself slipped from his fingers. After setting up a new anti-pope and being re-crowned emperor, Henry V left the city before the summer swelter in the face of yet another Norman relief army. However, other than exposing his men to malaria in the vicinity of Rome, nothing of consequence had been accomplished. Henry would eventually be forced to make major concessions to the Reform papacy on the issue of lay investiture in the Council of Worms in 1122, which formally ended the investiture controversy.

The reign of the next German emperor is perhaps best understood as a temporary intermission in this long drama of papal/imperial conflict. Emperor Lothair III owed his election in part to the work of papal legates in Germany, who sought the election of an emperor who was "obedient, humbly devoted and useful to [the] Holy Church."[20] In Lothair, they were not disappointed. When Lothair met Pope Innocent II in Liège, he agreed to act as the Pope's *strator*—someone who holds the stirrups of a pope's horse when the pope dismounted—an act which the papacy would later portray as a sign of imperial submission to the papal office.[21] What is more, when Pope Innocent II published a bull claiming that the emperor's authority derived from the papacy, Lothair ignored it. Many contemporary Germans were angered by his silence, which they saw as a tacit acceptance of the Pope's humiliating decree.

Worst of all, when Innocent II demanded that the emperor declare war on the Normans of Sicily, who had become unreliable allies, Lothair once again jumped to obey the Pope's command. Marching into south Italy with a large army, Lothair forced the Normans to retreat almost entirely from the Italian peninsula. By July, however, his fever-fearing army was in a state of near mutiny and clamoring loudly to return to the north. Lothair was thus compelled to withdraw to the healthy hills north of Rome, after which the Normans and their Islamic allies swiftly re-took all the territory Lothair had occupied, rendering worthless Lothair's battlefield successes.[22]

As for Lothair himself, he never made it back to Germany, perishing in a small hut in an Alpine pass in early December 1137. It is quite possible that Lothair's death, and perhaps those of many of his followers, can be attributed directly or indirectly to the malarial fevers of the Italian south. Gregorovius would later speculate that "like so many of his German predecessors and successors," Lothair had brought the "seeds of death back with him from Italy."[23] Given the paucity of sources on Lothair's reign, however, there is no way now to be sure.

Barbarossa, Rome and Malaria

Unfortunately for the papacy, Lothair's brand of pliant and accommodating emperor died with him. His death signaled the start of a second act of the struggle between papacy and empire, and thousands more transalpine Europeans would follow their leaders up a steep disease gradient into central and southern Italy as a result.

With Lothair's death, the German throne fell to Conrad III, the first king of the Hohenstaufen dynasty. Conrad himself never found time in his busy reign to be crowned in Rome, in part because his kingship was challenged from the start by the Welf dynasty of Bavaria, stirring up nearly a decade of civil war in Germany. Nonetheless, Conrad insisted on styling himself *rex romanorum*, or "King of the Romans," probably as a signal that he did not believe that his sovereignty was in any way subordinate to that of the Bishop of Rome. And indeed, many Europeans of the time shared Conrad's sentiment. Although best known today for his *Divine Comedy*, Florentine author Dante Alighieri was an active participant in 12th-century politics and his influential *De Monarchia* contains the best surviving defense of the pro-imperial position. Kingship, Dante insisted, was "indispensable for the best ordering of the world," and he argued that political authority should be unitary, with a single emperor ruling over all humanity.[24] The fact that the current line of emperors was German rather than Italian was of no consequence to Dante since in his mind all emperors were virtual demigods, "lifted high above national passions" by virtue of their office. In any case their coronation in Rome served as a "mystic rebirth," a baptism of sorts that freed the emperor from any remaining vestiges of their barbaric Germanic origins.[25]

Although the emperor was customarily crowned by the pope, Dante contended that imperial power did not arise from the papacy. Rather, the emperor's universal sovereignty emanated directly from the providential will of God himself. And how could it be otherwise? The imperial office, after all, was older than either Christianity or the papacy; in fact, the first emperor was none other than the "divine Monarch Augustus" himself, heir to Caesar. For Dante, it was no coincidence that "Christ willed to be born in the fullness of time when Augustus was Monarch," perhaps so that the seed of Jesus might be planted in ready soil. The authority of all emperors therefore "derives immediately from the summit of all being, which is God."[26]

In keeping with this theory, Dante systematically dismantled any papal claim of superiority over the Imperial office. While conceding that "Jesus is the rock on which the church is founded," Dante insisted that the "foundation of the empire is human right," and thus the "temporal power receives from the spiritual neither its existence, nor its strength … nor even its function." The proper role of the papacy, therefore, is not to claim control over the empire but rather to support the empire's sacred mission, while in turn "Caesar" should "honor Peter as a first-born son should honor his father."[27] Those Italians who bought into this vision of empire would come to be called Ghibellines, a word that owes its origin to the Hohenstaufen castle of Waiblingen combined with Italian inability to pronounce the letter W. Italian supporters of the papacy, on the other hand, were called Guelfs, an Italianization of the name of the Welf dynasty, the Hohenstaufens' main German rivals.

While Dante's defense of the power of the emperor was rooted in philosophic argument, other Europeans were moved to support the emperor by doomsday religious fervor. Only the prophesized "Emperor of the Last Days," many believed, could protect Christians from the imminent threat of the Antichrist. According to this legend, which was based on a hodge-podge of biblical quotes, Jewish millenarian beliefs, and the uncanonical *Revelation of Pseudo-Methodius*, a Last Roman Emperor would soon arrive to reunite east and west and re-conquer Jerusalem from the heretic Arabs, thus triggering the Day of Judgment.[28] Some German emperors actively embraced this notion of the Last World Emperor, in particular Otto III, whose reign coincided with the millennium and who bedecked himself at coronation with "ceremonial cloaks embroidered with cosmic symbols" proclaiming his messianic status.[29] Indeed, Otto's dream of "*renovation imperii Romanorum*," or "Renewal of the Roman Empire," may reflect Otto's belief that the German Empire was fated to play an important eschatological role in the coming apocalypse.[30]

These grandiose visions of imperial destiny were embraced fervently by the next German emperor, Frederick I, whose red beard earned him the nickname Barbarossa. Like Otto III, Barbarossa believed that he was the foretold Last Emperor with a divinely-sanctioned mission and he re-named the German monarchy accordingly, declaring it henceforth to be the *sacrum imperium Romanum*, or the "Holy Roman Empire."[31] In keeping with his elevated understanding of his prophesied historical role, Barbarossa's eventual ambition was to reign in Holy Jerusalem after leading a victorious new crusade, thus hastening the End of Days.[32]

Nonetheless, given the realities of the age, Barbarossa realized that his road to Jerusalem by necessity began in Italy, since only Italy contained the resources that Barbarossa needed to enact his grand imperial designs. This was an unintended consequence of the Council of Worms, which made it more difficult for a German emperor to rely on the support of ecclesiastical vassals. Barbarossa hoped to make up for this deficiency by re-asserting imperial rights to taxes and tribute from the Kingdom of Italy. Since these Italian subjects would inevitably appeal to the pope against imperial exactions, however, the Council of Worms had the ironic effect of stirring up further papal/imperial conflict.

Barbarossa began his Italian adventures in October 1154, just a year after being crowned king in Charlemagne's cathedral in Aachen. While his German force wintered in the plain of the Po near Roncaglia, Barbarossa dipped his beak into Italian politics, siding with the cities of Como and Cremona in their war against Milan, the strongest city of the Italian north. In an effort to bring the Milanese to heel, Barbarossa launched a spring-time siege of the city and fortress of Tortona, an ally of Milan. When Tortona refused to yield quickly, the frustrated young king resorted to brutal tactics, hanging Tortonan prisoners of war and poisoning Tortona's wells with corpses. Tortona finally surrendered around Easter, and Barbarossa's troops systematically put the town to sack before razing it to the ground. While some historians believe that Barbarossa's siege of Tortona was an unnecessary diversion from his main mission in Italy, Peter Munz has argued that Frederick Barbarossa was all but forced into conflict with the Italians by the material needs of his enormous army, which required both daily rations and occasional spoils of war. As a result of his army's constant "clamor for loot," Munz argued, Barbarossa had little choice but to pick fights as he progressed through the Italian peninsula.[33] While the German Empire may have gained some short-term booty from these fights, in the long term they stoked Italian enmity towards the German "barbarians" and thus undermined the very imperial authority in Italy that Barbarossa was hoping to establish.

Following the sack of Tortona, Barbarossa continued southwards, and on June 8 the stage was set for Barbarossa's first meeting with Pope Hadrian IV. At this point, Frederick Barbarossa made it clear that he was no Lothair. When Hadrian arrived at Sutri on horseback, Frederick refused to hold the Pope's stirrup, which in his mind would have signaled acceptance of the Pope as his liege lord, an act of submission incompatible with the imperial dignity. Hadrian, in turn, interpreted Barbarossa's refusal as an outrageous act of disrespect against Saint Peter and the papal office. Frederick Barbarossa was later persuaded to agree to the *strator* ceremony to Hadrian's satisfaction but the affair left an aftertaste of distrust between the papacy and the Hohenstaufen emperors that would only grow with the passage of time.

Frederick Barbarossa's original plan, after being crowned, was to take his troops still further south and to seize Sicily from its Norman overlords. By July, however, his homesick soldiers began to murmur fearfully about the forthcoming fever season. Those fears soon turned into reality. Despite placing his summer quarters in the healthier heights of the Alban hills the "oppressive heat and heavy noxious air infected many soldiers with a languor," bringing with it fevers and stomach cramps.[34] As a result, Barbarossa gave his princes leave to return home and his army more or less disintegrated. Still, Frederick Barbarossa probably regarded his first Italian campaign a success: he had come to Italy as King of Germany, but left as Emperor of the World.

Frederick Barbarosa's coronation campaign into Italy proved to be just the first of many. In all, Barbarosa would launch six more Italian expeditions over the next two decades, eventually spending all or part of 12 of the next 20 years on Italian soil. Since his men were loath to travel south of the Apennine Mountains, Frederick focused for the most part on restoring imperial control and taxation over the long-defunct Kingdom of Italy, the old Lombard domain centered in the plain of the Po. His main opposition there was Milan, Lombardy's strongest state, but after several years of marches and sieges Barbarossa managed to put the town to sack in 1163.

By this point, however, renewed trouble was brewing in Rome. In the conclave that followed Pope Hadrian's death in 1159, a Ghibelline faction amongst the cardinals openly flouted the will of the majority and bestowed the papacy on Octavian of St. Cecilia, who reportedly tore the purple papal mantle out of the hands of the rightful victor in the election. Worse yet, Frederick Barbarossa was himself blamed for this outrage, since one of his own ambassadors, Otto von Wittelsbach, played a suspected role in the papal coup. In protest against Octavian's effrontery, the majority of cardinals assembled later to pick their own pope, meaning the papacy was in schism, divided between adherents of Victor IV, as Octavian now called himself, and Alexander III.

Barbarossa declared Victor the rightful pope, as did (initially) most of the princes of Europe. To further bolster his pet pope's claims of legitimacy, Barbarossa held a council in Pavia in 1160 to judge between two popes. Since Alexander refused to attend this rigged council, a judgment for Victor was a conclusion. In response, Alexander let loose the dogs of propaganda war, labeling Octavian as the son of a devil

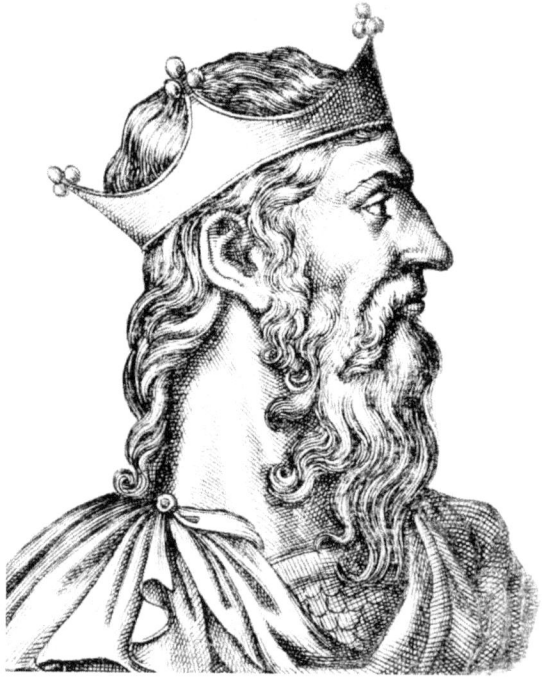

Frederick Barbarossa, from a 1583 book of Effigies of Emperors. Giovanni Battista Cavalieri and Tomasz Treter, *Romanorum Imperatorum Effigies* (1583), p. 135.

and Barbarossa as a persecutor of God. Alexander's anti–Barbarossa message found particular resonance in North Italy, then groaning under the weight of new imperial taxations and exactions imposed by the German emperor.[35] For the moment, Barbarossa could do little more than ignore Alexander, who was safe in French territory. In 1165, however, shortly after Victor IV's death Alexander III returned to Rome and Barbarossa, sensing opportunity, judged that the time had come to defeat this gadfly pope once and for all. In July of 1167, Barbarossa hurried to Rome with a large army and directed a siege of the city from the nearby heights of Monte Mario. By July 29, his forces had seized the Leonine City, and on August 1, the victorious emperor was re-crowned in Saint Peter's Basilica by his own client pope.

Just days later, however, Barbarossa's triumph dissolved into disaster. In the early days of August, a "severe pestilence attacked the army and in large measure destroyed it," claiming the lives not only of many of his men, but also numerous princes and "countless barons" amongst the imperial army.[36] Even Barbarossa himself fell seriously ill. Decimated by disease, the imperial army had no choice but to scurry back north. Upon reaching the north Italian plain, however, Barbarossa found his path to Germany blocked by a league of Lombard cities who, jubilant at the news of Barbarossa's misfortunes, had risen in rebellion against him. Frederick Barbarossa was only able to get to safety by donning a disguise, crossing the Mount Cenis pass in the raiment of a servant while one of his friends stayed behind to play the part of the fugitive emperor.

Was Barbarossa's army destroyed by malaria? Most historians have argued exactly that, noting that both the location and the season support a diagnosis of malaria infection. The fact that a similar epidemic apparently swept through the city of Rome at the same time complicates the issue somewhat, since Rome's Italian defenders would presumably have had greater intrinsic and genetic immunity to malarial fevers, not to mention local cultural knowledge that helped them avoid infection. This last line of defense, however, was likely weakened by the war itself, which forced thousands of Romans to stay at the fortifications of the half-deserted city well into the season of the Dog Star, which as we will see in Chapter 11 was the traditional time for *villeggiaturas* into the healthier countryside.[37]

In a recent biography of Frederick Barbarossa, however, John Freed has attacked the conventional wisdom that Frederick's army succumbed to an outbreak of malarial fevers. Freed notes that contemporary sources date the outbreak of disease to "within hours" of a torrential downpour of rain on August 2. This chronology, according to Freed, suggests that some sort of gastrointestinal disease triggered by the contamination of water sources with fecal matter was to blame for the epidemic, not malaria. As Freed points out, "the eight-day incubation period of malaria precludes it from being the primary cause of the epidemic that began killing a large number of men within hours of the storm."[38]

However, there are several problems with Freed's argument. For one thing, his thesis that the latrines of the German military camp overflowed during the downpour cannot explain the near-simultaneous outbreak of disease within Rome, which would have been using entirely different water sources. Even more damning for Freed's argument is the fact that most diarrheal diseases also have their own multi-day incubation period. Typhoid, the gastrointestinal infection most closely associated with epidemics in marching armies, shows no symptoms from between six to 30 days after exposure, and bacterial dysentery requires two to ten days to show symptoms. In all likelihood, the intense summer rainstorm that Freed and the chroniclers make so much of was entirely unrelated to the fever outbreak and was only remembered because it happened to coincide with the first outbreak of malarial fevers amongst Barbarossa's forces, most of whom had been encamped in the moist lowlands surrounding the city since late May.[39] Malaria, most likely of the *P. falciparum* variety, remains the best available explanation for the epidemic that devastated Barbarossa's army in 1167.

Despite his near-fatal brush with Roman Fever, Frederick Barbarossa was not yet done with Italy, though the remainder of his reign has an air of anticlimax to it. In 1172, he contemplated another expedition across the Alps, though this time the dukes and princes of Germany, mindful of the 1167 disaster, were reluctant to follow him.[40] As a result, when Barbarossa did belatedly return to Italy in 1174, he did so with such a small army that he was defeated on the battlefield by the papal-backed Lombard League, forcing the emperor to agree to major concessions to both the Italian cities and the papacy. Humbled but unbowed, Barbarossa returned to Italy once again in 1184. This time, the older but wiser king attempted to accomplish through matrimony what he had been unable to achieve by force of arms, negotiating a marriage alliance between his son Henry and Constance, the heiress to the Norman Kingdom of Sicily. With his dynasty's future now secure, Barbarossa was finally ready to march on the Holy Land and at age 66 he joined with the kings of England and France in the Third Crusade. His dreams of reigning in Jerusalem as the Last Roman Emperor, however, died with him in the Saleph River in Turkey. Chroniclers reported that Barbarossa fell from his horse and drowned in waist-high water, probably pinned to the bottom of the riverbed by the weight of his own armor.

Notwithstanding Frederick Barbarossa's death in a Syrian stream, the papacy's Hohenstaufen problems were far from over. Barbarossa was succeeded by his adult son Henry, who arrived in Rome for coronation in 1191. Shortly afterwards, Henry VI marched to Naples in an attempt to seize Sicily from a usurper, Tancred, the illegitimate son of the Norman King Roger III. However, Henry's troops did not thrive in the Italian south: repeated disease epidemics reportedly "swept away" both "troops and captains" alike. Contemporaries blamed these deaths on "too liberal indulgence on the delicious fruits of the south," which suggests some sort of diarrheal infection, but malaria may have played its usual role as well.[41] Henry and his men therefore hurried back north of the Alps, where he found new troubles brewing with the Welf family, who had forged an alliance in his absence with both the papacy and the King of England.

Several years later Henry renewed his efforts in Italy, and this time they were crowned with success, in large part due to Tancred's unexpected death in late 1194. To the dismay of the papacy, which had long dreaded the prospect of imperial annexation of Sicily, Henry proclaimed himself King of Sicily on Christmas Day of 1195. The papacy had traditionally relied on the King of Sicily, who since Norman times was a papal vassal, to counterbalance the power the German emperors. If the Emperor of Germany and the King of Sicily were one and the same, however, Rome would be enclosed by enemies and the vassalage of Sicily might be permanently lost.[42] Making matters worse, Constance bore Henry a son and heir, Frederick, shortly afterwards. At this point, Henry VI was at the height of his power: he claimed overlordship of England and France as well as Italy and Germany, was in diplomatic contact with kings as distant as the ruler of Armenia, and was publicly planning both a new Crusade and a possible war of conquest against what remained of the Byzantine state.[43]

In 1197, however, Henry's grand plans came crashing down. Outrageous Hohenstaufen fiscal demands in Sicily sparked a revolt which Henry suppressed with great brutality, to the point of hammering a red-hot iron crown onto the head of one Sicilian rebel who was rumored to have coveted the kingship. Henry's cruelty, however, only fanned the flames of rebellion, and even his estranged wife Constance joined the rebels. By summer Henry and his loyalists found themselves virtual prisoners in the highly malarial city of Messina. Henry was able to sign a treaty with the rebels to save his kingdom, but he could not save himself: shortly after a hunting trip near Messina, Henry VI fell ill and by September 28 was dead at only 32. Some historians have alleged poison, but given the time and place of his death, it is quite possible that Henry was just one more unacclimated German to fall prey to *P. falciparum* in the Italian south.[44]

After Henry's death, the infant Frederick II inherited the Kingdom of Sicily, while a papal-supported Welf candidate took the German imperial throne as Otto IV. However, by the time Frederick came to the age of majority the papacy had soured on Otto, who had proven himself to be more Barbarossa than Lothair, investing Italian lands upon his vassals in defiance of papal complaints. In desperation, Pope Innocent III threw his weight behind Frederick instead. Spurred on by the papacy, Frederick left Sicily in 1212, was formally crowned King of Germany in Mainz, and then rallied Staufen supporters to his cause. Two years later, in the decisive battle of Bouvines in Flanders, Frederick and his French allies crushed forces of the Welfs and the English king, cementing Frederick's claim to the German throne.

Frederick II and Italy

For the next five years, it looked as if the papacy had backed the right horse in the Hohenstaufen/Welf conflict, since Frederick focused his attentions on Germany. It would not be until 1220 that Frederick finally crossed into Italy, where he received both the Lombard and imperial crowns. Unfortunately for the papacy, however, Frederick did not scurry home afterwards but rather remained in Italy for a total of nine years, steadily solidifying his position in South Italy. There is little indication that Frederick or his troops suffered much from malaria during these years, which is understandable, since much of Frederick's army was drawn from his Sicilian and Italian possessions rather than from Germany and like the Italian-born Frederick these men would have enjoyed some resistance to the disease due to childhood exposure. However, Frederick's Spanish-born first wife, another Constance, was not so lucky. To Frederick's dismay, Constance succumbed to malaria in Catania, Sicily, in July of 1221.[45]

During this Italian interlude, Frederick was dogged by a rash promise he had made at coronation to go on a crusade to Jerusalem. For years, Frederick tried to delay the inevitable. First he claimed that he needed to settle his affairs in Germany before setting out. Then he had trouble getting the Northern Italian cities, who deeply distrusted the Hohensaufens, to provide troops. Finally, Pope Gregory IX decided in 1227 that enough was enough and threatened excommunication if Frederick delayed any further. Frederick therefore took himself and his army to Brindisi in Apulia to await transport to the Holy Land. But there, on the very eve of embarkation, Frederick and countless other crusaders were struck down by a horrific epidemic which "converted the camp into a pest-house."[46] Frederick set sail regardless, but his condition grew so serious that his ship returned to port days later to seek medical attention for the ailing emperor.

Was this yet another example of malaria spoiling the best intentions of an imperial army? Quite possibly, though the exact cause of Frederick's illness is the matter of some scholarly debate. While some historians believe it was malaria, others blame gastrointestinal diseases like dysentery, typhoid, or even cholera, though the latter diagnosis is an anachronistic impossibility since *vibrio cholerae* bacteria did not reach Europe until the 19th century.[47] It may be that the closely-packed crusader camp suffered from a variety of different ailments. Nonetheless, both the location and the season point to malaria as a major factor in the outbreak: the epidemic began in August, high season for *P. falciparum*, and Brindisi would later gain the reputation of being single most malarial spot in the entire Italian peninsula.[48]

Upon reaching shore, Frederick wrote to the pope explaining his predicament but Gregory excommunicated him regardless. Angered by the pope's intransigence, Frederick decided to go on crusade to spite the pope and landed in the Levant with a modest military force in late 1228. Rather than risk his troops to the vagaries of warfare, Frederick sought a diplomatic solution and by dint of flattery and bluff convinced the Sultan of Egypt, who had other problems to contend with, to surrender Jerusalem without a fight. As a result, Frederick achieved what his namesake grandfather had never been able to accomplish: he sat as a crowned (albeit excommunicated) emperor within the city of Jerusalem. Despite the doomsday predictions of the Last Emperor legend, however, the

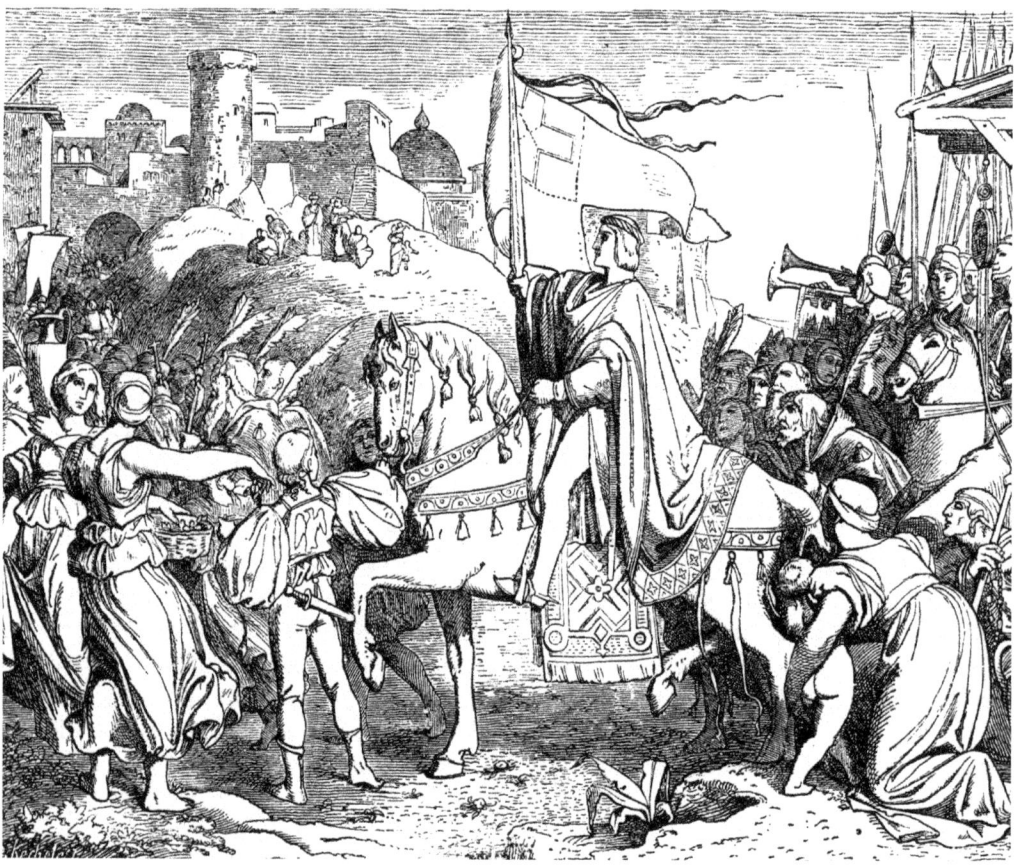

A storybook scene depicting Emperor Frederick II's entry into Jerusalem (INTERFOTO/Alamy Stock Photo).

antichrist did not appear to challenge him. Or perhaps the excommunicated Frederick was himself the antichrist. That was certainly the position of the papacy, which by this time was resolved to exterminate the Hohenstaufen dynasty, that "race of Herod" and "brood of vipers," once and for all.[49]

Upon returning from the Holy Land, Frederick first turned his attention against the papal-backed Lombard League, which had been an annoyance since the start of his reign. In November of 1237, Frederick's German troops and Ghibelline Italian allies won a decisive battle against the allied forces of Northern Italy at Cortenuova, but lost momentum during a disastrous siege of Brescia, during which Frederick himself was nearly captured in a night raid. Heartened by Frederick's failure before Brescia's walls, Gregory IX renewed its decree of excommunication against the emperor, throwing Frederick into open war with the papacy. For the next several years Frederick, unwilling to challenge the fortifications of Rome directly, was forced to "run circles" around the walls of Rome, trying to scare or starve the pope into negotiating a settled peace.

To counter Frederick's threat to the Eternal City, Gregory decided to summon a council in Rome for Easter of 1241 in order to muster support against the hated Hohenstaufens. In response, a pro–Ghibelline priest penned a remarkable letter which evoked Rome's malaria problems to discourage non–Italian clergy from attending the council. "How can you enjoy safety," the imperial propagandist asked his transalpine brothers, in a city where

> The heat is insufferable, the water foul, the food is coarse and bad; the air is so heavy that it can be grasped with the hands, and is filled with swarms of mosquitoes; the ground is alive with scorpions, the people are dirty and odious, wicked and fierce. The whole of Rome is undermined, and from the catacombs, which are filled with snakes, arises a poisonous and fatal exhalation.[50]

As for Frederick himself, he tried to avoid these "fatal exhalations" by camping his army each summer upon the cooler slopes of the Alban hills, from which (in the words of Gregorovius) his army could look down upon the distant city of Rome, "veiled in the malarial mists of summer."[51]

Those malarial mists may have played a supporting role in Gregory's death: unable to leave Rome for the healthier countryside due to the imperial siege, Pope Gregory IX breathed his last in the stifling heat of Rome in August of 1241. However, the passing of his old enemy brought Frederick no respite. Gregory was succeeded by Innocent IV, who fled to Lyon in France. Safe from Frederick's grasp, Innocent excommunicated the emperor anew and meddled in German imperial affairs. In the meantime, the war continued in Italy, though it was increasingly directed by Frederick's legitimate and illegitimate sons rather than the aging emperor himself. Frederick finally died of natural causes in 1250 and was buried in the cathedral of Palermo.

While the popes were unable to achieve their goal of the extermination of the Hohenstaufens during Frederick's own lifetime, they had better luck after his death. Frederick's son Conrad came south to claim his Italian inheritance in 1252, but due to his German upbringing he lacked the acquired malaria resistance of his father, which might explain his death by fever (possibly *P. vivax*) in southern Italy in late May of 1254. Fredericks' bastard son Manfred then took control over the Kingdom of Sicily's territory, only to be defeated and killed by a Charles of Anjou, a French prince backed by the papacy, who with his victory assumed the Sicilian throne as Charles I. The Hohenstaufens and their

Ghibelline allies still had one more card to play, Frederick's young son Conradin, who followed the "voices of sirens" into Italy, the "historic paradise of German desire," as soon as he came of age.[52] But Conradin's large army was defeated decisively in southern Italy at the Battle of Tagliacozzo by Charles I and his Guelf allies. Conradin himself fled the scene of slaughter in disguise, only to be recognized and captured by partisans of the Guelfs, and died under the axe of Charles I's executioner.

Conradin's death brought to an end not only the Hohenstaufen line of kings, but also a century of sustained German imperial interference into Italian affairs. However, the extirpation of the Hohenstaufens did not mean the end of transalpine military campaigns into the feverish battlefields of Italy. Far from it: as we will see in later chapters, the void left behind by the Germans was increasingly filled by the French, who had their own ambitions and interests in the Eternal City.

9

IMPERIUM'S PRICE

With the fall of the Hohenstaufens, the imperial impulse into Italy slackened considerably, but it did not die. Fifty years after Conradin's death the Ghibelline cause in Italy enjoyed a brief Indian summer during the calamitous reign of the ill-fated Henry VII.

Henry VII, Ghibelline Revival and Maremma Malaria

Truth be told, Henry should never have been emperor at all. No member of Henry's House of Luxembourg had ever before held the Imperial office, and his land holdings as Count of Luxembourg were so modest in scale that while still a provincial count he was obliged to become a vassal of the powerful King of France.[1] Despite this, Henry managed to get himself elected King of Germany in 1309 largely because the imperial electors of that year were split almost equally between pro–French and pro–German factions, opening the way for Henry to take power as a dark horse compromise.

As we saw in previous chapters, it had been customary before the mid–13th century for newly-anointed German kings to march on Italy and receive the imperial crown, but by Henry's time the office of emperor had become atrophied by a half-century of disuse. Henry's immediate predecessors in the German royal throne had been weak nonentities, including the forgettable Rudolf I and Albert I, who barely had any control within Germany itself much less south of the Alps. Other "German" kings of this era had been foreigners, including Richard of Cornwall, the wealthy second son of the English King John, who had bribed four of the seven electors into supporting his candidacy for the kingship. Once elected, Richard treated the imperial office like a prize upon the mantelpiece, barely setting foot into his supposed German domain. No doubt many of the German electors preferred it that way—a purely titular king, unable to assert his rights over the German high nobility, was their monarchical ideal.

Unlike his predecessors, however, the ambitious Henry craved the power that had once come with the German crown and thus followed the footsteps of the Ottonian and Hohenstaufen emperors across the Alps into Italy. In part, he was seeking Rome, the traditional fountainhead of imperial legitimacy. He also had a nose for gold, which the rich city-states of Northern Italy had in abundance: in the 14th century the annual revenue of Milan and nearby Lombard cities alone almost equaled that of France.[2] As a result, barely a year after his election, Henry entered Italy at the head of a modest army.

Once there, Henry received a rapturous welcome from Italian Ghibellines, including Dante, who proclaimed Henry "Augustus" and "lieutenant of God," the "new offspring of Jesse" and the "consolation of the world."[3] Despite this Ghibelline adulation, Henry

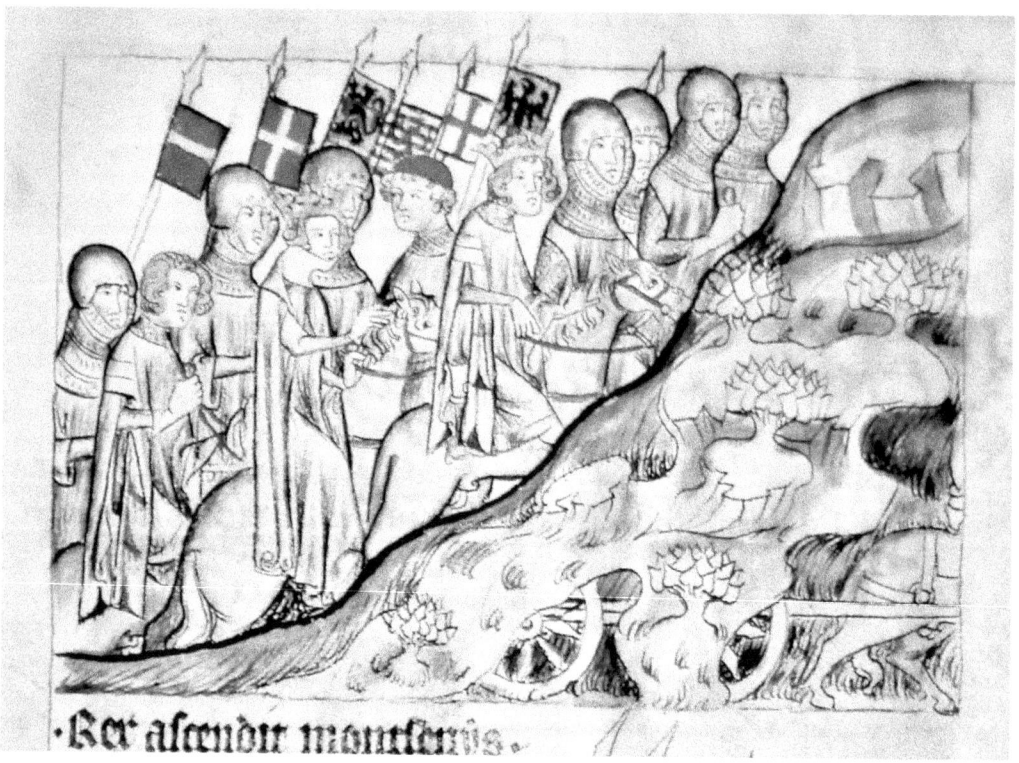

Henry VII marching over the Alps. Codex Balduini Trevirensis, c. 1340, taken from George Irmer, *Die Romfahrt Kaiser Heinrich's VII im bildercyclus des Codex Balduini Trevirensis* (Berlin: Weidmannsche buchhandlung, 1881), between pp. 36 and 37.

initially presented himself as a neutral peace-maker in Italy and actually convinced the Guelf stronghold of Milan to allow him entry to the city to be crowned King of Italy. By mid–January, however, Henry's coffers were almost empty, and in an effort to fill them Henry extorted oppressive fees from Milan. The predictable result was the Guelf uprisings throughout Lombardy against the cash-hungry Henry, who in response showed his true Ghibelline colors and compelled the submission of pro–Guelf Lodi, Cremona, and Crema and seized the arch–Guelf city of Brescia. But success came at a heavy cost: while besieging Brescia, Henry lost half of his men to disease. Chroniclers blamed "plague" for Henry's losses, but the fact that the campaign was conducted during the high summer and that unacclimated transalpine troops suffered disproportionate disease casualties suggests that malaria may have been fighting on the side of Brescia's defenders.[4] In any case, since his forces were depleted by disease and desertion to the North, Henry was forced to delay his trip to Rome until the following year.

When Henry finally arrived in the *caput mundi* for his coronation in May of 1312, the city he discovered bore little resemblance to the storybook seat of the Caesars. In the words of Gregorovius, Rome in the early 14th century

> ... resembled a huge field, encircled with moss-covered walls, with tracts of wild and uncultivated land, from which rose gloomy towers or castles, basilicas and convents crumbling to decay, and monuments of colossal size clothed with verdure; baths, broken aqueducts, colonnades of temples, isolated columns, and triumphal arches surmounted with towers; while

a labyrinth of narrow streets, interrupted by rubbish heaps, lead among these dilapidated remains, and the yellow Tiber, passing under broken stone bridges, flowed sadly through the ruinous waste.[5]

Henry arrived at this post-apocalyptic scene with a fairly small army, just 2000 mounted knights and an unknown number of infantrymen. There was no pope in Rome at the time, since the papacy had by this point moved to Avignon due to constant political tumult in the Eternal City. Henry had brought with him papal legates for purposes of coronation, but they were only empowered to crown Henry in Saint Peter's Basilica. Upon arriving in Rome, however, Henry found that his access to Saint Peter's was barred by troops loyal to the heir to the House of Anjou, Robert of Naples, who had decided that Henry's ambitions in Italy were incompatible with his own. As a result, Henry was forced to slog his way through the half-deserted ruin of Rome street by street, rubble-pile by rubble-pile, fighting for a crown that marked him as ruler of the world.[6] Even by the standards of the Middle Ages, the scene of many bizarre events, this was a ludicrous spectacle.

And in the end, it was all for naught. While Henry did manage to seize the heights of the Capitoline from its Angevin defenders, his troops were unable to storm the all-important castle of St. Angelo, the key to the Leonine City. Having accomplished little except for painting the streets of Rome with the blood of hundreds of men, the humiliated emperor was eventually compelled to take his crown in the burnt-out shell of the Lateran Basilica, which had been badly damaged by fire in 1307.

The remainder of Henry's ill-starred Italian adventure proves the validity of Mark Twain's old adage that history doesn't repeat itself, except in rhyme. Unwilling to give up the Roman hill he had won at such great cost, Henry left a garrison of 400 knights there and retired to the hillside Ghibelline town of Tivoli to avoid the stifling summer heat and its accompanying malarial fevers. By August, however, his army had been so depleted—mainly by desertion—that he was forced to flee Rome and its surroundings entirely. The remnants of Henry's army slouched back north and spent much of the next year conspiring fruitlessly with Ghibelline Pisa to seize the Guelf stronghold of Florence.

By summer of 1313, however, it seemed that the wheel of fortune was turning in Henry's favor. New reinforcements had arrived from Germany, swelling his army to 4,000 horsemen and many more infantry. With this strengthened force came a more ambitious objective: Henry was now determined to overthrow the Angevin King Robert of Naples, whose dynasty had murdered young Conradin and had made a mockery of Henry's own Roman coronation.[7] To that end, Henry set out from Pisa on August 8, hoping to reach Rome by mid-month. Fate, however, had other plans. By the time his army neared Siena, Henry was already gravely ill, and by August 24, the 38-year-old emperor was dead. With his passing, the imperial expedition dissolved in disorder, much to the relief and delight of Robert of Naples.

What had happened? Contemporaries speculated that Henry had died of poison, administered to him along with the Eucharist by an Italian monk near Siena. Henry thus joined a long line of emperors and other august personages whose sudden deaths have been ascribed to Italian treachery. Indeed, during the late Middle Ages the Italians had the sinister reputation of being the most skilled poisoners in Europe.[8] However, malaria scholar Corrado Tommasi-Crudeli has dismissed such stories of "secret assassinations" and "poisoning" as a false trope; in actuality, Henry's death and many more like it were "purely and simply cases of death caused by deadly malaria."[9] The real killer was almost certainly *P. falciparum*, which Henry probably contracted during his summertime march through the notoriously malarial Maremma coastal plain of Tuscany south of Pisa.[10]

Imperial Engagement in Italy: Scale and Scope

Henry's Italian fiasco was not quite the swan song of imperial adventures into Italy. In the two centuries that followed, crowned kings of Germany would lead 11 more campaigns into the Italian peninsula, four of which would climax in imperial coronations. One of these later expeditions, that of Louis IV, was perhaps even larger in scale and ambition than Henry VII's last campaign. For the most part, however, these latter-day Imperial excursions were modest affairs, involving small numbers of men and limited objectives. Case in point was Charles IV's 1354–1355 expedition into Lombardy to receive the Iron Crown, during which Charles and his paltry escort of 300 knights was escorted from place to place by Milanese forces "like a merchant journeying to mass."[11] Charles would later take a larger force with him to Rome when seeking imperial coronation but didn't spend even a single night in Rome before "hurry[ing] like a fugitive" back through Milanese territory "with the imperial crown in his travelling chest."[12]

As it turned out, Charles was the last emperor whose trip to Rome was truly necessary. To the dismay of the papacy, and perhaps the plasmodia of Rome as well, the electors of the empire agreed in 1356 to the so-called Golden Bull: the empire was declared to be a domestic German institution and the papacy was henceforth denied any role in selecting or crowning the emperor. Two more emperors did seek imperial coronation in Rome in the 15th century, Sigismund and Frederick III, but such trips were now a matter of preference and prestige rather than a constitutional requirement. While the emperors still styled themselves the *Rex Romanorum*, or (in German) the *König der Römer*, the direct imperial link between Rome and empire had at last been severed.

For some historians of Germany, however, the Golden Bull came far too late. Since at least the 19th century German scholars have been openly hostile to Medieval Germany's "pointless dream of re-creating the Roman Empire," an unachievable fantasy which squandered resources that could have been better spent on Germany's domestic development. This distraction turned the Germanic Empire into a "monstrosity," an irregular kingdom with no defined central authority which James Madison would later denounce as a theater of "general imbecility, confusion and misery."[13] By the modern era, 19th century German historian Jacob Burckhardt would argue, "the German crown, encumbered with its Roman Empire, [was] too weak either to live or to die."[14] Small wonder, then, that Germany was doomed to become a "delayed nation" and would not emerge as a centralized national state until the late 19th century, long after the unification of other European powers such as England and France.

Did Medieval Germany's *Romegedanke*, or obsession with Rome, really delay German historical development as Burckhardt and others contend? Quite possibly, though it is hard to be sure, since there is no real metric we can apply to assess the issue. What is certain, however, is that the repeated German imperial campaigns must have represented a considerable demographic drain on German society, since they served to expose of thousands upon thousands of unacclimated Germans and other transalpine Europeans to Roman Fever.

Indeed, based on my reading of the relevant primary and secondary source materials, the German Empire's entanglements with Italy were extensive in both scale and scope. All told the German Empire launched at least 88 major imperial campaigns in Italy from 800 to 1509. Most of these expeditions were led by a crowned emperor, though a number of them were headed by rival claimants to the throne (such as Frederick the Fair, the Habsburg Duke of Austria) or by proxies (such as Pepin son of Charlemagne). Another 16 were imperial in nature but largely Italian in origin, such as the many southward campaigns by the Lombardy-based Kings of Italy or by imperial vassals such as Berengar of Ivrea. To this number could be added reinforcement expeditions, such as the three bodies of troops sent from Germany to bolster the campaigns of Frederick II between 1229 and 1250 and the German reinforcements that Henry VII received in 1313. Similar reinforcement expeditions no doubt arrived from Germany to bolster other imperial campaigns in Italy but are invisible from the historical record.

The German Empire, therefore, launched expeditions into Italy at a rate of about one every eight years, but this average conceals considerable variations over time. No less than 15 expeditions were launched during the chaotic 9th century due to of the progressive fracturing of Charlemagne's domain and the resulting rise in the number of claimants to imperial title. The following half century saw a prolonged fifty-year hiatus of imperial expeditions across the Alps, but the empire's Italian ambitions revived with the Ottonian dynasty after 950. The pace of imperial expeditions remained rather steady thereafter, with 11 expeditions in the 11th century and 13 in the 12th; as Horst Furmann pointed out in his 1994 article exploring the Medieval German Empire's entanglement with Rome, "from 962 to 1190 ... all the German Kings from Otto I to Frederick Barbarossa [with the exception of Conrad III] marched on Rome and had themselves crowned by the pope."[15] By the 13th century, however, the imperial impulse into Italy fell off considerably, and the next three centuries would see only 6, 6, and 7 expeditions respectively.

How many troops do these 88 expeditions represent? That is a hard question to answer, since the evidence on this point is extremely scanty. When describing imperial expeditions into Italy contemporary Medieval chroniclers made little attempt to estimate the size of armies, perhaps because they took this information for granted and assumed the reader would as well. Even descriptive adjectives are generally absent: most chroniclers limit themselves to noting that a given emperor entered Italy in a given month and year, and modifying details, such as Theitmar of Merseberg's description of Otto I's "powerful army," and Regino of Prüm's comment about Arnulf's "strong army," are exceptional.

Modern historians have been somewhat more willing to guess at imperial army size. Drawing on earlier work by Ernst Oehlmann, J.E. Tyler has estimated that the average imperial army must have included "from ten to fifteen thousand" heavily armed mounted troops and the size of such armies, "with their followers," must have "totaled well on to thirty thousand" exclusive of "reserve forces which might be called over the Alps into Italy over the course of a campaign."[16] Of course, not all expeditions reached this size, especially in the later Middle Ages. Henry VII entered Italy in 1310 with only "5000 men, chiefly mercenaries and insignificant people" since "none of the great princes of the empire had come forward as on previous expeditions to Rome."[17] Other expeditions numbered in the hundreds, such as Charles IV's foray into Italy to fetch the Iron Crown, and Louis IV's small force of 800 German knights dispatched in 1323 to help defend Milan, which was then under imperial control, from an advancing Guelf army. Given this wide range of army sizes an average force size of about five to ten thousand for these imperial expeditions seems reasonable. If these numbers hold, then well over half a million soldiers and hangers-on must have passed south of the Alps to fight for the German Empire during the 800–1508 period.

Not all of these combatants were Germans, of course. For the most part, we get only a dim picture of the rank-and-file soldiers of these campaigns; while the chroniclers often mention the number of armed horsemen and the names of elite participants in the expedition, they usually have little to say about the about the ethnic composition of imperial armies. There are, however, some exceptions. In one revealing passage Otto of Freising notes that Frederick Barbarossa's army at the eve of his ill-fated fourth campaign included not just Germans but also soldiers from Lorraine who may have been French speakers as well as Bohemians and Carinthians who were most likely Slavs. Frederick also brought "six hundred picked archers" from Hungary.[18] Henry V's large army was similarly multiethnic, containing "vassals from a hundred provinces of German, Slavic, and Romance lands."[19] Despite the diversity of customs and languages, these transalpine Europeans would have had one major trait in common: having never paid their tribute of children to the Minotaur, they were all extremely vulnerable to malarial fever, in particular the heat-loving *P. falciparum* of Rome.

Hills and Seasons: Imperial Patterns of Malaria Avoidance

Nonetheless, the actual exposure of these expeditions to malaria would have varied widely. For one thing, not all expeditions to Italy visited the *caput mundi*. Quite a few expeditions confined themselves to Italy north of the Apennines, either by design or by necessity, and a few others bypassed Rome entirely and concentrated on Sicily and the Italian south. Still, more than half (49 of 88) the expeditions spent at least some time in or around Rome, spending all or part of at least 141 months in Rome's immediate vicinity.

What is more, German armies campaigning near Rome took a number of steps to protect themselves from the fatal exhalations of the dragon's lair. German expeditions to Rome tended to cling to the heights, such as the Capitoline and Aventine hills within Rome and the Vatican Hill and Monte Mario just outside the city. Armies perched on these hilltops would not have been entirely immune to Rome's malaria, but they would have enjoyed at least some protection against plasmodia infection: *Anopheles* mosquitos are poor uphill flyers and would have found few places to breed amongst the hill's windy slopes. The same was even more true of the Alban hills, a favored summer retreat for imperial forces besieging the city, where summertime temperatures might be 2–4°C lower than the surrounding lowland plains. These temperature differentials could prove crucial, especially when it comes to *P. falciparum*, which develops much more slowly in mosquitos when temperatures stay below 30°C.

In addition to adapting to Rome's malaria by means of topography, imperial armies also tried to avoid malaria by carefully choreographing their visits to Rome. Following Charlemagne's example, the preferred time for imperial coronation in Rome was December or January and imperial armies tended to leave the vicinity of Rome in April or May. To some degree, this preference for spring probably reflected a desire to spend the two most important religious holidays, Christmas and Easter, in the holy city of the holy church. However, a conscious desire to avoid malaria infection probably played a role as well. To test this hypothesis, I counted the total number of months spent by imperial

9. Imperium's Price

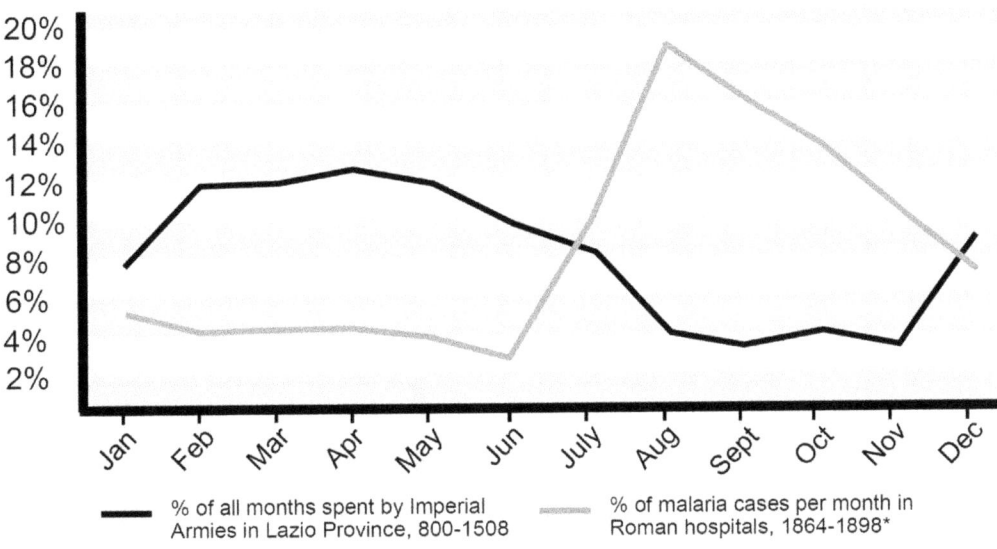

Imperial Expeditions and Malaria Prevalence by Month. Angelo Celli, *Malaria, According to the New Researches* (New York: Longmans, Green, 1900), p. 149.

expeditions spent in in the modern Lazio province (Rome and its environs) from 800 to 1508, and plotted this data alongside seasonal malaria statistics taken from Roman hospitals from 1863 to 1898. The results are striking: as is clear from the chart below, the German imperial presence in Rome is almost perfectly inversely correlated with malaria prevalence. It is surely no coincidence that the month of the sharpest drop-off in German presence in Rome, August, is also the first month of Rome's high malaria season.

Still, despite their best efforts, logistical problems or political contingency did occasionally force various German emperors to risk their troops to the "bad air" of the Italian summer. As Otto Kestner has pointed out, the campaign season of imperial armies was sharply limited by the Alpine passes, which were usually impassable by a large force until mid-May. Thus, imperial forces had barely two months in which to operate in Italy before the malarial season set in.[20] This problem could be addressed by marching over the Alps in fall and wintering in relatively healthy northern Italy, where *P. vivax* would have been a danger in the spring and early summer but *P. falciparum* was mostly or completely absent. However, provisioning a large army for months at a time was a difficult task, and emperors found themselves obliged to feed their troops with forced tribute and occasional plunder.[21] Nor did wintering in northern Italy guarantee arriving in Rome on time, as Frederick Barbarossa found out in 1154–55: his march on Rome was fatally delayed by a three-month siege of Tortona and thus he did not arrive in Rome for his coronation until June, the very cusp of the malarial season. In addition, we should keep in mind that even those imperial armies that avoided Rome did not necessarily avoid malaria. This is especially true if they were campaigning in the Italian south, some parts of which were even more malarial than Rome and its environs.

As a result of these factors, malaria epidemics seem to have been a fairly frequent occurrence amongst imperial expeditions to Italy. In all, I was able to identify 22 incidents in which either an imperial army or an imperial leader may have been afflicted by malaria in the years between 810 and 1313.[22] Five crowned emperors may have been killed by malaria in Italy during this period, namely Lothar II, Otto II, Otto III, Conrad VI, and Henry VII, and the latter two deaths were particularly consequential since both were young men at the height of their power when fever cut them down. In addition, malaria may also have taken a toll upon various potential imperial heirs, including Pepin, son of Charlemagne, Luidolf, son of Otto I, and Conrad, who died suddenly in Florence in July 1101 while rebelling against his father Henry IV. I should point out that this diagram shows only the *known* disease cases amongst imperial troops in Italy and thus may represent just the point of the spear. Some minor or moderate outbreaks of malaria amongst imperial armies probably went unnoticed, especially if they confined

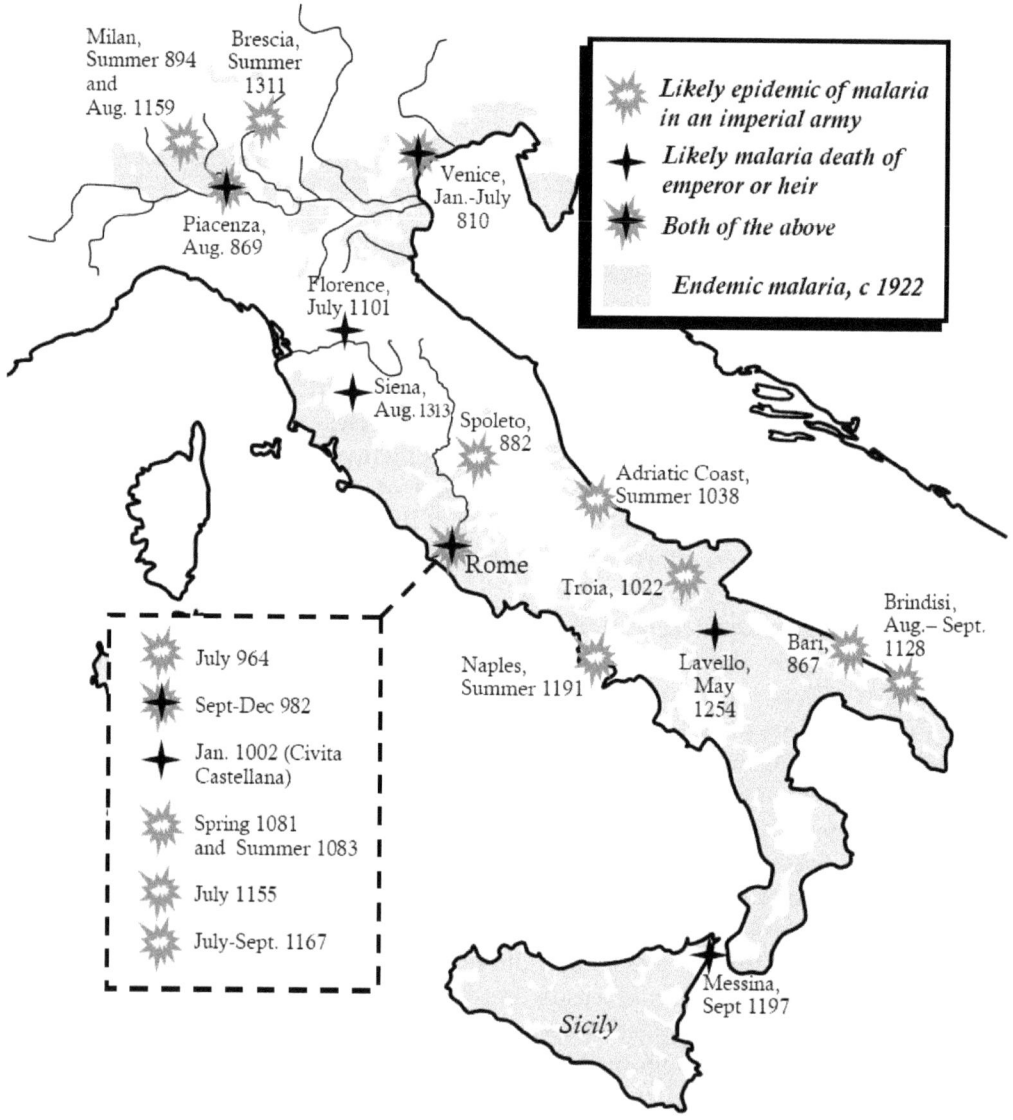

Malaria Outbreaks and German Imperial Expeditions. W. O. Blanchard, "Malaria as a Factor in the Italian Environment," *The Scientific Monthly*, Vol. 27, No. 2 [August 1928], pp. 172–176.

themselves to rank-and-file soldiers and spared the imperial elites. It is impossible now to try to estimate the overall number of imperial deaths to malaria over these five centuries, but given the scale of these expeditions and the danger that malaria posed, the cumulative death toll was probably in the tens of thousands.

Shock, Awe and Malaria

The impact of malaria on the empire, however, goes far beyond any crude calculation of body count. One of the ironies of history is that the very tactics used by German monarchs to limit malaria deaths rebounded against the empire itself, fatally weakening it and transforming its successes into failures. Malaria cut short the campaign season, dissuaded the empire from establishing permanent garrisons in Italian territory, and hastened the deaths of unacclimated German appointees to the papal office. As a result, imperial successes in Italy often proved fleeting and subsequent emperors were unable to build upon each other's accomplishments but instead were repeatedly forced to return to square one. A few emperors did try to maintain constant presence in Italy, including Otto III, who made Rome his capital, and Henry IV and VII, both of whom tried to maintain garrisons in Rome through the summer season. However, these exceptions proved the rule. Otto III ultimately succumbed to malarial fever and the garrisons the two Henrys left in Rome quickly melted away. The only emperor who managed to successfully maintain a presence in Italy over a long period of time was Frederick II, and once again, the exception proves the rule: Frederick was more of a Norman King than a German one and thanks to his childhood in Palermo he probably had some acquired malaria resistance, as did many of his locally-recruited soldiers.[23]

The threat of summertime death also weakened the empire in a second way—by predisposing it to shortsighted, tyrannical behavior. As most German emperors campaigned in Italy, a clock was no doubt ticking in their heads, counting the months and days until the start of the unhealthy season. As a result, these emperors often relied on brute force, which could achieve goals quickly, rather than diplomacy, negotiation, and institution-building, which were far more time-consuming enterprises. In his recent book on the Holy Roman Empire, Peter Wilson argues convincingly that malaria may have forced the empire to rely on "violent shock and awe" in Italy.[24] Case in point was Frederick Barbarossa's barbaric treatment of the city of Tortona, but other imperial campaigns fit the bill as well, including Henry V's strong-arm actions against the papacy in 1111 and the reign of terror that Henry VI inflicted upon rebels while pacifying his newly-won Kingdom of Sicily.

These methods might yield valuable short-term gains, but they were inherently self-defeating. Indeed, many imperial campaigns into Italy resembled William McNeill has called "epidemic warfare": parasitical military operations, sustained largely through plunder, which devastated the territory through which they passed.[25] Such operations might collect bribes or tribute, but not annual taxes. Cities were taken, but looted and dismantled rather than garrisoned, meaning they quickly rose again to challenge the empire anew. German emperors in Italy gained crowns, but not enduring provinces; they defended their rights and prerogatives, but did not create lasting institutions.

What is more, whatever ephemeral authority the German emperors gained from their battlefield successes was soon lost as soon as the Germans, inevitably, turned their backs on Italy and its resident fevers. In their absence, fear of the emperors was replaced by bitter resentment against German barbarism, undermining everything that the previous round of epidemic warfare had accomplished. As a result, each successive emperor was forced to start from scratch each time they attempted anew to realize their Roman Imperial aspirations. In large part because of malaria, therefore, the dream of empire proved to be a recurring nightmare for Germans and Italians alike.

10

Jubilee

While imperial soldiers were a frequent Medieval visitor to the *caput mundi*, such men were by no means the most numerous variety of European visitors to Rome. That pride of place undoubtedly belongs to the pilgrims, spiritual warriors of staff and scrip. Unfortunately for historians, however, these pilgrims have left only a faint imprint upon the pages of history. As Christopher Cheney points out in his work on Innocent III and England, "one category of visitors to Rome we cannot hope to discover in any quantity, for they do not figure in papal letters or other official correspondence or in chronicles, [are pilgrims]: they are the lost witnesses to the eternal attraction of the Eternal City."[1] In a similar vein, Brian Barefoot quipped that "the sandaled footprints of these innumerable travelers have left very little trace in the sands of history."[2] Of all the sparks that streamed towards Rome in the Middle Ages, then, the pilgrims are the dimmest cinders. Other than a few exceptional travelers whose itinerary was preserved for history, pilgrims are usually seen only in aggregate if they are seen at all.

Pilgrims and Pilgrimage

The tradition of pilgrimage has deep pre–Christian roots. In ancient Greece, all travelers were under the protection of Zeus and the feeding, clothing, and housing of such men and women was a religious duty. Odysseus found it useful to take on the guise of an anonymous pilgrim-traveler, a "no-man" and "every-man," when he returned to his home in Ithaca, then besieged by hostile suitors seeking to make a bride of his wife.[3] The later Western European tradition that pilgrims must be treated as Christ in disguise is probably a just a Christian continuation of this hallowed Greek custom.[4]

Christian pilgrimage was not necessarily synonymous with Rome, of course. From the founding of the faith, the most popular pilgrimage site was Jerusalem, where pilgrim sandals could walk upon streets that had been blessed by the dripping blood of a living god. Nonetheless, records of pilgrimage to Rome go back to at least the 3rd century, when the Greek cleric Eusebius of Caesarea toured the holy sites in Rome.[5] Transalpine Europe probably sent very few pilgrims to Rome during this time period, except perhaps from heavily Romanized France. Over the course of the Dark Ages, however, as Europe steadily Christianized, pilgrims would flock to Rome from the newly-converted territories, first in a popular wave and later in a sustained steady stream. In Anglo-Saxon England, where missionary work began in the late 6th century, the flood of initial pilgrims crested in the 7th century and 8th centuries. Next to come were Frisians, Germanic peoples of the modern-day Dutch coast, who were converted by missionaries from Rome in the later 7th century. By the 8th and 9th century, so many Frisian pilgrims flooded to Rome that they built their own *schola* to support (and to some degree, exploit) the incoming travelers. In later years, still more pulses of pilgrims descended upon Rome, including a wave of pilgrims from newly-converted Saxony. The Hungarian wave washed into Rome in the early 11th century following the gradual conversion of Magyar pagans to Christianity after Hungary's defeat in the battle of Lechfeld. In the following century, it was the turn of the Danes, the Poles, and the Icelanders.[6]

Although pilgrims hailed from diverse countries, their experiences were similar and became increasingly so over time due to standardizing regulations set by various councils of the Church. Sir Walter Raleigh immortalized the typical Medieval pilgrim in the following verses:

> Give me my scallop-shell of quiet,
> My staff of faith to walk upon,
> My scrip of joy, immortal diet,
> My bottle of salvation,
> My gown of glory, hope's true gage;
> And thus I'll take my pilgrimage.[7]

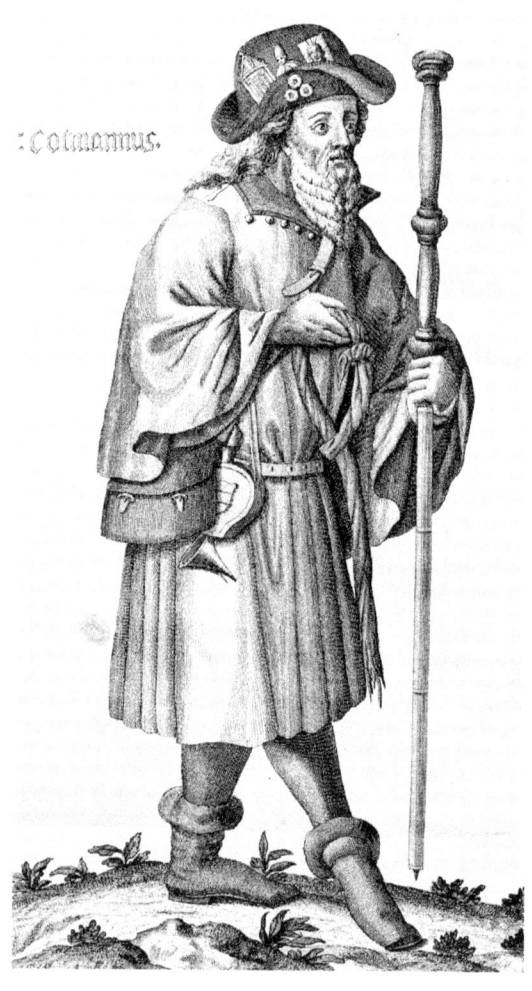

Although the meaning of this text is largely obscure to modern readers, Raleigh's contemporaries would have easily decoded the imagery. The "staff of faith" was not just a walking aid for a wayfarer but the trademark symbol of pilgrimage, carried even by pilgrims who mainly travelled by sea. The "gown of glory" was a pilgrim's hooded robes, generally grey in color, which evoked the sheepskin raiment of Hebrew holy men.[8] The "scallop-shell of quiet," in turn, suggests that Raleigh's pilgrim was destined for Santiago de Compostela in Spain, where pilgrims received a distinctive seashell plucked from local beaches as a physical memento of their spiritual journey.

As for the scrip, it was a leather satchel containing the pilgrim's documents, usually including an authenticating permit from the bishop of the

Medieval illustration of a pilgrim with staff and scrip. This seems to have been an experienced pilgrim, as his hat is decorated with numerous pilgrim badges. Gottfried Deppisch, *Geschichte und Wunder-Wercke des heiligen Colomanni Königlichen Pilgers und Martyrers* (Vienna: Frantz André Kirchberger, 1743).

pilgrim's home diocese. Pilgrims armed with a scrip could demand special treatment, such as free food and lodging in monastic hospices along the way as well as exemptions from river and bridge tolls. This scrip also allowed ecclesiastical authorities to distinguish genuine pilgrims from frauds, including merchants claiming pilgrim status to avoid tolls and taxation, peasants seeking to escape exploitative feudal relationships, and spies hoping to keep a low profile.[9] Still other ersatz pilgrims were pure moochers, including the famous George Psalmanazar, an 18th-century wandering Frenchman who claimed to be an Irish pilgrim to acquire free food and lodging during his various travels. When his ruse was discovered, Psalmanazar cooked up a still more audacious scam, declaring himself to be a "Japanese heathen" from Taiwan who had been kidnapped and carried to Europe by a Jesuit missionary.[10]

After receiving staff and scrip, an aspiring pilgrim was supposed to settle their affairs, repay their debts, and provide for any dependents. Pilgrims also tended to write their wills before travelling, since many pilgrims never made it home. For the supporters of pilgrimage, however, the spiritual rewards earned by a pilgrim on his or her journey were well worth the many risks of the road. "What fool, what laggard," asked Jacopo, Deacon of Rome,

> …would not set out, not count as cool the summer's heat,
> Warmth winter's ice, parching dry the drizzling damp….
> Let not hunger of fasting, thirst through choking,
> Height of mountains, depth of valleys, dripping sweat….
> Rivers, the journey, expense, the sea, a haughty host,
> Weakness of age or sex, sleepless nights, or searing wind
> shatter your spirit; to these does the Kingdom of Heaven lie open.
> Yet none of these could cure our disease. The gracious, the lofty
> Apostle's See [Rome], based on Christ's crimson blood,
> 'tis she who dispenses riches received from the wounds of Christ
> And these holy fathers, and thus she remits your sins.[11]

Interestingly enough, while Jacopo mentions disease in this catalogue of possible pilgrimage perils, he does so metaphorically, likening disease to a longing for redemption—and prescribing Rome as the cure. Perhaps as an Italian Jacopo did not fear the bite of Roman Fever. Alternatively, Jacopo may have felt that reminding readers of Roman Fever might have discouraged potential pilgrims from visiting the Holy See, which was the opposite of his intent. We will return to the theme of pilgrimage and malaria later in this chapter.

It is important to note that not all pilgrims braved the hazards of the road voluntarily. During the Middle Ages many criminals were sentenced to penitential pilgrimage, either because their crimes could only be forgiven by the papacy or because their communities simply wanted to be rid of them: as Jonathan Sumption points out, such pilgrimages were "little more than the traditional penalty of banishment re-named."[12] Our best evidence about these pilgrimages comes from a 1922 study by Étienne Van Cauwenbergh on Medieval penitential pilgrims from his native Belgium. Not all Belgian penitent-pilgrims travelled to Rome, of course. The destination and duration of judicially-imposed pilgrimages depended upon the nature and the severity of the crime. Nonetheless, van Cauwenbergh identified a large number of infractions punished by pilgrimage to Rome in the late Middle Ages including murder, heresy, forgery, violence against your parents, eating meat on fast days, blocking ship traffic on the River Seine, and in one case, "permitting dangerous words to be said about the Duke of Brabant."[13] Unlike regular pilgrims, penitents were expected to travel barefoot in a rough tunic and keep to a diet of beans, bread, and water. What is more they were entirely dependent on charity, being forbidden to practice any trade, and unless they were ill they could not sleep in the same place for two sequential nights. After a specified time such pilgrims could return home, but only after procuring a certificate of completed pilgrimage from the "Grand Penitentiary" of Rome, the church official in charge of rehabilitating these wayward souls.[14]

Patterns of Pilgrimage to Rome

Whether their pilgrimage was voluntary or forced, most pilgrims followed similar itineraries and timetables. European pilgrims from northern lands usually set out for Rome in the early summer, when food was beginning to ripen in the fields and the roads had dried out from the downpours of spring. What is more, the Alps were at their most passable at that time, as they were free of snow and mountain torrents were at a low ebb.[15] For the most part pilgrims did not travel alone but rather formed large companies for the sake of safety and companionship.[16] On the way to Rome these companies often stayed in hospices, including the famous 11th-century guesthouse in St. Bernard Pass founded by the saint of the same name.

By mid- to late autumn, the excited pilgrims would have been approaching Monte Mario on the outskirts of Rome, a spot later immortalized in Dante's *Divine Comedy* as the "small hill" where Virgil, in his role of spiritual guide, met a sinful pilgrim and led him on a tour of Hell.[17] Dante called this hill the Mount of Joy, a name derived from the traditional cry of "Montjoie" that pilgrims would cry out upon their first glimpse of the Eternal City. Pilgrims typically raced up this joyful mountain with pell-mell abandon since by custom the first to reach its summit would become honorary king of his pilgrim company. Indeed, many royalty-evoking modern European family names—King, Koenig, Leroy, etc.—may be founded upon the pilgrim feats of their distant ancestors.[18] From Monte Mario onwards, pilgrims would swap their shoes for sandals and descend from their mounts, if they had any, as signs of Christian humility.[19] Typically pilgrims would remain in Rome until late March or April, partly out of desire to spend the Holy Week in Holy Rome, but also in order to wait for the thawing of the Alpine passes. They would then return home, lighter in wallet but richer in spirit as a result of their experiences.

In his immortal *Canterbury Tales*, Geoffrey Chaucer left us a satirical depiction of one such returning pilgrim, "the Pardoner," recently arrived "straight … from the court of Rome." The Pardoner had removed his pilgrim's hood "for jollity," and to advertise his recently-completed travels he sported a cap decorated with Rome's pilgrim badge, the vernicle. He carries neither staff nor scrip but is laden down instead with supposed Roman relics, including a bag crafted from Virgin Mary's own veil, supposed scraps of sailcloth from St. Peter's fisherman days, a decorated brass cross, and a jar full of pigs' bones. The loathsome Pardoner sells these dubious souvenirs to local country bumpkins with "flattery and japes," thus earning himself more money in a day than his gullible marks made with two month's work.[20] It is important to note, however, that Chaucer's Pardoner was not meant to be understood as a typical pilgrim. Here as elsewhere in Canterbury Tales, Chaucer tried to delight his reader by deliberately exaggerating his subject's faults and follies for humorous effect.[21] Chaucer most likely invented the Pardoner to parody the cupidity of those Romans who lined their pockets by exploiting the religious fervor of naïve foreign pilgrims.

By the 12th century, however, pilgrimages to Rome had entered a period of sharp decline. Muslim raids into Italy dissuaded many potential pilgrims, as did the repeated clashes of popes and emperors, not to mention the papacy's chronic inability to keep a lid on Rome's internal political turmoil. What is more, other major pilgrimage destinations were coming on-line, most notably Santiago de Compostela in Northern Spain in the 10th century and Jerusalem in the 12th century following its recapture from the Muslims during the First Crusade.[22] Rome also faced fierce competition from a plethora of local cult centers, often touted by provincial bishops trying to increase their status and revenue by encouraging pilgrimage to their own see while disparaging the efficacy of pilgrimage to other destinations. In the words of Diana Webb, during the Middle Ages it became commonplace for the custodians of regional saints' shrines to claim that their relics could cure sufferers "who had come away empty-handed from every other shrine he or she had visited, even from St. Peter at Rome."[23] As a result, by the 12th century the various foreign *scholae* in Rome were falling into disrepair, reduced to skeleton crews or dissolved entirely.[24]

By the 13th century, however, Rome was coming back into style as a pilgrimage destination. Jerusalem had fallen to the Muslim general Saladin in 1187, and although Christian pilgrimage to Jerusalem was still possible it was rendered less popular by perceived infidel danger.[25] And why go to Jerusalem in any case? Returning crusaders had filled Rome with artifacts related to Christ, including perhaps the famous Veil of Veronica, a piece of fabric boasting a distinctly savior-shaped stain. Many now considered Rome to be the New Jerusalem, equal in sanctity to the old, and much more conveniently located.

Rome and the Jubilee

In the later years of the 13th century the flow of pilgrims once again slackened due to the bitter conflict between the papacy and Frederick II. However, pilgrimage to Rome experienced a spectacular and unexpected revival at the century's end. On Christmas Eve in 1299, the Basilica of Saint Peter was besieged by an unexpectedly large crowd which included numerous foreigners to the city. In subsequent days pilgrim numbers swelled further and by January and February it was "scarcely possible to walk through the city, vast and large though it was."[26] Rome's bridges became so choked with pilgrims that authorities had to place dividers down the middle to direct traffic into eastbound and westbound lanes, a detail later incorporated by Dante into the special hell he designed for panderers and seducers.[27] These pilgrims were a multinational lot. While the English were notable mainly for their absence, French and Germans were numerous as were visitors from the "far North and from the East."[28] Contemporary chroniclers claimed that 10,000–30,000 pious pilgrims entered and left the city each day and that they swelled the city's population by as much as 200,000.[29] Indeed, the pilgrim-thronged streets were in such a state of chaos that the Chronicler of Asti remembered seeing "both men and women trodden under foot in the press, and I myself more than once was hard bestead to escape the same danger."[30]

What was going on? When Roman officials asked these pilgrims why they had come to Rome, most claimed they were drawn by the promise of complete remission of sins, though it is not clear who had made that promise in the first place. Martin Luther would later point a finger at the papacy itself, claiming the popes had invented a new pilgrimage tradition out of avarice and lust for coin. However, there is no evidence to support this notion, and in any case most of the additional revenue collected by the church in 1300 had to be spent providing food, housing, and other services to the innumerable and unexpected foreign visitors.[31] A more likely explanation for the 1300 mass pilgrimage was millenarian religious excitement at the dawning of the 14th century. As those of us who lived through the 2000 millennial and its accompanying Y2K panic clearly remember, the coming of a new century evokes both high expectations and doomsday fears. What is more, the Church itself had recently set the precedent that visits to certain pilgrimage sites, such as Francis of Assisi's Church of Santa Maria of the Angels and the Canterbury Cathedral shrine of the martyred Saint Thomas Becket, could expunge the stain of sin.[32]

At first, Pope Boniface VIII did little to encourage the mass pilgrimage of 1300. A worldly pope in the aristocratic tradition, Boniface had little time for popular piety and had recently shown his hostility towards the idea of pilgrim indulgences by cancelling his predecessor's decree granting absolution to visitors of Francis of Assisi's shrine.[33] Nonetheless, faced with the massive crowds of 1300, Boniface decided to jump on the bandwagon rather than stand in its path. On February 22, the pope announced that a new

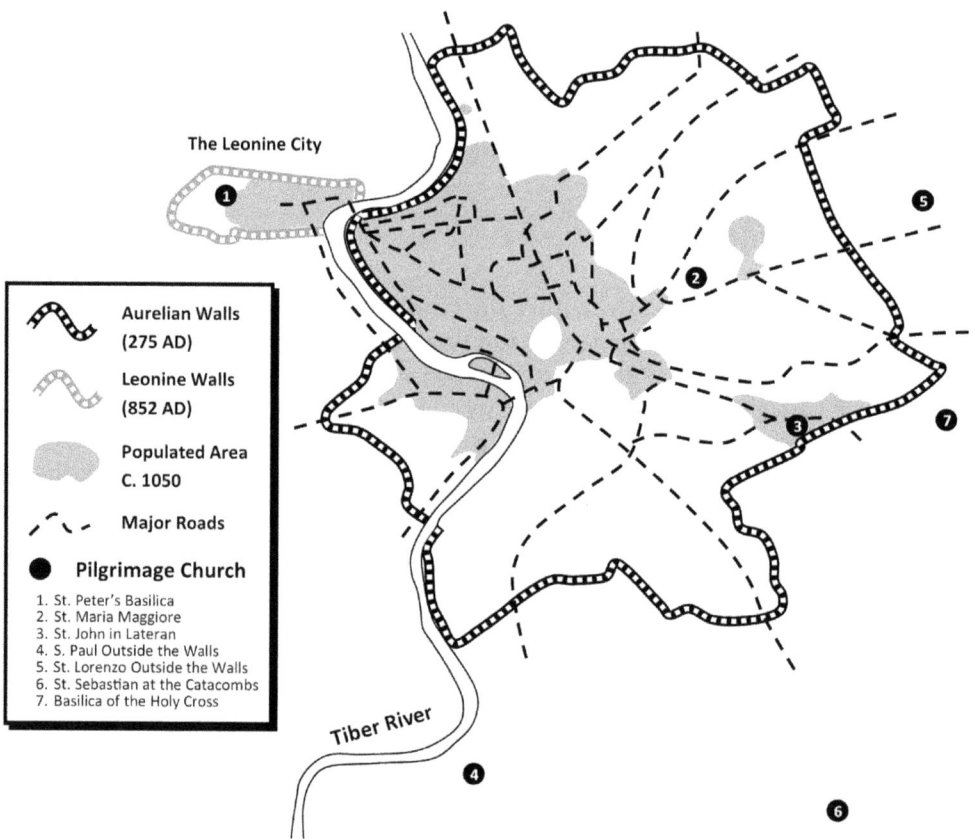

Rome of the Medieval Pilgrim. Adapted from Richard Krautheimer, *Rome: Profile of a City, 312–1308* (Princeton, NJ: Princeton University Press, 2000), p. 245.

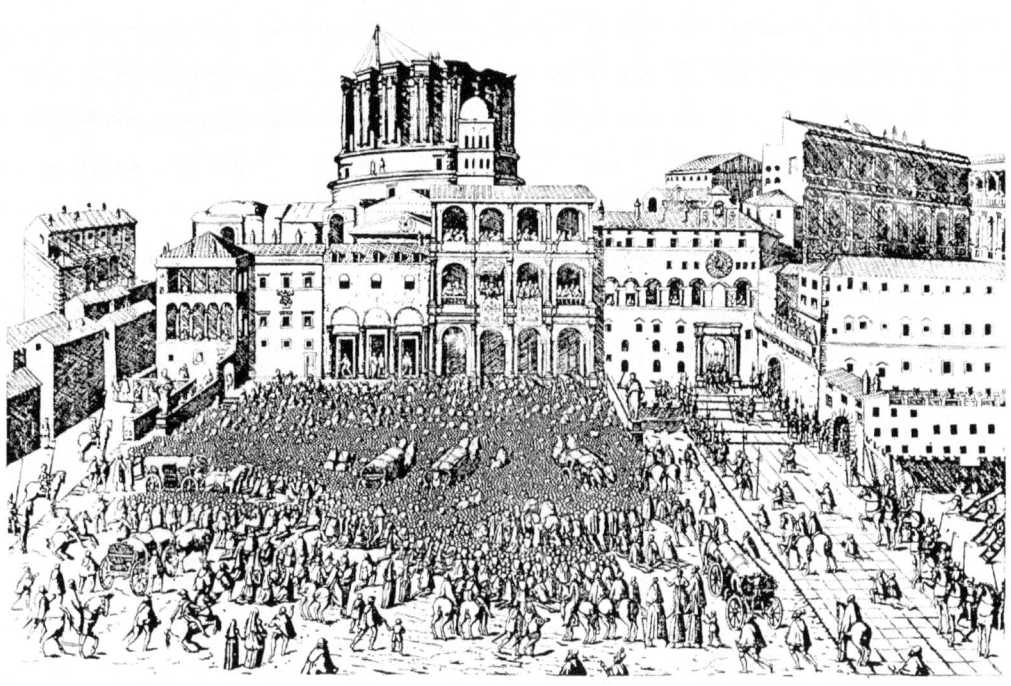

Crowds in Rome during the 1575 Jubilee. Herbert Thurston, *The Holy Year of Jubilee: An Account of the History and Ceremonial of the Roman Jubilee* (London: Sands and Co., 1900), p. 359.

indulgence, "the most full pardon of all their sins," was available to that year's pilgrims to Rome. To receive it, the pilgrim must be penitent and fully confessed and must spend 30 days visiting the seven major basilica churches of Rome, or 15 days if they were "foreigners or strangers."[34]

Following Boniface's decree, still more pilgrims flooded to Rome, though there is some evidence that the religious enthusiasm of these pilgrims did not entirely blind them to the dangers of Rome's malarial fevers. According to Cardinal Stefaneschi, a contemporary of Boniface who wrote a history of the 1300 pilgrimage, each nation of visitors to Rome was careful to arrive in Rome only during the season when temperature conditions conformed to that of their own country. During the high summer, the people most likely to visit Rome were the Puglians, Corsicans, and Sardinians, who came from territories with high levels of endemic malaria—for such peoples, Rome's summertime climate might have actually represented an improvement over what they left behind.[35] As for the French, German, and Hungarian visitors to the city, they "wait[ed] for a season of the year when the climate of Rome is somewhat similar to the cold of their own country," and thus arrived at the start of autumn or in winter, when Roman Fever was at a very low ebb.[36] No doubt some transalpine visitors deviated from this schedule and paid for it with their lives, but there is no way now to know; very few surviving pilgrims told their stories, and dead men tell no tales.

The 1300 mass pilgrimage proved to be just the first of many. In his authorization of the 1300 indulgence, Boniface had established that centennial pilgrimages would henceforth occur regularly on a hundred-year schedule. Forty-three years later, however, the

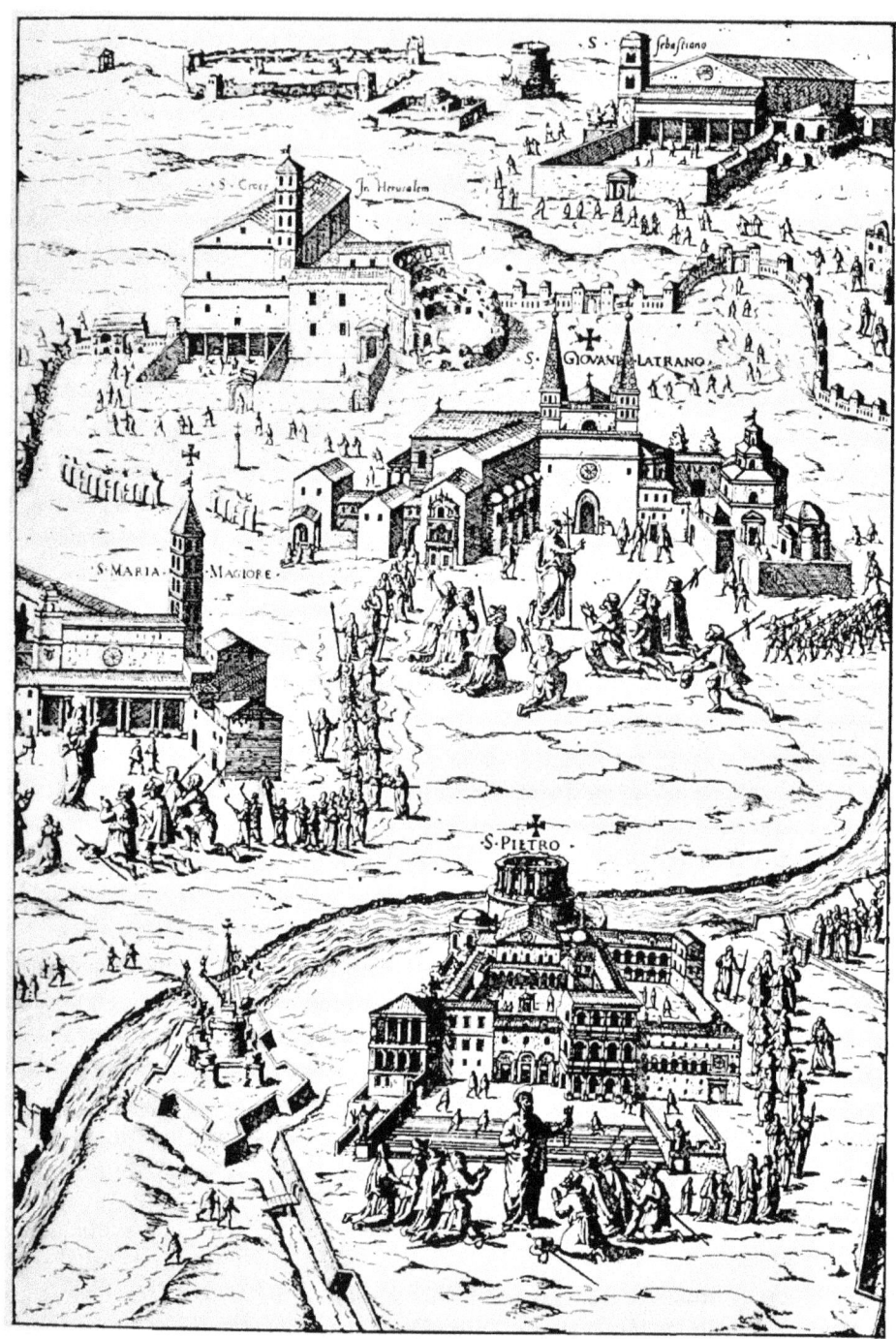

Illustration from the 1575 Jubilee showing five of the seven holy-year basilicas of Rome. Depicted: Saint Peter's, Saint Maria Major, the Lateran, Basilica of the Holy Cross, and Saint Sebastian outside the Walls. Not shown: Saint Lawrence outside the Walls and Saint Paul outside the Walls. St. Angelo fortress can be seen in the lower left corner. Herbert Thurston, *The Holy Year of Jubilee: An Account of the History and Ceremonial of the Roman Jubilee* (London: Sands and Co., 1900), p. 135.

papacy changed its mind and decided on a 50-year schedule instead. In part, this was a sop to the generation born in the early years of the 14th century, who were unlikely to survive until 1400. The shift to a half-century cycle also drew upon Old Testament tradition of designating every 50th year as a holy Jubilee year in which debts were forgiven, slaves were freed, land was left unplowed, and God was particularly merciful towards wayward sinners.[37] Indeed, although Boniface did not use the term "Jubilee" in his papal bull granting an indulgence to pilgrims in 1300, the term was already on the lips of many pilgrims.

The second Jubilee proved to be even better attended than the first, despite or perhaps because of the recent horrors of the Black Death, which had killed a third to a half of Europe's population just two years earlier. In 1350 a contemporary chronicler exclaimed that "all of Christendom flocked to Rome to get the indulgence" and the number of visitors to Rome may have peaked at 1.2 million during Holy Week.[38] On Sundays and feast days, the stained napkin of Saint Veronica was displayed to such large crowds before the Basilica of Saint Peter that "many were suffocated or trampled to death."[39] Since the number of visitors far surpassed the accommodation capacity of the city, some foreign visitors were forced to sleep under the arched porticoes of Rome's buildings or else huddled for warmth around outdoor huge campfires. The crowds thinned somewhat in the heat of the summer, but "a great multitude remained," much to the delight of Rome's resident plasmodia species.[40] By Christmas of 1350 the crowds swelled once again. Chroniclers reported that pilgrims threw so much money upon the altar in Saint Paul's Basilica that two priests were employed, day and night, to collect it into baskets with rakes. Overall the papacy earned about 1700 florins a day during the 1350 Jubilee, which means the Papacy's take from that pilgrimage year was equal to three times the normal yearly expenses of the Church.[41]

After 1350, Jubilee years followed in regular succession, though not all of them enjoyed 1350's success. In 1389, Pope Urban VI decided to shorten the Jubilee schedule still further to 33-year intervals—the life span of Jesus Christ—so a Jubilee was held in 1390, though it was not well attended due to an ongoing schism in the church.[42] Despite this new schedule, pilgrims descended on Rome for an unofficial Jubilee in 1400, further proof that the Jubilee tradition owed as much to Christian Europe's centenary hopes and fears as to papal proclamations. In 1423, another official Jubilee year, Rome was again "inundated by Barbarians [non–Italians]" who "filled the whole city with dirt and confusion."[43] Overall, however, the revenues generated by this jubilee seem to have been disappointing, perhaps because 1423 was not a number likely to fill anyone with a sense of millenarian dread.

In contrast, the 1450 Jubilee was a triumph, at least from the standpoint of pilgrim numbers. Chroniclers reported that 40,000 pilgrims entered Rome daily over the course of that year and witnesses likened the incoming pilgrims to "flights of starlings or the march of myriads of ants."[44] Rome's inns and lodgings became so crammed with humanity that latecomers were forced to camp out in the fields and vineyards enclosed by Rome's Aurelian walls. By mid–May, however, the "plague" came to Rome and "all the hospitals and churches were full of the sick and dying." As a result, pilgrims fled the city, but so many died along the way that "graves were seen all along the roads even in Tuscany and Lombardy." According to the Roman chronicler Paolo di Benedetto di Cola dello Mastro, the epidemic did not die down until the coming of cold weather in late September, after which "the pestilence ceased and the pilgrims once again poured in."[45]

Was the disease that disrupted the 1450 Jubilee malaria? It is certainly possible, though there are other suspects to consider. *Y. pestis*, which recurred repeatedly in Europe after the great plague years of 1347–1351, cannot be ruled out. Nor can gastrointestinal diseases, fostered by poor sanitation and water source contamination in the overcrowded city. However, many of the available facts point strongly to malaria, perhaps *P. vivax* in late spring and *P. falciparum* during the summer heat. Observers agree that the disease disproportionally afflicted visiting pilgrims, which is only to be expected given both the greater malarial vulnerability of transalpine Europeans and the fact that many such pilgrims were camping out in the highly malarial orchards, fields, and wastelands encompassed by the city walls.[46] The fact that the epidemic declined with dropping autumn temperature is also what we would expect from a malaria outbreak. Even if malaria did not play the lead role in the 1450 disease outbreak, then, it likely was at least a supporting actor. Much the same drama played out during the next Jubilee, in 1475, which coincided with heavy floods of the Tiber that "rendered the roads impractical and the flooded area [of Rome] unhealthy."[47]

Unfortunately, blessed few pilgrims of the period left written records of their travels, but the experiences of Arnold von Harff, a late 15th-century German pilgrim, were probably at least somewhat typical of the bunch. Von Harff's ultimate destination was the Holy Land but he made time for a Holy Week detour to Rome, which he described as "very large and spacious" but "more than half destroyed."[48] During his stay in the Eternal City, Von Harff dutifully prayed at the pilgrim basilicas and noted for his readers the relative spiritual efficacy of Rome's many shrines, quantified in terms of how many years of each shrine could subtract from a sinner's posthumous suffering in purgatory. What seemed to interest Von Harff most, however, was Rome's smorgasbord of relics. By the late 1400s, Rome's various churches sported a bewildering bric-a-brac of sacred remains, including Jesus's cradle, the grill on which Saint Lawrence was roasted, the suicide noose of Judas Iscariot, Saint George's dragon-slaying spear, a tuft of St. Peter's beard, and vials purporting to contain the blood of Jesus and the milk of Mary.[49]

Malaria and the Pilgrim

Although amazed by Rome's relics, Von Harff and other pilgrims were not blind to Rome's malaria dangers, as is clear from curious tale Von Harff recorded about a haunted tree which supposedly stood near the northern wall of Rome. In former years, Von Harff tells us, the people passing the gate were imperiled by "many devils ... and no one knew whence they came." The pope at the time eventually traced the problem to a certain nut-tree standing near the old Flaminian Gate. Upon striking the accursed tree, which was "at once rooted up," the pope discovered the coffin of the wicked tyrant Nero "who slew St. Peter and St. Paul and many other martyrs."[50] In order to exorcise the devils from the site, the pope ordered that the tree be destroyed and that a church be founded in its place. While this story swaps the dragon for a tree, overall this tale follows the same format as the dragon legends described in Chapter 5 above in which saintly intervention banishes a devilish presence from a malarial natural location. In this case, however, the cure was not very effective. The Flaminian Gate district, later re-named the Piazza del Popolo, remained one of Rome's most malarial districts well into the modern area and

French troops stationed there during the Napoleonic-era occupation of Rome would suffer repeatedly from the ravages of Roman Fever.

At this point, it is impossible to determine exactly how many visiting pilgrims fell prey to the miasmic dragons and devil-haunted trees of the Eternal City. We know the flow of pilgrims to Rome was heavy, especially in the 13th to 16th centuries of pilgrimage, when contemporary sources estimated that 50,000 pilgrims flocked to Rome in normal years and numbered a million or more during the holy Jubilees.[51] These numbers may be exaggerated, however, and it is not clear in any case how many such pilgrims were from across the Alps. Nor is it possible to say what fraction of such pilgrims caught malaria. History has preserved the names of a few bright sparks who suffered from fever while on pilgrimage to Rome, including the colorful Rahere, an English court jester whom Rudyard Kipling would later describe in verse as a standing deep in "dark [King] Henry's crooked councils."[52] Such references, however, are very few and far between.

We do, however, have one piece of hard data that is relevant to the question of pilgrims and malaria, namely documentation collected by George Parks about registrants in English hospices in Rome from 1500 to 1525. While this tells us little about overall numbers of English pilgrims in Rome—not all English registered with these hospices—it does give us a tantalizing glimpse of the seasonality of such travel. As the diagram below suggests, some English were present in the city every month of the year, including the summer malaria season. Nonetheless, overall English travel to Rome exhibited marked seasonality, peaking between March and May, and trailing off sharply thereafter.

Undoubtedly, some of this seasonal variation can be explained by the Christian liturgical calendar. Both then and now, the preferred time for pilgrimage to Rome was

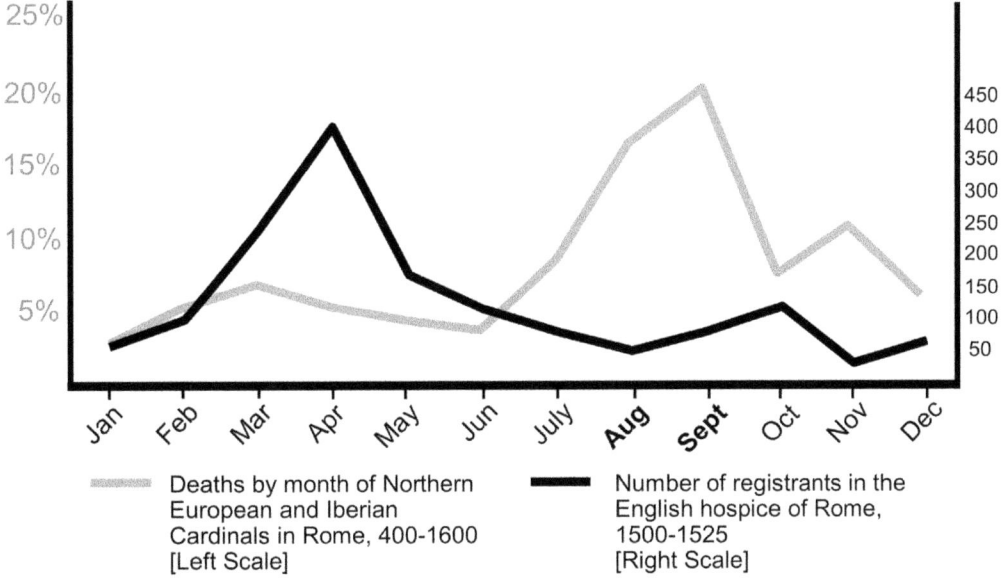

English Hospice Registration 1500–1525 and Seasonal Mortality Risk in Rome. Benjamin James Reilly, "Cardinal Numbers: Changing Patterns of Malaria and Mortality in Rome, 494–1850," *Journal of Interdisciplinary History*, Vol. 49, no. 3 (2019), p. 415, © The Massachusetts Institute of Technology and The Journal of Interdisciplinary History, Inc.; and George B. Parks, *The English Traveler to Italy* (Stanford, CA: Stanford University Press, 1954), pp. 370–371.

the Easter Holy Week, which typically falls between late March and mid–April. However, it is clear that climate also played an important role in determining English travel patterns. To illustrate this fact, I overlaid the hospice registrant numbers provided by Parks with data drawn from my own 2019 study on northern European and Iberian cardinals' death rates, 400–1600. As the resulting composite diagram indicates, the presence of pilgrims in Rome, much like the presence of imperial armies in the vicinity of the city, was strongly inversely correlated with malaria risk. The most popular months for pilgrimage, March to May, are also amongst the healthiest months for northern European visitors to Rome, while the summer ebb in visitors corresponds nicely with the worst of the malaria season. Undoubtedly, some pilgrims to Rome succumbed to malaria, but based on Park's data, it appears that English pilgrims were cognizant of the malaria risk and timed their travels accordingly.

While some pilgrims no doubt suffered from Rome's malarial fevers, the ability of pilgrims to time their travels to the healthier season in Rome probably kept their malarial death toll to a minimum. However, the same could not be said for a second group of travelers to Rome of the time period, the numerous litigants that were drawn to the papal court during and after the era of the reform popes. It is to such travelers we now turn.

11

Fullness of Power

In the early 13th century, the roof of Evesham monastery in Worcestershire sprung a leak that would eventually trickle all the way to Rome. The abbot of this poorly-maintained monastery, Roger, was no monk but rather a courtier who had been granted Evesham for services rendered to the English king. Roger "loved feasting," was "boastful at the table," and showed little respect for his monkish subordinates, calling them his "vassals" or "puppies."[1] What is more, in the tradition of Christian of Mainz, Roger was accused of keeping "concubines in his chamber from morning to night." Due to Roger's systematic mismanagement and embezzlement of monastic funds, the roof and walls of the monastery were in a dire state of disrepair and the monks were going unclothed and unfed. Upon hearing of these problems, the local bishop of Worcester decided to visit the monastery to allow the monks to lodge a formal complaint against their abbot.

At this point the story of Evesham takes an unexpected turn. Although Roger was by all accounts a terrible abbot, Evesham's monks decided that allowing the bishop of Worcester to investigate the matter would only make matters worse by setting a precedent for future local interference into Evesham's internal affairs. Citing Evesham's charter, which put it under papal protection, the monks refused to open their monastery to the bishop. The miffed bishop responded by excommunicating the monks, prompting an immediate appeal to the Archbishop of Canterbury, who ordered a panel of local judge delegates to look into the matter. However, the bishop of Worcester feared this panel would find against him so he countered with an appeal directly to the papal court. Both sides of the dispute were now bound to present their case in person before the pope and his cardinals in Rome.

Evesham first sent a monk called Ermefred, "a man of good sense, well educated and a very good notary" to present their case in Rome. After making his initial arguments before the papal court, however, Ermefred died unexpectedly.[2] As his replacement the Evesham monks selected Thomas of Marlborough, who, because of his university studies in Paris and Oxford, understood the workings of the ecclesiastical courts better than most of his brothers. Upon arriving in Rome, Thomas gifted the pope a cup of fine silver, just the first of many presents that both sides of the case would lavish upon papal officials. Roger himself soon arrived to distribute far more generous largess, and presumably the lawyers for the bishop of Worcester did the same. The case then bogged down, and as the litigation dragged on into summer, Thomas left Rome for the healthier air of Bologna to the north where he studied law to aid his case. Upon his return to the papal court in the October of 1205, Thomas drew upon these Bologna connections to hire all the best lawyers in Rome. Outgunned in the courtroom, the Worcester contingent complained to the pope about inadequate legal representation. However, their complaint was dismissed by the pontiff, who joked that one thing Rome was never short of was lawyers.

After formally presenting his arguments and bestowing his bribes, there was nothing left for Thomas but to wait for a final judgment, so he spent his time appealing to a still higher authority through prayers, fasting, charity, and visits to Rome's holiest shrines. Finally, in December of 1205, the papal court ruled in favor of Thomas and the Evesham monastery. In large part, this verdict was a tribute to the guile and cunning of Nicholas of Warwick, a notorious English forger who had most likely fabricated the Evesham monastery's bogus papal charter 80 years before. However, this court decision was also testimony to Thomas' skills as a lawyer, not to mention his perseverance; in all, Thomas spent over a year and a half in Italy pursuing the case.[3]

The same could not be said of his courtroom rivals, the representatives of the bishop of Worcester. "Frightened by the unhealthiness of Rome" and mindful of the fate of Ermefred and many other transalpine visitors in the *caput mundi*, the men of the bishop's contingent "did not pursue their case against Evesham vigorously."[4] Evidently, the bishop was willing to gamble their money on bribes to the Roman court, but was less willing to gamble the lives of his subordinates to the threat of Roman Fever.

"Constant Diligence" and the Papal Court

What gave the papacy jurisdiction over such a minor matter in distant England, nearly 1600 kilometers as the crow flies from Rome? In general terms, the papacy based its claims of ecclesiastical superiority on the so-called Donation of Constantine, a forged document that granted the popes vaguely-defined sovereign rights over "Rome and Italy and all of the regions of the West."[5] More specifically, the popes relied on the Pseudo-Isidorian Decretals, a compilation of genuine and fraudulent documents cobbled together in the 9th century by a team of Frankish ecclesiastical officials who invented a tradition of papal authority over the Frankish church as a means to wriggle free from the control of their immediate ecclesiastic superiors.[6] By 11th century, however, the papacy had begun to turn the Pseudo-Isidorian Decretals against their original creators, using the Decretals to support the pope's claim to be "judge of the whole church" with authority even over local ecclesiastical affairs.[7]

Supporters of the supremacy of the papacy further bolstered their arguments with quotations from the *Dictatus Papae*, a document promulgated by Gregory VII in the midst of the investiture controversy. Drawing upon the Pseudo-Isidorian Decretals and other sources, Gregory laid out a bold vision of papal supremacy in the west. The pope, according to the *Dictatus Papae*, was a living saint, universal and "Catholic" in his authority, and entitled to the imperial insignia. Princes should kiss his feet, and no one may judge a pope. To the pope alone belongs the right to depose or reinstate bishops and even to enthrone or dismiss emperors. What is more, "the most important cases of every church" should be submitted to papal authority for adjudication, since "the Roman Church has never erred, nor ever, by the witness of Scripture, shall err to all eternity."[8] At the time they were written in 1075, these words must have seemed like an empty boast. Two years later, however, after Gregory VII had humiliated Henry IV in the snow of Canossa, the *Dictatus Papae* seemed less like an abstract theory and more like a statement of fact.

In the two centuries that followed, the papacy increasingly asserted the right to oversee ecclesiastical matters throughout Europe, however minor or inconsequential. From the standpoint of Rome these renewed and heightened ties between Rome and local parishes were an unmitigated benefit for all Europe. Pope Adrian IV, who reigned 1154–1159, likened the papacy to a "diligent mother" who "provides for the individual churches with constant vigilance: all must have recourse to her, as to their head and origin, to be defended by her authority, to be nourished by her breasts and freed of their oppressions."[9] Constant vigilance over church affairs allowed the reform papacy to fight injustice, cleanse the church of corruption, and protect clerics from lay interference.

As a result of strong papal encouragement, the number of appeals to Rome skyrocketed over the course of the 1100s. By mid-century, Rome was inundated with court cases, in large part because litigants increasingly bypassed the lower courts and took their cases directly to the papal curia.[10] During the High Middle Ages, the papacy tried to establish itself not only as an appeals court, but as the "omnipotent court of first instance for the whole of Christendom," at least for cases that touched on ecclesiastical matters.[11] According to R.W. Southern, in the mid–12th century "papal jurisdiction emerged as a perceptible fact in everyday European life," penetrating even "the lowest strata of the ecclesiastical structure as a matter of ordinary routine.... Business rushed upon them; they had only to invent the rules and reach the decisions."[12] By the time of Celestine III (1191–1198), appeals to Rome swelled still further largely because of Celestine's stated belief that "anyone who felt that he was threatened by others could and should seek justice in Rome."[13] Not surprisingly, many popes of the period were trained not as theologians but as lawyers.

During this litigious time even laymen pled their cases before the pontiff and his cardinals, especially on matters where religious and secular concerns overlapped. Certain crimes, such as striking a cleric, could only be forgiven by the pope, forcing accused laymen to come to Rome to adjudicate their cases.[14] What is more, despite the settlement of the investiture dispute, lay and ecclesiastical authorities continued to squabble over real estate, in part because many monasteries were still quasi-controlled by the royal or aristocratic families which had founded them. In addition, since marriage was a spiritual institution many laymen came to Rome to be absolved of the stain of bastardy or else to dissolve their marriages, usually on specious grounds of consanguinity. One such appellant was the Norman Count Hugh of Molise who brought lavish gifts to the papal court in 1050 in hopes of obtaining a divorce from his barren wife. He was treated instead to an impassioned defense of marriage from the somewhat simple-minded Eugenius III, who, overcome with emotion, "prostrated himself before the count so utterly that his miter, slipping from his head and rolling in the dust, was found after the bishops and the cardinals had raised him [from] under the feet of the dumb-founded count."[15] Needless to say, Hugh failed in his quest for divorce, but he would not be the last heir-minded European ruler to petition the pope to for permission to break an unwanted bond of matrimony.

Hugh's marital problems notwithstanding, most litigation before the papal court centered around ecclesiastical issues, including contested episcopal elections, jurisdictional squabbles, and simple property matters. Not content to wait for cases to come to Rome, the papacy also exercised its growing judicial power within the church by sending judge-legates north of the Alps. In some cases, however, these legates from Rome had the paradoxical effect of drumming up more business for Rome itself. Case in point was the disastrous visit of two papal delegates to Germany in 1150, one of whom was Octavian of St. Cecilia, the same cardinal who in the reign of Barbarossa would rip the papal robes out of his rival's hands during the contested 1159 conclave. These cardinals came at the invitation of King Conrad, who wanted them to settle a number of ongoing disputes. Once in Germany, however, the two men ignored established law and brazenly traded bribes for favorable rulings. This would have been less of a problem if Rome had sent only one legate, but the papacy sent two, and as a result for every court case "one [litigant] would approach one legate, the other the other; and whoever was acquitted by one was condemned by the other in contradiction." Germany's coffers were emptied, but nothing was definitively settled, so "in consequence swarms of appellants flew off to the papacy" like bees from an angry hive.[16]

The papacy used other tools to tighten its control over the church as well. From the year 1053 onwards, all archbishops were required to come to Rome to receive their symbol of the office—the pallium—and to promise fidelity to the pope.[17] Even after being installed in their offices, archbishops were expected to visit Rome every few years, though the frequency depended on how close their diocese was to the Eternal City. The archbishops of Canterbury and Rome as well as the abbot of the monastery of St. Augustine in Canterbury were expected to visit Rome once every three years; French and German archbishops were presumably expected to visit Rome still more frequently. By the 12th century, these enforced visitations on Rome were required from the growing number of bishops, abbots, and other prelates who were appointed directly by the papacy. The stated goal of these trips was to establish personal ties between the popes and their ecclesiastical underlings, though there was a financial element as well: each of these visiting ecclesiastics were expected to make generous payments to the papal court.[18]

The papacy also flexed its muscle over ecclesiastical affairs by calling church councils, many of which took place in Rome. The first of these was the Lateran Council of 1123, convoked to ratify the compromise over investiture reached between the papacy and the German Empire at Worms in 1122. All told, the First Lateran was attended by 300 bishops and more than 600 abbots, each accompanied by a large retinue of clerical and lay followers. Three more Lateran councils followed over the course of the next century and the Fourth Lateran was the largest of all, attracting 71 patriarchs and archbishops, 412 bishops, and 900 heads of monastic orders, as well as the representatives of several European monarchies. The majority of the participants in these councils were undoubtedly Italian—not surprising, given both the location of the council and the structure of the Western Church—but delegates from beyond the Alps came in substantial numbers as well. The Fourth Lateran, for example, attracted 11 English and Welsh bishops along with 13 monastic leaders, plus a number of individual monks and church lawyers[19]; 17 Irish ecclesiastics attended as well, along with four from Scotland.[20] Since each of these delegates would have come with a retinue of servants and scribes, the contingent to the Fourth Lateran from Britain alone probably was upwards of 300–400 people. If the delegations from France, Germany, and other parts of the Northern European world were added in, the total would be far higher.

The Scope of Papal Jurisprudence

These various initiatives on the part of the papacy drew large numbers of transalpine Europeans to Rome. It would strain both the page count of this book and the patience of the reader to try to summarize all such contacts for a 200-year period. I will focus instead on data from a single source, the relations between England and Rome in the age of Innocent III (1198–1216), which are the subject of a magnificent 1976 book by historian Christopher Cheney.

During the reign of Innocent, Cheney tells us, a "steady trickle" of English laymen arrived in the Eternal City. In addition to pilgrims, Rome received a number of secular English criminals whose crimes—attacking a clerk, forging a papal letter, and arson—could only be adjudicated by the pope. Still other laymen came as royal agents, first to represent royal interests in court cases that interested the crown, and later to try to convince the papacy to lift the spiritual sanctions that the papacy had placed on England due to King John's continued insistence on interfering with ecclesiastical elections within his domain. Another wave of royal agents streamed to the papacy in 1212 when John caved in to papal pressure and agreed to become a vassal of the pope, and then again in 1215, when John sought papal support against his own barons following the signing of the Magna Carta.

The majority of the English litigants during Innocent's papacy, however, were men of the cloth, bishops, monks, and the like, who filled the courts of Rome with "mundane and often trivial bickering over ecclesiastical property."[21] According to Cheney, the number of such legal cases "increased enormously in number in the last third of the twelfth century" and in the pontificate of Innocent alone "about 270 lawsuits are recorded." For Cheney, however, these cases were just the tip of the iceberg, since he suspected that about two-thirds of the documents of the era have been lost over time. The real number of cases, he guessed, "may have amounted to 800."[22] This number represents appeals from a single European country during the pontificate of a single pope; the number of cases adjudicated by the papacy over the entire Middle Ages was certainly far higher.

In Cheney's survey of the surviving court records, a few major themes predominate. Cheney noted relatively few cases in which ambitious clerics went to Rome seeking papal help in getting appointments to ecclesiastical office, a practice that was far more common amongst the contemporary French.[23] Rather, the typical English case argued in Rome concerned elections to episcopal or monastic office and most commonly pitted the principle of *libertas ecclesastica*, or free election to office, against the English king's customary prerogative to make his own ecclesiastical appointments.[24] Other legal proceedings revolved around the prohibition against holding ecclesiastical office by bastards, including a certain Morgan, illegitimate son of English King Henry II. Still other cases, including the Evesham affair cited above, involved monks, who in Cheney's judgment were particularly likely to appeal to Rome rather than seek justice in local courts.[25] These monastic cases often contested the jurisdiction of bishops over the affairs of monasteries within their dioceses but could touch on other matters as well, such as the rights of noble patrons of monasteries to appoint abbots, or clashes between a monastic mother-house and a local chapter. A few more cases involved individual monastics, including two prodigal monks who pled to the pope to be let back into their old orders and one nun who claimed to have been placed in a convent by her wicked stepmother without her consent, to deprive her of her inheritance.[26] In the high Middle Ages, then, whether you were a monk, a nun, a murderer, a royal agent, or even the bastard son of a king, all roads led to Rome.

Popes and Parasites: Malaria and the Papal Court

Were these delegates, appellants, new ecclesiastical appointees, and lay defendants before the papal court putting themselves at risk from Roman Fever? Not necessarily. Many litigants followed the example of Thomas of Marlborough and timed their residence in Rome with the "summer heats" in mind.[27] What is more, going to the papacy did not always mean going to Rome. During the 12th century, the papacy was repeatedly forced to flee to Viterbo, Anagni, or some other nearby central Italian town after being ousted from Rome by ambitious aristocrats or by the commune movement, a middle-class coalition that sought to revive republican governance over Rome. Largely as a result of such political pressures, the papacy spent

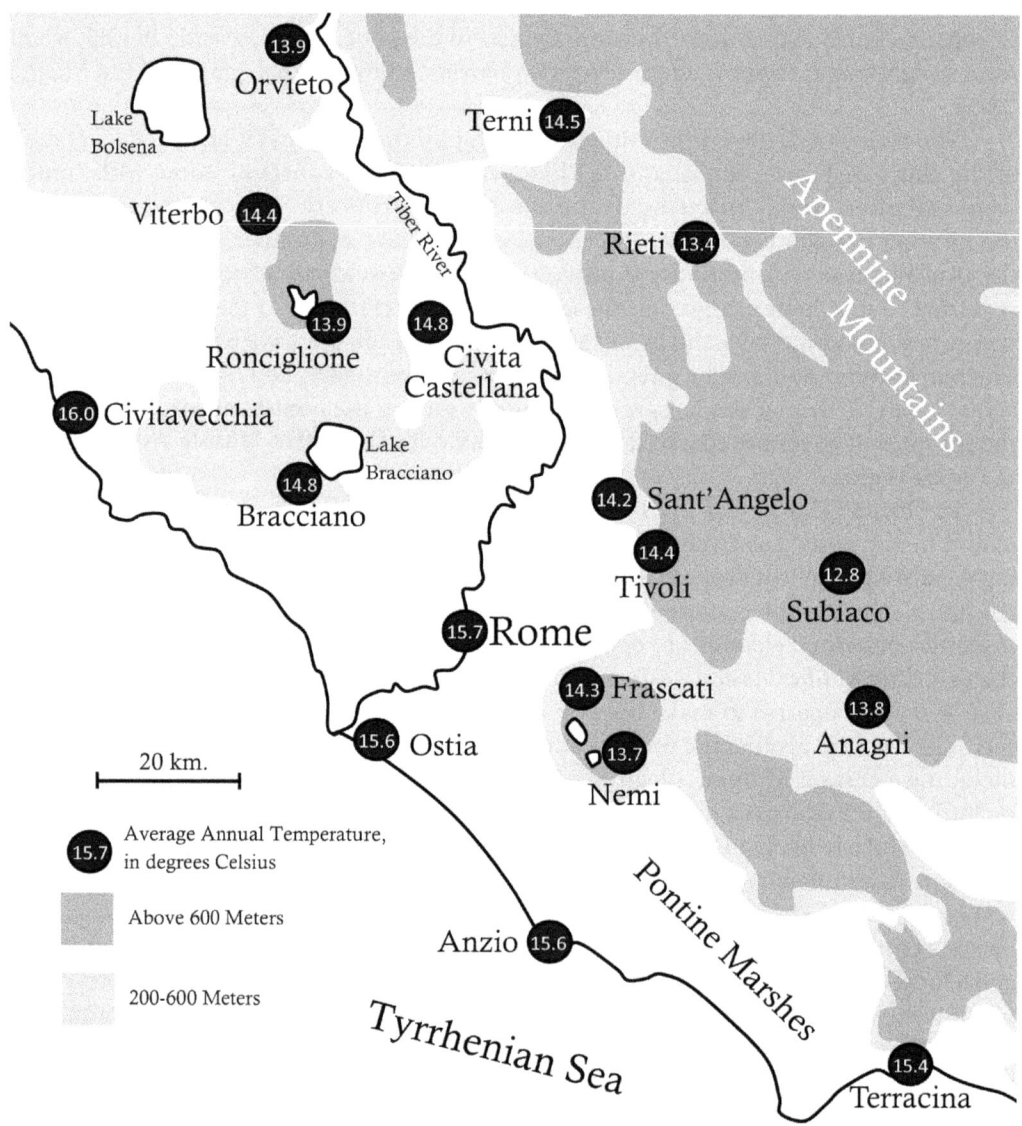

Average Annual Temperature, Rome and Environs.

approximately 122 years outside the city between 1100 and 1304 and only 82 years in Rome itself.[28]

In other cases, popes and cardinals absented Rome voluntarily as part of their own malaria avoidance mechanism, the *villeggiatura*, the practice of taking country holidays during the heats of the summer. When going into *villeggiatura*, Rome's clerical elite vacated Rome but didn't necessarily go very far. From the standpoint of topography, Rome's Lazio province is extremely varied, ranging from hot coastal plains, volcanic hills topped by caldera lakes, the sloping fields and low ridges of the Roman *campagna*, and finally the foothills of the Apennines, which rise so steeply above the surrounding Tiber Valley that modern-day paragliders can leap into the sky directly from their slopes.

As a consequence, even a small journey in Lazio province can lead to dramatic temperature changes. In one of my own *villeggiaturas* into the Alban Hills, I remember that the temperature had already reached 29°C in the lowlands near Rome by about 11 a.m., but by the time I reached the old papal palace at Castel Gandolfo on the lip of a caldera lake a half-hour later, the temperature had dropped to 25°C. In the early afternoon, my car's thermometer bottomed out at 22°C at Rocca di Papa, a town high in the Alban Hills that earned its name by being a *villeggiatura* retreat for Eugenius III, the same pope who had wept inconsolably at the feet of the divorce-seeking Hugh of Molise. So great was the temperature differential between Rocca di Papa and Rome that, in the age before air conditioning, snow was collected from northern slopes of the Alban Hills during the winter and stored near Rocca di Papa in wells and ice caves so that it could be sold to overheated Romans during the torrid summer months.[29]

The *villeggiatura* tradition of Rome dates back to pre-imperial times, when elite Romans routinely abandoned the *caput mundi* in the hot months in favor of "the more pure air in the vicinity of Mount Albani, Tusculum and Tivoli."[30] Nonetheless, the first known papal *villeggiatura* dates to 1079, the year that Gregory VII and his cardinals "left the heat of the City to travel to the cooler banks of the river Liri at Ceprano [in the Apennine mountains], there to live under canvas."[31] As for Innocent III, he preferred to camp out in the breezy foothills town of Subiaco along the banks of the Aniene River, known today as a destination for whitewater rafters. Other favored *villeggiatura* retreats included Frascati in the Alban hills, Anagni, and Viterbo, another location favored by Innocent III. When William, the abbot of Andres, visited Viterbo to petition Innocent in 1207, he "found Rome there." So many Romans had followed the pope on *villeggiatura*, William reports, that Viterbo's population swelled to several times its normal size and the abbot had trouble finding somewhere to stay.[32] Since the malaria risk in these windy and cooler hilltop towns was considerably less than in Rome or its surrounding *campagna*, litigants to the papal court may have enjoyed some protection against the region's resident malaria even if their cases dragged on into summer.

Despite this, we do know of a few cases in which appellants to the papal court succumbed to Roman Fever. In 1186, prior Honorius of St. Augustine's monastery in Canterbury appealed to Rome against the exactions of the Canterbury archbishop, who was "making free with monastic property." Taking a party of monks with him, Honorius entered Italy in early 1187, initially staying in Verona, where the papacy was then residing due to an ongoing conflict with the Roman commune and the German emperor. The monks received an initial decision on their behalf in Verona, but the Archbishop of Canterbury refused to honor it, leading to another round of litigation.

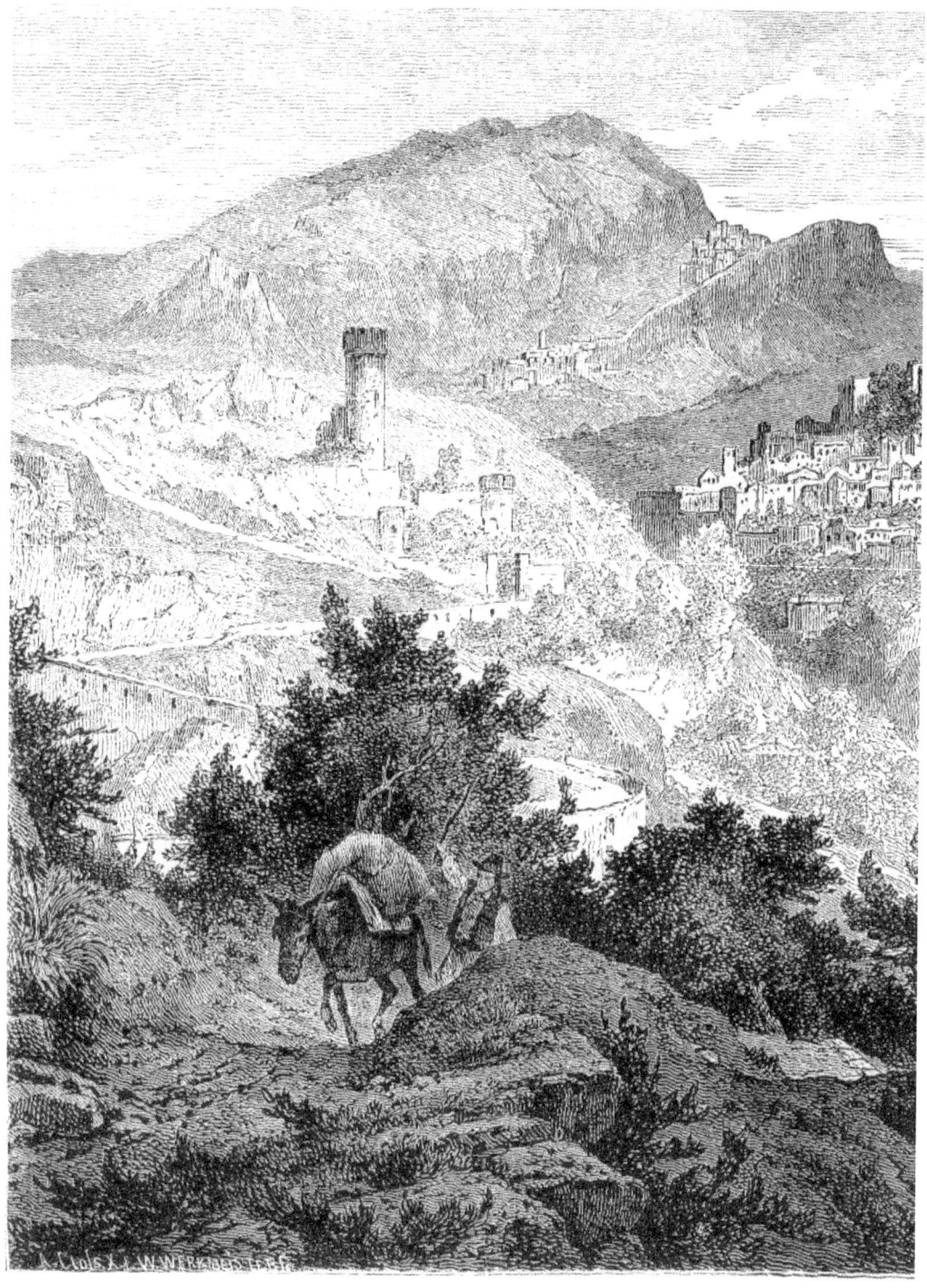

A late 19th-century engraving showing a somewhat idealized view of Subiaco, focusing on the fortified abbey of the hillside town. Jules Gourdault, *Rome et la Campagne Romaine* (Paris: Hachette, 1885), p. 243.

By December 1187, both the papacy and the legal proceedings moved to Rome. Finally, in summer of 1188, the papacy decided in favor of the monastery and resolved to send a legate back to England with Canterbury's monks to enforce the papal decision.

Before this deputation could set out, however, disaster struck. In July, a "horrid pestilence from the heat of the summer" settled over Rome, killing "foreigners especially and some thousands of clerks." As for the Canterbury monks, they were so badly afflicted that "none could even serve cold water to the others." Some died quickly, but Honorius lingered on, and was moved in late summer to the "hills of Velletri [in the Alban Hills] to breathe more freely in that air" in hopes of improving his health. But the cure proved inefficacious: Honorius died on October 21 from "the corrupt air" that had "already taken hold of his vitals." When Brother John of Canterbury arrived in Rome to take the place of the dead monks, he found only a few survivors, including one monk he described as "thin and weak and rather dead than alive, so that one might say he lacked only a tomb."[33] John himself lived to accompany a papal legate back to Canterbury, and the monastery's case ultimately prevailed, though the human and financial and human cost of Canterbury's appeal to Rome had been heavy. Nor was this a one-off event: other clerical missions to Rome suffered the ravages of Rome's malaria parasites as well. When a party of monks from Sempringham Priory in Lincolnshire returned home alive after litigating in Rome in the summer of 1201, it was "accounted a miracle."[34]

The parasitism most resented by appellants to Rome, however, was that of the papal court itself. Papal oversight came with a hefty price tag. Burchard, the chronicler of Ursperg, lamented that

> There remains hardly any bishoprick or ecclesiastical dignity, or even a parochial church, which is not made subject of litigation and its cause carried to Rome: but not with empty hands. Rejoice, Rome, our mother, because cataracts of treasures are opened in the land so that brooks and piles of money flow to you in great abundance.[35]

Other authors made the same complaint more succinctly. William of Malmesbury complained that the Romans were "the most fickle of men, bartering justice for gold and selling the rule of the canons for a price." Similarly, Peter of Blois, a French cleric in English royal service, noted ruefully that royal officials typically returned from Rome "relieved of silver [and] loaded with lead."[36]

Some of these critiques were probably born in the sour grapes of failed litigation, but by the mid–12th century even some high church officials were becoming unhappy with Rome's growing role as Europe's supreme ecclesiastical court. The most articulate such voice was that of Bernard of Clairvaux, an intellectual lion of his age and the mentor and confidant of Pope Eugenius III. In his letters to the latter, Bernard acknowledged that popes held a fullness of power over all the churches of the world but cautioned Eugenius that this spiritual coin was being debased rather than augmented by the constant flow of appellants to the papal court. After all, the pope was the heir of Jesus, who did not claim to be a judge of man but who was himself put on trial. Why then did the popes seek to preside over the complaints of "men full of ambition," "sacrilegious keepers of concubines," and other "human monsters," whose avaricious demands threatened to transform the pontiff into the "slave of men in their acquisition of filthy lucre?"[37] "How long," Bernard demanded of his former pupil,

... before your consideration awakes to this gigantic confusing and abusing of appeals? They are contrary to laws human and divine, contrary to custom and established order ... these frivolous, and in most cases, useless [appeals]... are themselves a terror, and that to good men. The antidote is turned to poison.[38]

In the end, Saint Bernard's plea went unheeded. Over the next several centuries the poison would spread, transforming the papacy into ever-more secular institution. The eventual result of this process, as we will see in subsequent chapters, was a dramatic alteration of the relationship between Rome and Europe. While some parts of Europe would become even more closely tied to Rome in coming centuries, many areas in the north would escape the orbit of the papacy—and with it, the deadly spell of *P. falciparum* malaria.

12

From Scandal to Sack

By the start of the 14th century, the prestige and power of the popes seemed to be approaching its peak. With the extermination of the Hohenstaufens, the establishment of the papal court as the *de facto* high court of Europe, and success of the 1300 Jubilee year, the pope of Rome could justifiably claim to have replaced the German emperor as the natural head of Christendom. However, a yawning chasm was about to open beneath the papacy—and the resulting crisis would lead to important and lasting changes in the relationship between Rome, European visitors, and malaria.

The pope was Boniface VIII of Anagni, a worldly cleric from high aristocratic stock and the grand-nephew of another pope. Not surprisingly, the high-born Boniface had a rather lofty conception of papal powers. When delegates of the newly-elected German King Albert descended on Rome in 1298 to seek papal recognition of his election, Boniface haughtily informed the German envoys from atop his throne that "I, *I* am the Emperor."[1] This was par for the course for Boniface, who during his rule treated foreign princes and kings not just as subjects but as menials.[2] In Boniface's mind, the pope was the natural sovereign of Europe and Rome was its rightful spiritual and temporal capital.

The agent of Boniface's undoing was Philip the Fair, King of France, who had run afoul of the pope by collecting a special tax on the French clergy in 1296 to pay for the ongoing Hundred Years' War between France and England. Anxious to humble the French sovereign, Boniface took advantage of the imprisonment of a papal legate in France in 1301 to demand the legate's immediate release in imperious terms. What is more, he summoned an ecclesiastical council in Rome that rubber-stamped his *Unam Sanctam* decree, which declared that both spiritual and temporal power were under the pope's jurisdiction and that no one could be saved unless they subjected themselves to papal authority. The lesson was clear: if Philip continued to resist papal decrees, he was jeopardizing both his kingship and his soul.

In response, Philip appealed to a growing sense of nationalism in France by summoning the French estates-general, a traditional body made up of noble, commoner, and clerical delegations. In an affront to the pope, all three estates—even the church contingent—declared loyalty to Philip during their 1303 meeting at the Louvre palace in Paris. Worse yet, Boniface was accused at the estates-general of multiple crimes including "heresy, tyranny, unchastity, intercourse with the devil."[3]

Furious now, Boniface issued a blanket excommunication against the French government and demanded that Philip appear before the papal court to explain his behavior. But the ground was crumbling beneath Boniface's feet. In early September of 1303, French troops allied with Boniface's main Italian rivals, the Colonna family, surprised Boniface during his *villeggiatura* at Anagni and demanded his immediate resignation.

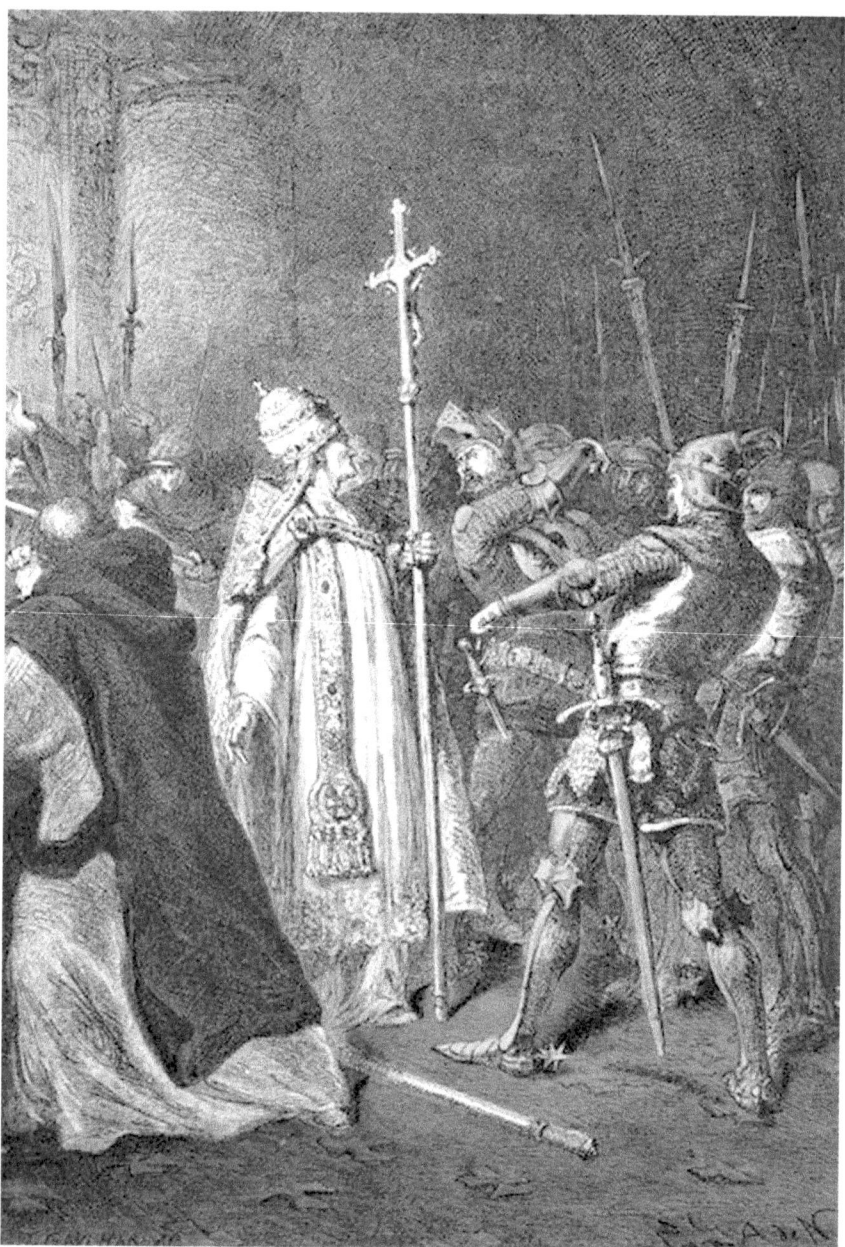

The "Anagni Slap." Pope Boniface VIII, surrounded by French troops and Colonna family forces, is struck full in the face by Sciarra Colonna during the height of the papal conflict with Philip IV, the French king. Picture Art Collection/Alamy Stock Photo.

When this was refused, one of the Colonnas slapped the heir to Peter full in the face. French troops then took the pope into custody, keeping him prisoner for three days. By the time the populace of Anagni roused themselves to rescue their native son from French and Colonna captivity, something had broken in the old man. According to Florentine Chronicler Giovanni Villani, upon being freed the pope "did not … rejoice in any wise" but rather seemed to suffer "a strange malady so that he gnawed at himself as if he were mad."[4] Humiliated, and reduced to a "phantom who no one feared," Boniface "shut himself up in his room, refused food, and beat his head in frenzy against the wall."[5] Finally, on October 11, the pope died from a violent fever. While it is possible that the fever was related to Boniface's injuries at Anagni, it may be that that Boniface was suffering from *P. falciparum*: after all, Boniface's three-day flight through the *campagna* from Anagni to Rome took place during the tail end of the summer malaria season.

Even if Boniface had not succumbed to fever and madness, it is doubtful that he could have done much to resist Philip in 1303. Boniface's arrogance had already alienated him from the would-be German emperor, not to mention Italy's leading aristocratic houses. What is more, little help could be expected from the Angevins, the French dynasty that the popes had invited to become kings of Naples in order to counter the Hohenstaufens. While Roger of Naples, Charles of Anjou's grandson, did not actively participate in the joint French-Colonna plot, he could hardly be expected to take up arms to defend the pope against his distant French relations. What is more, Boniface faced a potential enemy within: despite recent attempts by Boniface to stack the papal curia with Italians, a substantial number of his cardinals were French or pro–French in their sympathies due to recent pressure from the powerful Angevins. As Gregorovius quips, Boniface had so little support that his papacy "stood, so to say, in the air."[6] Small wonder then that the papacy was sucked into the wake of the increasingly powerful French state after Boniface's death.

The Avignon Papacy

Boniface's downfall was a disaster for the papacy, but worse was to come. For the French, Boniface's death was not the end of the matter—Philip insisted on exhuming the dead pope and placing him on trial.[7] In response, the council of cardinals opted to elevate Raymond Bertrand de Got to the papal chair as Clement V. This was an attempt to pour oil on troubled waters; as Bishop of Bordeaux de Got already enjoyed a good working relationship with the French king, so the cardinals probably believed de Got was their best bet to convince Philip to drop his outrageous demands. However, the papacy eventually paid a high price for peace with the French. Rather than return to Rome, the papacy under Clement only got as far as Avignon, a town belonging to the Angevin dynasty in modern south France. And there it stayed. To the dismay of many Christians, the "Bishop of Rome" was now a Frenchman and a former confidant of the French king, holding court nearly 700 kilometers from his pastoral flock in the Eternal City and from the sacred grave of Saint Peter.

The papacy's stay in Avignon was supposed to be temporary, but as the years passed the popes made themselves at home in an expansive fortress-like palace on the banks of the River Rhône from which they ruled the Western Church in a style more becoming of royalty than men of God. Under the guidance of these popes, Avignon developed into a substantial settlement whose imposing city walls enclosed "fine palaces and mansions built for cardinals and ambassadors, the bankers and merchants, [and] the architects, painters and craftsmen who came from all over Europe to make their fortunes."[8] Historians would later call the papacy's long stay in Avignon their "Babylonian Captivity," but the truth of the matter was that the French pope and his mostly French cardinals were comfortable in their supposed exile and had little desire to return to the chronic political turmoil of Italy and the *caput mundi*.[9] True, the French kings were able to exert some influence on the nearby Avignon popes. But the papacy had been no less subject to French pressure while in Rome, where (as we shall see below) they were under the eye and influence of the Angevin dynasty. At least in Avignon, the popes were no longer troubled by the endless intrigues of the Roman aristocracy.

What is more, the creature comforts of Avignon could not be denied. John XXII supposedly held a feast so luxurious that it required "nine oxen, fifty-five sheep, eight pigs, four wild boars," over 2000 birds and rabbits, and a "three hundredweight of cheese" to fill the party platters.[10] The poet Petrarch, who served the papal court, conceded that Avignon offered enough wine, soft beds, and good food, and pretty young girls to "try the limits of debauchery." For Petrarch, however, the "feather-cushioned shade" of Avignon was itself a betrayal of the mission of the papacy, which should follow Christ's example of poverty and live "bare to the wind, shoeless among thorns."[11] Petrarch thus advocated that the papacy leave Avignon, that "nest of treachery," and return as soon as possible to Rome, the mother of all nations.[12] Indeed, Petrarch likened the papacy to the bridegroom and Rome to a pining bride counting the days until her husband's return.[13] Neither Rome nor the papacy, in Petrarch's mind, was complete without the other.

In Rome, many shared Petrarch's longing for the papacy's return. While the town of Avignon grew rich from the presence of the popes, Rome was impoverished by their absence—Roman money-lenders, lawyers, innkeepers, grooms, servants, clerks, scribes, and prostitutes all found themselves unemployed. Some transalpine pilgrims still came to Rome, especially during Jubilee years, but the traffic of diplomats and litigants from across the Alps to the papal court dried up entirely during the years of Avignon papacy. What is more, the bleak descriptions of Rome that foreign pilgrims brought back with them probably dissuaded others from following in their footsteps, since by the second half of the 14th century Rome had reached the very nadir of ruin. According to Gregorovious, by the age of Petrarch the wreckage of Christian Rome was scarcely distinguishable from the rubble of the ancient city, since the Lateran was a burned-out husk and Saint Peter's was in dire need of repair. Indeed, "almost all the basilicas and convents were deserted and were scarcely frequented by priests" while "swamps and rubbish took the place of squares and streets, where shattered towers, burnt houses, and ruins of every kind furnished a terrible chronicle of all the wars from which the city had suffered." Malaria alone still prospered within Rome's depopulated shell. Small wonder that contemporary Frenchmen referred to Italy as the "land of the dead."[14]

Angevins, Mercenaries and Malaria

The Avignon popes were also dissuaded from returning to Italy by the continued intrigues of the Angevin dynasty, which they had invited into Italy to provide political support to the papacy but who proved to be a cure worse than the disease. When the Angevins were strong, as they were at the start of the reign of Charles I, they constantly meddled into Roman affairs. During the papacy of Martin IV, a Frenchmen deeply unpopular in Rome, Charles forced the Pope to select four new French cardinals immediately after his elevation to the papal throne; as Michel Grenon put it, the "servant of the servants of god" had become to a mere creature of Charles of Anjou.[15]

The situation for the papacy became even worse after Angevin power began to weaken, since it triggered new cycles of warfare—and renewed exposure of European soldiers from north of the Alps to the resident fevers of Italy. Problems began late in the reign of Charles I, who lost control of Sicily in 1282 to the Sicilian Vespers, a popular anti–French insurrection. Repeated Angevin attempts to re-take the island were unsuccessful, in part because unacclimated French troops were "decimated by the torrid Sicilian summer."[16]

The Angevin political situation in Italy worsened further following the 1343 death of Robert the Wise, grandson of Charles I. Although Robert had enjoyed a long and fairly prosperous reign, he never produced a male heir, so after his death he was succeeded by his politically naïve 17-year-old granddaughter Joanna. She intended to rule Naples in her own right but was forced by her relations to take a young husband, Andrew, a scion of the Hungarian branch of the Angevin family. However, Joanna's followers worried that Andrew's family would snatch the crown from Joanna's own head once Andrew came of age. As a result, they murdered the young king shortly before his planned coronation.

In retaliation, Andrew's brother Louis of Hungary led a large military force into Italy in an attempt to acquire by force what his family had failed to gain by marriage. Landing on the west coast of Italy in the 1347, his Hungarian troops summered in the relative cool of the Apennines near L'Aquila and then seized Naples in the winter of 1348. At that point, his army was decimated by disease, and for once malaria cannot take the blame: Louis's campaign happened to coincide with the start of the Black Death. Joanna fled to France and persuaded the pope to declare her innocent in Andrew's murder in return for surrendering formal control over Avignon to the papacy, which served only to further entrench the popes in their French exile.

Joanna later returned to Naples, but unfortunately for her—and fortunately for south Italy's various malaria species—Joanna's ambitious male relatives refused to let her rule in peace.[17] In the early 1380s, Joanna faced another major threat to her rule in the form of Charles of Durazzo, her first cousin and a potential heir to the Kingdom of Naples. To counter the threat Joanna adopted yet another relative, Louis of Anjou, as her formal heir, but by the time Louis showed up in south Italy with a relief army, Joanna had already been captured and killed in prison, possibly by suffocation between two feather mattresses. As for Louis, he and his troops were cornered in the south Italian city of Bari by Charles' forces. Predictably, by mid-summer, disease began to beset Louis' mostly French army, including Louis himself, who died at the age of 45 in late September. The illness in question may have been an aftershock of the Black Plague—the plague had raged through Rome earlier that year—but given the season and location, not to mention the unacclimated nature of Louis' troops, malarial infection may have played a role as well.[18]

While malaria may have played a supporting role in destroying Louis' army, the real architect of Louis' defeat was John Hawkwood, one of the many British, French, Spanish, Hungarian, and German soldiers-for-hire who mobbed Italy in the 14th century. Indeed, a number of factors conspired to make Italy in the 1300s a golden age for foreign mercenaries in Italy. The Italian peninsula was rich but extremely decentralized, riven into feuding Guelf-Ghibelline factions.[19] In addition, the Avignon papacy relied mainly on mercenaries to keep some degree of control over the distant Papal States, whose tax income helped pay for Avignon's "feather-cushioned shade."[20] What is more, this trade in military men was a buyer's market during this age: the ongoing Hundred Years' War between France and England had created legions of unemployed veterans, many of whom gravitated to Italy whenever that war was halted by a temporary truce. These mercenary companies eventually became so large that they effectively became "moving states" in Italy, selling their steel for gold, extorting tribute from the city-states of Italy even in the midst of conducting their campaigns. One chronicler compared Hawkwood's company to a "moving ant hill" since it stripped clean the countryside as it passed.[21]

Was mercenary work in Italy yet another way that transalpine Europeans were exposed to malaria in the Italian south? The answer is probably yes, though with several caveats. For one thing, many of these expatriate sell-swords came to Italy for a prolonged stay—Hawkwood, for example, had a 30-year military career in Italy—so if they survived their first bouts with malaria they would have enjoyed some acquired resistance. Secondly, these mercenary companies seem to have operated in Italy with malaria in mind. While Hawkwood's White Company hired out its services to various Italian states each year during the cold-weather campaign season, it tended to spend the summer in the healthier upcountry of the Apennines or Tuscany where it confined military operations to raids and extortion of bribes.[22] As for Hawkwood himself, he invested his blood-splattered profits into property in the Apennine foothills district of Romagna, an area famous for its healthy air.[23]

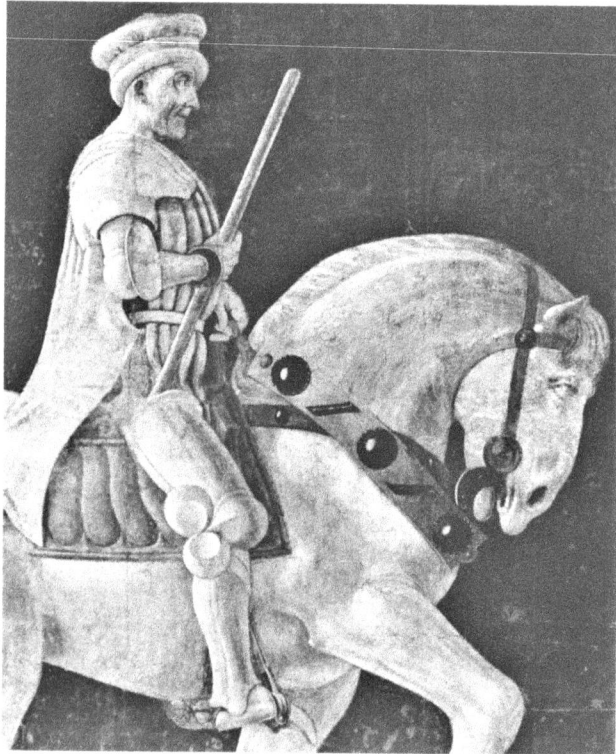

1436 Fresco of John Hawkwood by Paolo Ucello, in the Santa Maria del Fiore Cathedral in Florence. Although Hawkwood took contracts with many different Italian employers, he worked most closely with Florence, where he was buried. Yorck Project (2002), *10.000 Meisterwerke der Malerei*, distributed by DIRECTMEDIA Publishing/Wikimedia Commons.

In 1377, Italy got some rare good news in this century of troubles: the papacy was finally returning to Rome. The popes of Avignon had been under pressure to do so for years but chaos in Rome, war in Italy, and other factors had always conspired to keep the popes on the banks of the Rhône. However, the joyful reunion between bride and bridegroom soon turned into an ugly spat. In the papal election of 1378 the Roman populace, thoroughly sick of distant French popes, surrounded the conclave and chanted "we demand a Roman, or at least an Italian!"[24] Under pressure from the raucous mob, the intimidated cardinals picked an Italian pope, the Naples-born Urban VI. However, the hastily-selected Urban proved to be such a tyrannical and unstable pope that in August of the next year the majority of the cardinals met in the *villeggiatura* town of Anagni to demand his resignation and vote on a replacement.

12. From Scandal to Sack 131

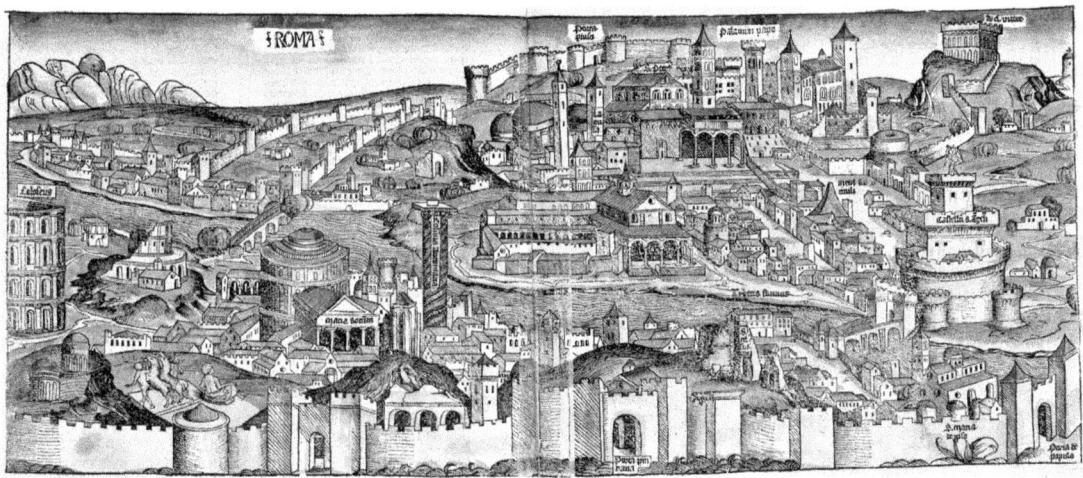

View of Medieval Rome which highlights the main tourist sites. The Colosseum is on the far left, Vatican Hill and its papal complex are in the center distance, and the papal fortress of St. Angelo is in the right foreground. The gate in the bottom right corner is the Porta del Popolo, the site of the Von Harff's malaria-haunted tree. Michael Wolgemut and Wilhelm Pleydenwurff, illustrators, *The Nuremberg Chronicle* (1493), p. 58.

Predictably, Urban refused to yield power to the new pope, so the newly-elected Clement VII was forced to flee with his cardinal partisans back to Avignon. The church was now once again in schism, with two popes, two Colleges of Cardinals, and two seats of the church, Rome and Avignon. Eventually a church council was convened in Constance in 1414 and resolved the matter by dethroning both existing popes and electing a new pontiff. However, neither of the other two popes backed down, so Europe briefly had *three* popes. The Western Schism did not completely end until 1429, when the last of pope of Avignon resigned his office for the sake of Christian unity.

With the return of the papacy to Rome, many Europeans had high hopes that the papacy would now be able to recover some of the power and prestige that it had lost during the Babylonian Captivity and the Schism. Under the first few post–Schism popes, it appeared that this goal might be achievable. A number of these popes were good men, including the Colonna aristocrat Martin V, who found Rome in ruins and thus inaugurated a much-needed program to rebuild the Eternal City. Another pope of the era, Nicholas V, was also a credit to his office. A scholar-pope of rather humble social origins, Nicholas organized the successful 1450 Jubilee, tightened papal control over the often-turbulent Roman civic government, and amassed more than 30,000 books, a collection that would later become the core of the Vatican Library. In addition, Nicholas rebuilt the city's fortifications—although not well enough, as it would turn out—and set about cleaning the streets and repairing the long-defunct Aqua Virgo aqueduct. What is more, in an effort to encourage pilgrimage Nicholas began ambitious restoration projects for Rome's major Basilica churches, including St. Peters. Unlike many of his successors, Nicholas himself lived a fairly frugal life. The only things worth spending money on, Nicholas believed, were books and buildings.[25] If Martin and Nicholas had a fault, it was that they joined with their fellow popes in ignoring the Council of Constance's decree that general councils of the church should continue to take place at regular intervals. As a result, the tradition of periodic church councils which might have served to check papal corruption slowly died on the vine, paving the way for Luther's more existential assault on the Roman Church.

During this era of rebuilding, many of the ties that had once bound Rome to the wider European world were now renewed. This was good news for Rome's impoverished shop-keepers, tavern, owners, and prostitutes; thanks to the dearth of visitors in the Avignon and Schism eras, Rome's population may have dropped as low as 20,000 in the early 1400s. Most of the few Romans who remained were huddled together, not within the ancient Aurelian walls, but inside the Leonine City on Vatican Hill, while Rome proper was virtually abandoned.[26]

Following the return of the papacy to the Eternal City, Rome's population buoyed upwards with the returning tide of travelers, but things were not quite the same as before. Pilgrims continued to arrive in large numbers, but imperial coronation expeditions to Rome petered out. In addition, due to the growth of stronger state governments and increasingly self-governing national churches during the later Middle Ages, Rome received fewer lay and ecclesiastical litigants to the papal court.[27] Furthermore, the weakened papacy of the 15th century was no longer strong enough to compel most non–Italian clergymen to make regular visits to Rome. The Archbishops of Canterbury are case in point. According to Parks, while nearly all the Archbishops of Canterbury from 1066 to 1300 went to Rome or at least Italy, only three did so in the 14th century, and only one in the 15th century.[28] Nevertheless, the overall flow of European visitors to Rome was certainly higher in the mid–1400s than it had been during the dark days of the Avignon papacy—and the potential exposure of such visitors to malaria increased correspondingly.

Papal Corruption in an Age of Foreign Invasion

Almost as soon as it resumed, however, the returning tide of travelers to Rome was imperiled by spiraling corruption at the highest levels of the Roman Church. The rot became noticeable during the reign of Pope Sixtus IV, best known today for commissioning the Vatican chapel that still bears his name. Sixtus was also, in the words of church historian La Due, an "egregious nepotist who made six of his nephews cardinals and bestowed great riches on untold numbers of his relatives."[29] To fund this largess Sixtus created and sold off ecclesiastical posts which despite being empty titles were eagerly snatched up by Rome's status-conscious aristocrats. Sixtus also began the practice of selling indulgences, or remission of sins, a problem that would only grow in the years to come. The sum result of Sixtus's seven-year reign was the "devaluation of the figure of the pope" from the spiritual leader of Christendom to "just another Italian Prince."[30]

The next pope was even worse. Cardinal Rodrigo Borgia was a scandalous figure even before his elevation to the papacy, having fathered no fewer than six illegitimate children. Women were reportedly attracted to the wealthy and charismatic cardinal like "iron to a magnet."[31] Borgia won his election as pope through widespread bribery and then showed his Spanish Valencian roots by celebrating his accession with a bullfight in St. Peter's square. Over the course of the next few years, Alexander VI (as he re-named himself) raised the number of his illegitimate offspring to nine and attempted to seize control over the Romagna province of Italy, the former haunt of Hawkwood, by ordering the murder of his aristocratic opponents and then seizing their property upon their demise. According to the Venetian ambassador in Rome "four or five men" were found assassinated every night, including "bishops, prelates and others, so that Rome trembles for fear of being murdered by the Duke."[32]

The "Duke" in question was Alexander's son Cesare. Although he was given a cardinal's hat at age 18 by his father, Cesare proved just as popular with the ladies as his old man, eventually siring his own brood of bastards. Cesare was also a brilliant tactician, equally at home on the battlefield and on the political stage. Machiavelli, who knew Cesare well, praised him as the very model of a successful commander. Machiavelli's famous dictum—that it is better to be feared than loved—was almost certainly written with Cesare in mind.[33]

Cesare's political skills would soon be tested by a new wave of foreign intervention into the Italian peninsula. By 1495, French throne was occupied by Charles VIII, a "young and licentious hunchback of doubtful sanity" in the words of H.A.L. Fischer. Charles was drawn into Italy by his ambition to rule the Kingdom of Naples, which had fallen into the possession of a Spanish dynasty in 1442 but was now in the feeble hands of a "bastard grandson of a usurper."[34] Charles VIII thought his own claim to Naples was better, since he was a distant relative of Charles of Anjou, so after securing an alliance with Milan he descended into Italy with both a large army and artillery pieces of the latest style. By December of 1442, Charles had entered Rome, where he took a tour of the principal churches. In the meantime his soldiers ran riot in the streets behaving more like "an occupying force" than a friendly army.[35] According to Christopher Hibbert, "houses were occupied; banks attacked; palaces ... were ransacked," especially those belonging to traditionally anti–French aristocratic families of Rome.[36] In desperation, Alexander himself retreated to St. Angelo for protection against the French.

To the relief of the Borgias, Charles VIII eventually continued southwards to Naples, where his thundering artillery secured the surrender of the town with astonishing ease. However, Charles and his generals knew that his cannons were useless against Italy's fevers, so most of the French troops hurried out of Naples by May 20 before the start of the unhealthy summer season. After defeating an army of allied Italian city-states on the way out of Italy, Charles returned to France. Three years later he was dead; bizarrely, he seems to have killed himself accidentally by whanging his head on a door lintel.[37]

Charles returned to France confident that Naples had been won, but the French position there collapsed just a year later when a joint Spanish-Venetian relief arrived to re-take the kingdom. The French prisoners were herded into an internment camp in marshy coastal town of Pozzuoli, where malaria took up the work that war had started. By the time the defeated French were allowed to return home, precious few remained. But fever also killed the heir to the Neapolitan throne, throwing the question of succession into question.[38]

As a result, Charles' 1495 expedition into Italy would prove to be just the first of a half-century of repeated French campaigns into Italy. To a certain degree, the root cause of these wars was Urban IV's fateful decision to invite a French fox, Charles of Anjou, to guard the henhouses of the papacy. Nonetheless, more recent political developments played a triggering role as well. By the start of the 16th century the Habsburgs were not only emperors of Germany but also kings of Spain, a country that was becoming fabulously wealthy due to plundered American gold. As a result, the German emperors were in better shape than ever to assert power in the Italian peninsula. The French, in turn, were fearful of encirclement by Habsburg possessions and thus made a determined effort gain territory in Italy, thereby driving a wedge between Hapsburg Spain and Germany. This required them to control not just Naples but also Milan, which lay at the crossroads of northern Italy and controlled French access to the Italian south.

The stage was thus set for a great power conflict where foreign kings dominated the Italian chessboard and the Italian city-states played the role of pawns. Contemporary Florentine historian Guicciardini lamented how "foreigners fearlessly range through our miserable Italy every day, assaulting cities, taking them with ease, sacking them without mercy and with little cost to themselves, then occupying them in happiness and security as long as it suits them."[39] For many Italians, it must have seemed that the dark ages of the Vandals, Visigoths, and Lombards had returned.

As for Cesare and Alexander Borgia, they survived the French invasion only to fall victim to malaria. The year 1503 was exceedingly hot and humid and fever stalked the streets of Rome. However, rather flee the city on *villeggiatura*, Cesare and Alexandria stayed in the *caput mundi* in order to keep tabs on the ongoing Spanish-French rivalry over Naples. Indeed, the ever-ambitious Alexander was reportedly plotting to get Cesare installed on the Sicilian throne. In early August, however, both Alexander and Cesare fell gravely ill. Rumors immediately spread that father and son had been poisoned at a dinner party they had attended at a cardinal's villa, though Alexander himself blamed Rome's "putrid air" for his affliction. Despite or perhaps because of the exertions of his doctors, who favored "copious bleeding" as a remedy, Alexander succumbed to his fever on August 18.[40] Cesare would recover, but due to his illness he was unable to prevent his mortal enemy, Cardinal Gulliano della Rovere, from rising to power as Pope Julius II, and as a result Cesare was eventually forced into Spanish exile.

Under Julius, the papacy continued even further down the path of being just another Italian regional power. Fearful that the papacy had become the plaything of the great powers, Julius sought to bolster the military potential of the Papal States to the point that it stood on an equal footing with the other main Italian powers, namely Milan, Florence, Venice, and the Kingdom of Naples. To this end, the warrior-pope Julius waged unremitting war on Venice, which he saw as the greatest threat to Rome's standing in Italy. The only real advantage that Julius held over the other Italian despots was his ability to excommunicate his enemies, though by the 16th century the sword of excommunication had become blunted by over-use and no longer filled opponents with anywhere near the dread it had commanded in the age of Henry IV. Julius eventually managed to extend papal territory at Venice's expense by joining forces with the German emperor, though only at the cost of thousands of German, French, Swiss, and Italian lives.

However, Julius is best known today for his building projects. Early in his reign, Julius employed Donato Bramante to replace the dilapidated Church of Saint Peter with a much more grandiose, dome-topped basilica. Julius did not live to see the completion of that project—and neither did any of his immediate successors, since the ambitious project was not finished until the mid–17th century. However, he did survive long enough to see another work that he commissioned, the ceiling that Michelangelo painted for the Sistine Chapel. Julius died soon after the Chapel's completion in 1313, probably from syphilis.

His place was taken by yet another Renaissance prince in papal robes, Leo X, the second son of the Florentine ruler Lorenzo the Magnificent. Although personally pious, Leo shared his predecessors' enthusiasm for unchecked nepotism, high living, and elaborate building projects designed to glorify his rule. Leo's "lavish life style and luxurious court," according to church scholar La Due, "were the talk of the continent."[41] But luxury costs money, and to secure the requisite cash, Leo continued the dubious financial practices of his papal forebears. He created no fewer than 31 new cardinals, each of whom paid handsomely for his red hat, and aggressively marketed indulgences north of the Alps, even to the point of ordering excommunication for anyone who opposed their sale.[42] Despite these income streams the papal treasury was so deeply in arrears at the time of his death in 1521 that the Papal Master of Ceremonies economized on candles during Leo's funeral ceremony, re-using candles left over from another funeral the day before.[43]

Leo was replaced by Hadrian VI, a Dutchman who had served as German Emperor Charles V's chaplain. Hadrian's election opened the doors to possible reform of an increasingly corrupt papal office. However, as with many previous transalpine appointments to the papal office, Hadrian succumbed to illness in Rome in mid–September of 1523. Contemporaries did not credit malaria for his death, but blamed stress, and heat exhaustion, or even poison.[44] However, there is good reason to think that Hadrian's death, like that of previous imperial appointees to the papal office such Clement II and Damasus II, may have been caused or at least hastened by malaria. My own analysis of papal death patterns using data from Wendy Reardon's study on the deaths of popes and antipopes found that more than 40 percent of non–Italian popes died during the peak *P. falciparum* months of July, August, and September, almost two-thirds more than would be expected from a normal distribution of deaths. In contrast, only 25 percent of Italian-born popes perished in the same months, exactly what one would expect if deaths were equally distributed throughout the calendar year. Whether by poison or plasmodia, therefore, transalpine popes seem to have been far more susceptible to death in the Roman summer than their Italian peers.[45]

The Sack of Rome

Poor unacclimated Hadrian was followed in turn by another Medici pope, Clement VII, whose ineptitude led Rome to its greatest disaster since the sack of Robert Guiscard—and yet to another close encounter between Rome's *P. falciparum* malaria and unacclimated foreign troops. In 1521, Emperor Charles V had joined forces with a papal army to chase the French out of Naples. However, German success inspired the formation of an anti-imperial alliance between France and various North Italian states, prompting Clement to break with the emperor in December of 1524 and join what came to be known as the "Italian League." But his timing was terrible. Just two months later, a combined German-Spanish imperial army won a dramatic victory over French and Italian forces in the battle of Pavia: the French army was almost obliterated and French King Francis I was himself captured on the field. The pope's position as now precarious, but rather than bend to the prevailing winds, Clement doubled down and rallied the Italian League against the emperor anew.

In response, the commander of the imperial army in Italy, the Duke of Bourbon, decided to march on Rome. In reality, he had little choice: his large army was in a state of near-mutiny due to unpaid wages so he was glad to have an excuse to point his army towards a city rich in potential plunder. The result was another round of what William McNeill would call epidemic warfare—the imperial army meandered southwards, scoured the countryside for supplies, extorted money from the towns it passed, and in the words of Judith Hook "[left] a trail of burning hamlets behind it."[46] Years of unpaid campaigning had transformed these imperial troops into hard men, "clothed, or rather half-clothed, in rags … desperate, deprived of the necessities of life."[47] Despite the misery of its men the army snowballed in size as it marched southwards, attracting Italian hangers-on with a nose for plunder. This motley force was followed by a second army, that of the Italian League, but the League army made no effort to engage the imperials in combat. Rather, the League's goal seemed to be to channel the imperial force towards Rome and away from the territory of the League members of the Northern Italian plain.

By May 4 the imperial force had reached Monte Mario, where it salivated at the thought of the loot awaiting it the Eternal City below. Heavily outnumbered, Rome's defenders put their hopes on cannons strategically placed on the city walls. Their plans, however, were spoiled by thick fog on May 6 which rendered the cannons almost useless. Rome's resistance crumbled quickly in the face of the imperial assault. As usual, the pope scurried to the safety of St. Angelo, but in the words of contemporary chronicler Luigi Guicciardini, the "rest of the Roman people, as well as the merchants, prelates, courtiers, and foreigners all ran back and forth in great confusion and terror looking for some refuge."[48]

The panic of the Romans proved to be entirely justified. During the short battle on the city's wall the Duke of Bourbon had been killed while leading scaling-parties, and with him died any chance that the rag-tag imperial army could be kept under any semblance of control. Leaderless and undisciplined, the imperial troops "began a terrifying slaughter … killing anyone they encountered." One Spanish solider estimated that the Habsburg army had buried 10,000 slaughtered civilians on the Vatican side of the river alone, while another 2,000 corpses had been unceremoniously tossed into the Tiber.[49]

The bloodbath in the streets of Rome only ended when the imperial troops realized that it was foolish to slaughter people who knew where concealed treasures were hidden and thus switched to a policy of imprisoning and torturing Romans rather than killing them. As a result, the screams of the dying were replaced by the "pitiful cries" of the barely living as rich Romans were vigorously questioned as to the whereabouts of their valuables. Guicciardini recorded that some well-to-do Romans were branded with hot irons, hung by cords over the Tiber, led about with "ropes tied to their testicles," or even "made to eat their own ears, or nose, or testicles roasted."[50] What is more, since it was common practice at the time to throw valuables in the latrine to safeguard them from looting, some high-ranking Romans were forced at knifepoint to "empty with their own hands the sewers and other disgusting places."[51]

Thanks in part to these brutal but effective methods of persuasion, the imperial forces reaped a tremendous harvest of treasure from the Holy City. "In the street," wrote Guicciardini, "you saw nothing but thugs and rogues carrying great bundles of the richest vestments and ecclesiastical ornaments and huge sacks full of all kinds of vessels of gold and silver."[52] Many soldiers who had previously worn nothing but rags were now decked out in "silks and brocades" with "huge gold chains" adorning their breasts, "their arms … covered with bracelets … dressed up like mock popes and cardinals, they went for pleasure rides through Rome on beautiful hackneys and mules" accompanied by their "wives and concubines, proud and richly dressed." In the meantime the cardinals and other high ecclesiastics who had survived the initial slaughter were reduced to "torn and disgraceful" vestments which barely covered the "cuts and bruises all over their bodies from the indiscriminate whippings and beatings that they had received."[53] As for Clement himself, he was forced to melt down all the treasures contained in St. Angelo in an effort to ransom his safety.

Predictably, the imperial army began to fall victim to disease by early summer, though it is not entirely clear what diseases, or diseases, the sources are referring to. Guicciardini blamed the outbreak of illness on the "terrible stench, which was spread through every part of the city," vapors that only became stronger and more poisonous as they were "heated up during the approaching summer."[54] By the start of June, the reek of poorly-buried corpses was so pungent that, according to a contemporary observer of the Sack, "one cannot set foot in the streets, without holding one's nose."[55] However, such statements speak more to the prevailing miasmic theory of disease—the idea that illnesses were caused by "bad air" and foul odors—than to the actual identity of the 1527 outbreak.

Surprisingly, some modern historians have not been able to overcome this

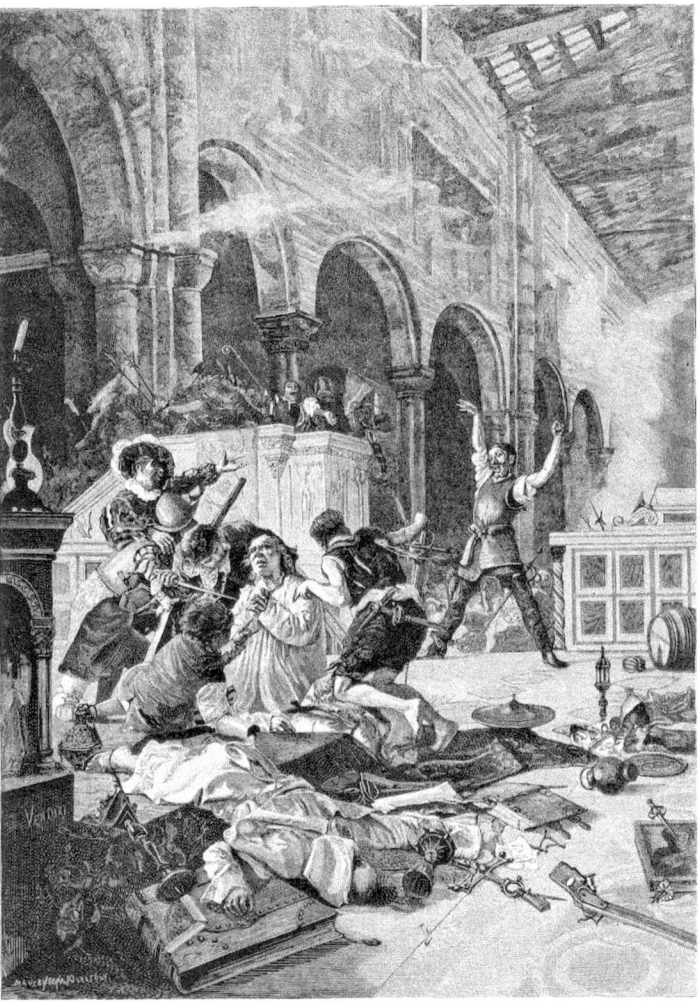

Looting and murder in a Roman church during the Sack, from a wood engraving by Roberto Venturi. Wellcome Library no. 4292li.

antiquated notion of disease. In his otherwise marvelous *Rome: A Biography of a City*, Christopher Hibbert speculated that the disease outbreaks of early June were "aggravated" by the "stench of ordure and of decaying corpses ... wafted by the early summer breeze ... mingl[ed] with the noxious smell of open drains and sewers."[56] Needless to say, this is not how real disease works. Hospital antiseptic is not used to mask odors but to kill germs, the actual cause of most human illnesses.

But what germs? One theory is that Bubonic plague was to blame for the disease outbreak that accompanied the Sack, and indeed the late 1520s coincided with a resurgence of plague in Europe.[57] The nearby city of Florence was ravaged by a continuous epidemic that killed up to fifty people a day from the summer of 1527 to the winter of 1528 so the presence of bubonic plague in Rome is a reasonable supposition.[58] However, malaria should not be discounted. Although some Spanish troops in the imperial army might have had some previous exposure to *P. falciparum* and other malaria strains, the Germans would have been immunologically innocent and highly susceptible to infection.

The imperial army certainly *behaved* as if malaria was the main culprit for the 1527 epidemics. Borrowing a page from the playbook of Hawkwood's White Company, the imperials abandoned Rome almost entirely in early July and spent the summer campaigning against Guelf towns in the hills around Rome, returning only in October after they had exhausted the opportunities for "rape, pillage, and arson" that the vicinity of Rome afforded.[59] In the process they avoided the worst of Rome's August–September malaria season.

The imperial occupation of Rome finally ended in the early months of 1528, when Habsburg troops abandoned Rome for Naples. The League army then turned its own attention to Naples, where it enjoyed some initial success, but as was often the case, the climate of the Italian South proved fatal to the transalpine soldiers that made up the bulk of the force. The French commander of the League army, Viscount de Lautrec, had encamped his men near Baiae, "a neighborhood where causes of endemic fever are never wanting" and his army, originally nearly 30,000 strong, declined to only 4,100 fit troops by mid–August.[60] Making matters worse, Lautrec and his second and command had died and not a single captain was healthy. The French and Italians of the League force were thus compelled to retreat back to Rome where their "sick and dying lay in the streets naked and unfed in their hundreds."[61] Rome's resident malaria parasites no doubt gave them a warm welcome.

In 1529, Clement finally lost his appetite for the Italian League and signed a formal alliance with Charles V. Their rapprochement was cemented in an imperial coronation ceremony at Bologna, where Clement offered Charles both the Iron Crown of Lombardy and the imperial diadem. Charles's coronation marked the end of an era—he would prove to be the last German emperor ever crowned by the pope. Unfortunately for both Rome and the papacy, however, a new era was starting in Europe, set in motion by the furious words of "one little Monk, weak in Strength, but in Temper more harmful than all the Turks, all Saracens, all Infidels anywhere."[62] It is to Martin Luther, and his role in severing a long-standing connection between transalpine Europe and Roman Fever, that we now turn.

13

THE SCARLET WHORE

Although few sources on him acknowledge the fact, it is likely that Martin Luther himself contracted malaria during his one visit to Italy. Luther had been dispatched to Rome—like countless litigious monks before him—to appeal an unfavorable legal decision to higher Roman authorities. After descending the Alps in the middle of 1510, he and a monkish companion crossed the plain of the Po, already simmering in the early summer. Despite the growing heat, locals advised the German travelers to "close hermetically every window, and stop up every chink and cranny" of their rooms at night—a common and highly protective cultural practice against the supposedly "pestilential air" of malaria-prone regions.[1] However, Luther and his travelling companion seem to have ignored the warnings. By the time they got to Pavia, both had fallen ill. Luckily for the young monks, they were still out of the normal range and normal season of *P. falciparum*. If their illnesses were indeed malarial, as seems likely given the context, they would have been the less dangerous "spring fever," malaria of the *P. vivax* or perhaps *P. malariae* variety.

Despite their afflictions, the young monks soldiered on, finally reaching Rome around the time of Saint John's Eve, June 23. Luther was overwhelmed at first by "holy Rome … made holy by the holy blood of martyrs." Like the countless foreign visitors who had preceded him to the Eternal City he and his companion "hastened to view the sacred places, saw all, believed all."[2] However, Luther's Roman sugar-high soon turned sour. Most of the actual Romans he encountered were crass and materialistic, to the point that he would later quip that "Christianity seems totally forgotten in this capitol of the Christian World."[3] When he sought solace in holy mass, he found that Roman priests hurried through the ceremony, delivering the service in an empty and formulaic manner. Luther's greatest disappointment, however, was the pope himself, the military-minded Julius II, who despite being the "father of the faithful" and successor to the Prince of Peace "breathed nothing but blood of ruin."[4]

As for his legal errand, Luther made little headway, since no one in Rome seemed interested in anything other than the ongoing war against the French. Luther therefore abandoned the *caput mundi* in early July—right before the worst of the *P. falciparum* season—and retraced his steps to Germany. But his voyage was not entirely in vain. Luther would later declare that "I would not for a hundred thousand florins have missed seeing Rome…. I should have always felt an uneasy doubt whether I was not, after all, doing injustice to the pope. As it is, I am quite satisfied on the point."[5] Luther's visit with Rome would ultimately leave him with a deep-seated antipathy, not just for the papacy, but for the Eternal City itself—an attitude that would later become a commonplace sentiment amongst his Protestant followers.

Rome, Seat of the Antichrist

The basic outlines of Luther's later rebellion against the Catholic Church are well known. While chairmen of Theology at the newly-founded University of Wittenberg, Luther became increasingly outraged by the papacy's sale of indulgences in Germany to fund Roman building projects. In response, Luther penned his famous Ninety-Five Theses, where he even took a swipe at papal corruption itself, asking "why does not the pope build St. Peter's ... with his own money—since his riches are now more ample than those of Crassus—rather than with the money of poor Christians?" That being said, the tone of Luther's 95 theses was more hopeful than confrontational, persuasive rather than combative. He still believed that the Roman church could be reformed from within.

However, Luther's hopes were misplaced. One year after posting his theses, Luther was put on trial in Augsburg where the papal legate, unable to defend his own pope's positions on the indulgences from a theological standpoint, sought instead to change the narrative and portray Luther as a heretic for his defiance of papal supremacy. Two years afterwards, Pope Leo himself ordered Luther to recant his views on pain of excommunication.

Instead, Luther went on the offensive, excoriating both the papacy and the city of Rome itself. In his *Open Letter to the Christian Nobility* of 1520 Luther attacked "unhappy, hopeless, blasphemous Rome," the "habitation of dragons, specters, and witches," whose court was a "swarm of vermin" and whose head, the pope, luxuriated in a "worldly splendor" entirely unbecoming to his office.[6] "It is horrible and frightful thing," Luther contended, that "the ruler of Christendom ... who claims the title of 'most holy' and 'most spiritual,' is more worldly than the world itself."[7] What is more, Luther complained that the sale of ecclesiastical offices had transformed the Holy City into a marketplace of "buying, selling, bartering, trading, trafficking, lying, deceiving, robbing, stealing, luxury, harlotry, knavery, and every sort of contempt of God." "Even the rule of the Antichrist," Luther contended, "could not be more scandalous."[8] The princes and lords of the Earth, Luther concluded, must rise up and resist the Roman pope, that "scarlet whore of Babylon," before Christendom itself was destroyed.[9]

Luther combined these theological critiques of papal authority with a strong streak of German nationalism. The Roman vampire, Luther charged, having already "sucked dry" Italy with its financial demands, was now turning its sights to greener pastures north of the Alps.[10] Each year the papal court was extracting "more than three hundred thousand gulden" from Germany for which the Germans received nothing in return but "scorn and contempt."[11] In one fascinating passage, Luther comes close to grasping the fact that the human parasitism of the Roman church was working in grim conjunction with the biological parasitism of Rome's resident malaria plasmodia. Traditionally, German clerical appointees either held a "free living," meaning they were elected by local authorities, or they were directly appointed by the pope. The Renaissance popes however asserted, in the words of Luther, that "if any one who holds a free living dies at Rome ... his living must forever belong to the Roman—I should say robbing—See."[12] The pope could then assign that benefice to support a cardinal in Rome, who would administer his German flock in absentia through an underling. Given the fact that the papacy still insisted that church officials come to Rome every few years, and given the high risk these transalpine Churchmen faced from malaria, Luther was in effect accusing the Roman church of using malaria as a silent partner in its campaign to transfer the wealth of Germany to Rome.

13. The Scarlet Whore

Clearly, Luther was becoming a problem, but all the Church's attempts to keep Luther in line through ecclesiastical courts had failed. As a result, the papacy now passed the buck to secular authorities. In 1521 Luther was ordered to appear before the Diet of Worms, which was a conclave of the general assembly of the estates of the German empire in the town of Worms on the River Rhine. There, Luther once again refused to recant his writings, telling his accusers that "unless I am convinced by the testimony of the Scriptures or clear reason" that his opinions were wrong "I cannot and will not recant anything." Emperor Charles V himself therefore declared the unrepentant Luther to be an outlaw and set upon him the Ban of the Empire. This ban was more or less an unexecuted sentence of death, since any imperial subject could now kill Luther without fear of retribution.

By this point, however, Luther was too big to fail. Persuaded by his words, or at least convinced of his right to speak them, Luther's aristocratic defenders offered him sanctuary and protection within Germany. With their help, Luther launched ever-more vehement assaults on the Roman Church. He was aided in this endeavor by the newly-invented printing press, allowing Luther to reach a mass audience by means of cheap prints and pamphlets.[13] In his many publications Luther began to lay the foundations of a German alternative to Roman Christianity by translating the Bible into the vernacular and re-writing the hymns and worship service. Luther also further escalated his rhetoric against the papacy and its seat, the city of Rome. In his last publication before his death, *Against the Roman Papacy*, Luther ranted that the pope was the

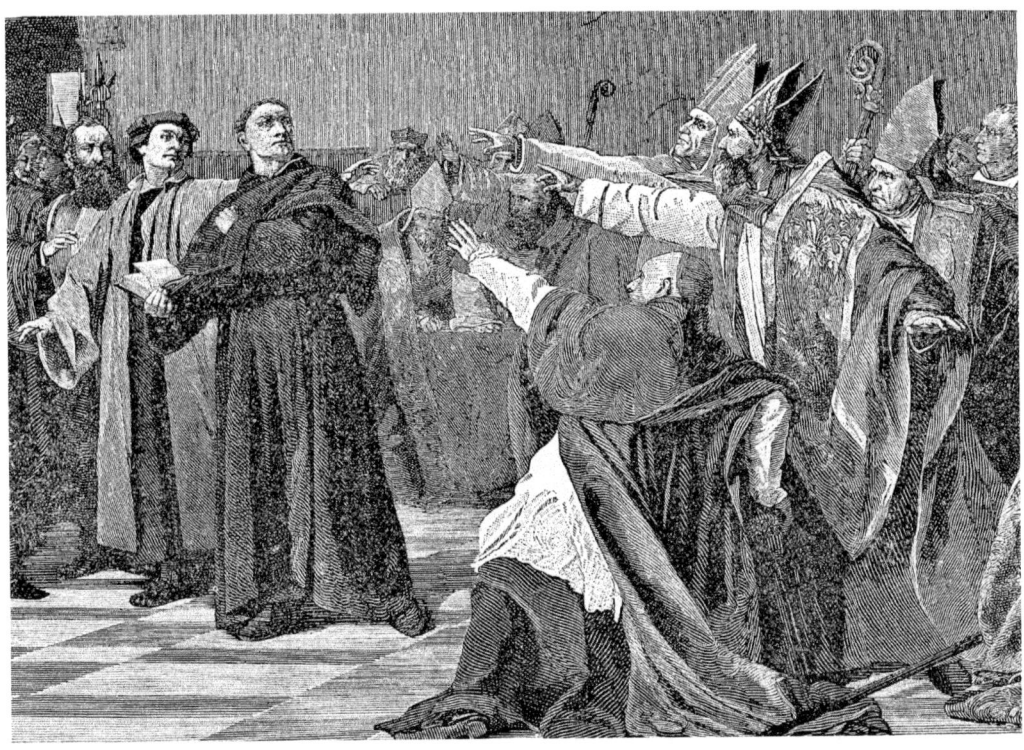

A rather dramatic woodcut of a heroic-looking Luther at the Diet of Worms in 1521, taken from an 1894 Protestant publication. Based on a painting by Emile Delperée, which is reproduced in "Belgian Art," *The Magazine of Art*, Vol. V (Cassell, Peter, Galpin and Company, 1882), p. 152.

"head of the accursed Church ... a vicar of the devil, and enemy of god, an adversary of Christ, destroyer of Christ's Churches, a keeper of lies ... a brothel keeper over all brothel keepers" and "an Anti-Christ."[14] "This farting ass in Rome," Luther charged, would rather "let the whole world bathe and drown in blood" than accept even the most desperately-needed reforms.[15]

In the coming years, Lutheran sentiment would spread rapidly throughout Germany. Indeed, a great many of the German soldiers who participated in the Sack of Rome were already Lutherans just ten years after Luther posted his famous theses. Guicciardini, the chronicler of the Sack, reported that the Lutheran contingent in the imperial Army behaved fairly well towards Rome's human inhabitants; unlike the Spanish, they did "not force their prisoners to undergo extensive torture" and were "both humane and respectful towards gentlewoman."[16] However, these Lutheran soldiers shocked the Romans and their Spanish comrades alike with their anticlerical sacrilege. At one point, a mob of Lutheran troops killed a Roman priest who refused to "administer the most holy sacrament to a mule in clerical vestments."[17] The Lutherans also reportedly gathered up "some of the most holy relics in Rome, which for centuries had drawn pilgrims to the city" and used them for target practice.[18]

Martin Luther himself rejoiced at the news of the Sack of Rome, which he interpreted as an overdue act of divine retribution. "Christ reigns in such a way," Luther chortled, "that the Emperor who persecutes Luther for the pope is forced to destroy the pope for Luther."[19] While Luther was not physically present in Rome during the Sack, he certainly was there in spirit. Lutheran soldiers even carved Luther's own name on a fresco in the Vatican, a Raphael work commissioned by the warrior-pope Julius II himself.[20]

While Guicciardini uses the term "Lutheran" as shorthand for German in his history of the Sack of Rome, in reality Luther's reform movement had already left its north German cradle by the time of the Sack and ventured out into neighboring states. In 1518, just one year after Martin Luther posed his theses in Wittenberg, the Swiss scholar Huldrych Zwingli began his own campaign against the Catholic Church and in the process took some theological positions that were too radical for even Luther to swallow. In 1530, the French theologian John Calvin joined the fray. Although forced to flee to Basel in Switzerland to avoid persecution, Calvin's theological ideas resonated strongly throughout Europe, especially Hungary, the Netherlands, Scotland, and his native France. Catholics called these men "Protestants" since they were joined in a common protest against the Roman church. Protestantism even spread clandestinely in the Catholic strongholds of Spain and Italy, though the movement eventually petered out in those countries in the face of intense persecution by the Inquisition and by secular authorities.

In other states, Protestantism became established not by popular pressure from below but by royal decree from the top. English King Henry VIII had initially championed the Catholic Church against the upstart Protestants, to the point that a thankful pope declared the English monarch to be the *Fidei Defensor*, or "Defender of the Faith," in 1521. In 1534, however, dynastic exigency forced Henry to make a break with Rome: the heirless Henry wanted access to younger wombs but was unable to convince the pope to grant him a divorce from his aging Spanish wife. Henry's break with Rome had financial roots as well. Nearly one-fifth of English land was Church property, and thanks to Henry's declaration of an independent English church, these land holdings could now be taxed or seized outright by the state.[21]

Catholic Europe did not take these defections from the true church lying down.

Over the course of the next century, European history was roiled by a series of wars and civil wars, most notably the Schmalkaldic War in Germany, the Wars of Religion in France, the Thirty Years' War in Germany, and the Civil War in England. By the time the dust had settled and the blood had dried, Christendom had been shattered irrevocably, and Europe was divided along confessional lines. Protestantism now prevailed in much of the European north—England, Scandinavia, the Netherlands, parts of Switzerland, and north-central Germany. However, the popes were able to hold on to Belgium, France and most of Europe's south, in part because the Papacy finally agreed to some much-need reforms at the Council of Trent between 1545 and 1563.

Rethinking Rome in the Age of Reformation

Needless to say, the victory of Protestantism in much of the European north profoundly changed that region's relationship to Rome. In the minds of many Protestants, the city of the popes was now the seat of Mammon rather than the *caput mundi*, a new Babel or new Babylon rather than a new Jerusalem. Protestant European rulers still sent diplomats to Rome, but only because the pope commanded an important Italian state, not because they regarded him as Christendom's head. In Protestant areas, clerical appeals to the papal court such as the one Luther himself carried out in 1510 dried up entirely. What is more, the flow of pilgrims to Rome from Protestant northern Europe declined drastically. Luther disliked pilgrimage in general and pilgrimage to Rome in particular, believing it to be yet another ploy by the perfidious popes to filch from the coin-purses of Germany. Luther was particularly critical of the tradition of the Jubilees, the "false, feigned, foolish 'golden years,' … by which people are excited, stirred up, torn away from God's commandments."[22] It was far better for a good Christian to stay at home, Luther advised, since pilgrimage leads only to "vagabondage," the "habit of begging," "endless knaveries" and a host of other moral ills.[23]

As a result, it seems safe to say that the number of Protestant-area European visitors to Rome dropped as a result of the Protestant Reformation. No historian I know of would dispute this claim. But how steep was the post–Reformation drop in such visitors to Rome? And how long was the drop sustained? If we are going to fully understand how the Protestant Reformation impacted Europe's connections with Rome and its resident malaria plasmodia, these are crucial questions to answer.

Back in 2011, making an attempt to address these questions, I was initially confounded by the problem of sources. In an ideal world a researcher on this topic would have access to a comprehensive database listing all non–Italian travelers to Rome over the centuries by name and nationality—but no such database exists. I was able to find a few sources that gave partial lists of foreign travelers to Rome, but these lists were all highly constrained in time, tended to focus on one or more geographical areas, or restricted themselves to certain types of travelers such as artists. What is more, even the authors of these studies admit that their own lists of travelers are woefully incomplete. Giles Bertrand's study of French "grand tourists" to Rome is case in point: while he is able to identify 212 travelers to the Eternal City in the 18th and 19th centuries, he admits that his list of names is probably only the "visible face of an infinitely more extensive planet."[24]

Unable to find a suitable data set for the study, I decided to create one myself. To determine whether the Reformation changed European travel patterns, I reasoned, we don't need the names of every possible traveler, just a data sample robust enough to allow for meaningful statistical analysis. While no existing archive or scholarly work covered the whole period of study, I suspected that the information we needed already existed in a raw form within the 32 billion web pages of the World Wide Web. The tricky part was accessing it. I initially tried the most obvious search term, "traveled to Rome," only to be inundated by modern-day travel and tourism web sites with little historical content. Eventually I settled upon on another search term, "died in Rome." While my inquiry was about travel and not mortality *per se*, "died in Rome" had the advantage of capturing mainly historical actors rather than modern tourists. What is more, *death* in Rome serves as a useful proxy for *presence* to Rome, insofar as one must either be born in Rome, or journey to Rome later in life, in order to die there.

Having decided on the search term, I entered it into Google's search engine and saved the full web addresses of the first 1,000 page hits. Then, in order to capture as wide a range of European travelers as possible, I searched for web sites containing the equivalent term in French (mort à Rome) and German (in Rom gestorben). Finally, I settled down to the time-consuming task of reading each of the nearly 3,000 web pages the search yielded, looking for the names, dates, and national origins of all listed travelers to Rome.[25] All told, this process yielded a total of 557 names, including 344 Italians, 71 Frenchmen, 38 Germans, 33 Englishmen (and women), 36 Spaniards, and 45 other individuals representing 17 other nationalities, all of whom died in Rome between 800 and 1930 CE. If we set the Italians aside and divide the non–Italians into their regions of origin, 76 (13.6 percent) came from parts of Europe that had become predominantly Protestant by the end of the wars of religion, while 137 (24 percent) of individuals hailed from locations that stayed majority Catholic.

So did these percentages remain steady throughout the entire 800–1930 period, or did the Protestant Reformation change previous patterns? If so, how long did the changes last? To test this, I re-grouped the individuals in the data sample into four periods: (1) the pre–Reformation era (800–1517), (2) the Reformation era (1517 to 1648), (3) the early modern era (1649-1789), (4) and the modern era (1790-1930). I selected 1648 and 1789 as landmarks points for the study because these were the dates of the Peace of Westphalia and the French Revolution respectively, each of which marked a turning point of sorts in the Protestant–Catholic conflict. The Peace of Westphalia brought the Thirty Years' War to a close and thus ended the worst of the struggle between Catholics and Protestants in Germany. The French Revolution, in turn, introduced Conservative vs. Liberal as the new fault line in European politics and reduced the importance of the old Catholic/Protestant axis of Europe.[26]

Going into this study I anticipated that my evidence would show that travel to Rome by Catholic countries would stay relatively constant throughout these four periods. Indeed, travelers from Catholic-majority lands are in some sense the control group of this study, the standard against which the Protestant numbers are judged. As for the travelers from the Protestant north, I expected that their numbers would decline sharply after 1517, rise somewhat in the early modern era after 1648, and then spike after the French Revolution due to the advent of the modern tourist age.

In the end, my guesses proved only partially correct. As is clear from the diagram below, the percentage of visitors to Rome from consistently Catholic areas increased over time but never deviates very far from the overall average, though there was a notable spike of such travelers during the immediate pre-Revolutionary period. Travelers from majority Protestant parts of Europe, however, followed a trajectory very different from the Catholics. While Protestant-region travelers represented 11 percent of all travelers in the pre–1517 period, their numbers dropped precipitously after the Reformation to only 5.9 percent of all travelers between 1518 and 1648. More surprisingly, the number of travelers from majority–Protestant lands stayed low all the way until the French Revolution, actually dropping further to merely 5 percent of all travelers between 1649 and 1789. One caveat is in order: some of the decrease in the 1649–1789 period might be accounted for by changes in European travel patterns in the post–1750 period. As we will see in Chapter 15 below, late 18th and early 19th century travelers to Rome would become increasingly aware of the seasonal dangers that Rome posed and tended to avoid the Eternal City in the unhealthy summer, potentially reducing the numbers of tourists who "died in Rome."

Be that as it may, the relative drop in Protestant-region travelers revealed by figure 13.2 remains striking, especially considering the continuing pattern of Catholic-area travel to Rome during the same time. All told, only 15 people from Protestant-majority territories found their way into my data sample between 1517 and 1789—and a close look at those 15 further underscores the notion that the Reformation fundamentally altered the relationship between Rome and the Protestant north. Of the 15, only three—Casper Van Wittel, Metz Hertzog, and Adam Elsheimer—were personally Protestant, and one, Elsheimer, would later convert to Catholicism. Five more of the 15 were Catholic political exiles from Protestant England, including two members of the exiled Stuart dynasty and Thomas Goldwell, the last Catholic Bishop of England. Two of the 15 were actually

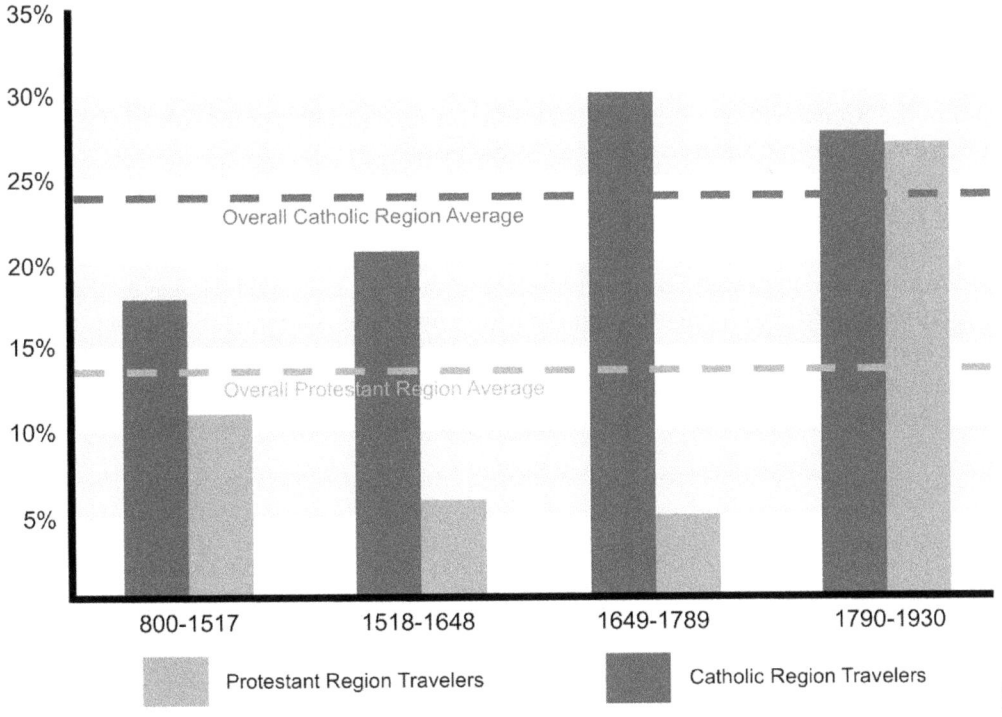

Protestant and Catholic Area Visitors to Rome as % of All Travelers, 800–1930. Modified from Benjamin James Reilly, "Malaria, Protestants, and Google," *Environmental History*, Vol. 16 (April 2011), p. 319.

popes, Hadrian VI and Clement VII, who hailed from Utrecht and Geneva respectively, cities that later became majority Protestant during the religious turmoil of the 16th and 17th centuries. The most colorful man of the 15 was Barthel Beham, an engraver banished from the Protestant Nuremburg for his apparent atheism. As I wrote in my 2011 article presenting these findings, post–Reformation Rome was clearly beginning to "attract outliers rather than mainstream representatives of the increasingly Protestant north."[27]

The Protestant Reformation therefore is overdue for reinterpretation, at least from the perspective of biology. We have already seen repeatedly throughout this book that Rome was a dangerous place for unacclimated foreigners, especially for travelers from across the Alps. Following Luther's diatribes against the Roman Church, the number of such vulnerable visitors shrank considerably and in a sustained manner. The Reformation, therefore, served as an inadvertent religious quarantine, protecting Protestant Europeans not only from the financial parasitism of the papacy but also from the tribute of lives previously exacted by malaria plasmodia from among these transalpine visitors to the Eternal City. It is surely no coincidence that the fortunes of much of Northern Europe, especially the Netherlands and England, begin to rise at exactly this historical moment.

Of course, no major event has only one cause. Other factors contributed to the rise of Europe's north as well, most notably the discovery of the Americas, which England and Holland were particularly well-positioned by geography to exploit. In the long run, England also benefited enormously from its large domestic coal deposits, which I suspect were probably a more important factor overall in the modern-era rise of England than the Reformation's inadvertent quarantine. Still, Protestant Europe's estrangement from Rome meant the reduction of a long-standing demographic drain that would have fallen disproportionately on that region's educated elite class. By reducing the tribute of lives paid to the Roman summer, the Reformation must have played some role in the growth of these states, even if the role is difficult to quantify.

What is more, as we will see in the next chapter, Protestant Europe's break with Rome occurred at an opportune moment. During the 16th and 17th centuries, Rome became more popular than ever as an international destination thanks to papal support for the arts and to renewed European interest in the classical world. However, these new attractions did little to reduce the danger posed by Rome's endemic plasmodia. Despite some incremental improvements over time, Rome remained a highly malarial city up until the modern era. As a result of the Reformation, however, it would be the Spanish and French that would bear the brunt of Roman Fever in the two centuries to come.

14

Fork in the Road

In spring of 1592, only 70 years after Luther incurred the Ban of the Empire for his defiance of papal authority, a black cap adorned with a "mighty blue feather" entered the Eternal City atop the head of a young Catholic German. Over the next month the dashing young man with the conspicuous hat "[drank] deep, in the German fashion" and took the typical tours of the town. But things were not as they seemed; in reality, the hat was an ingenious disguise. This apparent German lush was no German at all, but rather a Protestant Englishman named Henry Wotton who counted upon his hat's ostentatious display to render himself inconspicuous by comparison. Wotton hoped his ruse would allow him to ingratiate himself with the "English outlaws who congregated in Rome" plotting the overthrow of the English Queen. As an aspiring young courtier, Wotton knew that information of this sort could be traded for favors in the Elizabethan court.

Wotton's best-laid plans, however, were dashed by a "chance meeting" with an English acquaintance whom Wotton suspected to be a partisan of the Catholic cause. His cover now blown, Wotton risked being arrested and imprisoned by the Church. Even worse, Wotton feared that he might be accused of collaborating with the Catholics himself, thus opening himself up to prosecution or blackmail upon returning to England. Wotton therefore beat a hasty retreat to Florence where he put his tacky hat into retirement and resumed the life of a Protestant Englishman.[1] In the late 16th century, Protestant travel could be dangerous indeed—and not just because of Roman Fever.

The Perils of Rome

Wotton was not the only English Protestant to risk a trip to Rome in the unsettled century that followed the Reformation. Just two years later another Protestant Englishman, Anthony Munday, managed to spend several months in Rome masquerading as the son of a well-known English Catholic. Like Wotton, Munday hoped to collect valuable information in Rome about exiled British Catholics in Rome, whom he described as "practicing, and daily looking for, the overthrow and ruin of their Princess and Country."[2] Still another British Protestant, Fynes Moryson, visited Rome in 1594. Unlike Munday and Wotton, Moryson made no attempt to hide his Protestant identity, though he did seek the protection of an English cardinal in Rome. Despite the cardinal's promise of sponsorship, Morysons took fright shortly after Easter when a party of Roman priests came to the inn where he was staying and demanded to know if Morysons and his companions had taken Easter communion. Fearing that his Roman welcome had worn thin, Moryson like Wotton before him fled to the safety of Florence.[3]

Moryson's fear is understandable, since visits to Rome during this era were risky business for British Protestants. During Munday's own stay in Rome a Welsh visitor was imprisoned, tried, and executed for disrespecting the Eucharist. A few years earlier, English sailor Edward Webbe was released from Turkish galley slavery but discovered, as he passed through Italy on his way home, that he had fallen from the frying-pan into the fire. The Protestant Webbe was repeatedly imprisoned by Catholic authorities in Italy, first in Rome and then in Naples, where as a suspected spy he was subjected to months of horrific tortures.[4] Two decades later, an English tutor passing through Rome with his aristocratic charge was arrested and languished in jail for thirty years for refusing to abjure his Protestant faith.[5] Another Protestant traveler, William Lithgow, barely escaped a similar fate a few years later. After spending a month sight-seeing in Rome, Lithgow was threatened with arrest when his presence came to the attention of a crowd of "blood-sucking inquisitors, of which the most part were my own countrymen." Lithgow laid low for three days in a palace in the Borgo owned by a sympathetic English exile before escaping his pursuers by "leap[ing] the walls of Rome."[6]

Nor were physical dangers the only perils to be feared. According to the contemporary English scholar Roger Ascham, many Englishmen visitors to Italy of this era "returned Papists, or Atheists, experienced in newfangled vices, apt for treason, lying, and every form of swinish debauchery."[7] As the English Ambassador to Venice argued in 1616, such men left Rome "not only corrupted with their doctrine, but poisoned with their positions, and so return again into their countries, both adverse to Religion, and ill-affected to our State and Government."[8] A visit to Rome threatened not only your body, therefore, it corrupted your very soul.

Such perils ensured that the 16th and early 17th centuries marked the low ebb of Protestant travel to the Eternal City, at least for the well-documented English.[9] The years between 1570 and 1604 were particularly dangerous since they coincided with the military conflict between Queen Elizabeth of England and the arch–Catholic Kingdom of Spain, which controlled the Kingdom of Naples in southern Italy. Any Protestant Englishman in Rome risked being treated as a spy by the Spanish or prosecuted by the papal Inquisition. As a result, the English government estimated that there were "not above twenty Englishmen in Italy" during these tumultuous years.[10] English Protestant travel to Italy revived somewhat after a peace with Spain was signed in 1604. Nonetheless, continued religious tension in England served to politicize, and probably discourage, travel to Rome throughout the 17th century, especially during the civil war years of 1642–46, 1648, and 1688–1691.[11] As M.L. Clarke points out, some English Protestants still visited Rome throughout this era but "they did so in spite of discouragement and possible danger."[12]

Nor were English Protestants alone in avoiding Rome in the immediate aftermath of the Reformation. The Dutch had previously been enthusiastic visitors to the Eternal City, historian Gerrit Verhoeven claims, but following Holland's adoption of Protestantism, antipathy to popery and fear of the Inquisition all but severed this long-standing connection to the *caput mundi*. As a result, "Dutch travelers virtually ignored Italy in the early seventeenth century."[13] Those Dutch who did venture into Italy during this era rarely traveled south of Florence, largely because the place of primacy that Rome had once occupied in the spiritual life of the Dutch had been usurped by a new sacred destination: Geneva, the city of John Calvin.[14]

As for Northern European Catholics, they could venture to Rome in relative safety but might find themselves in mortal peril upon returning to Protestant-controlled territory. Following the establishment of the Anglican Church, for example, the British government formally forbade travel to Italy and most especially to Rome. Those who defied this prohibition risked being arrested, stripped of their properties, and even executed. Despite the danger, a number of English Catholics did visit Rome in the 16th century including hundreds of young men who were accepted into the Jesuit order's Roman seminaries. At least 41 of these would-be missionaries would become martyrs over the next few decades, either dying on their way back to England or else imprisoned and executed upon English soil after returning to preach the Catholic faith.[15]

A Catholic Capital

The relative absence of the English and other European Protestants did not discommode the Romans very much, however, as other European were pleased to take their place. In the immediate aftermath of the Sack of Rome, travel to the Eternal City slackened but by the late 16th century Rome was once again receiving "innumerable voyagers" from throughout Catholic Europe, especially from Southern Germany, France, and Belgium.[16] The motives of these voyagers varied. In the aftermath of the Trent reforms, Catholic bishops and archbishops were once again required to appear in person before the papal court, first to receive their offices, and later to make occasional reports about the well-being of their diocese.[17] Disputatious monks, priests, and bishops continued to come to Rome from throughout the still–Catholic portions of Europe to quibble about jurisdiction and bicker over revenues. What is more, Rome continued to attract an estimated 30,000 pilgrims a year during the 16th century, and during Jubilee years pilgrim numbers could swell to many times that amount.[18] Thanks to the Sack of Rome and the Protestant Reformation, the 1550 Jubilee was a disappointment, but the 1575 Jubilee was a spectacular success. Contemporaries estimated that 300,000 spectators were present in the piazza of Saint Peter's Basilica for the opening of the holy door ceremony and over the course of the year that followed there were rarely less than 100,000 foreign pilgrims in the city.[19] A more conservative modern estimate puts the pilgrim numbers of 1575 at 400,000, still an impressive total for a city of less than 100,000 inhabitants.[20] Twenty-five years later the 1600 Jubilee was better attended still, attracting an estimated 536,000 of the faithful.[21]

More secular-minded Catholics were attracted to Rome as well, in part because the city's ancient ruins and remains, which had become fashionable due to the rebirth of Classical scholarship during the Renaissance era. Some of these antiquities, such as Colosseum and the Forum, had to be appreciated *alfresco*. Still others could be seen within Rome's many museums; by 1556, Rome boasted 90 museums and private collections of ancient statuary and other antiquities.[22]

Whether they were ecclesiastics, pilgrims, or antiquarians—and some travelers were all three—visitors to Rome planned their trips using the guides that were produced in great abundance during the Renaissance era. All told, at least 127 different editions of guidebooks on Rome were published between 1475 and 1600 alone.[23] Printed maps of Rome circulated throughout Europe as well, creating a sense of familiarity with the fabled landscape of the *caput mundi*.[24] The publication of such works was driven in part by market forces. However, it also reflected a deliberate program enacted in the aftermath of the Council of Trent to advertise the marvels of Rome and thus defend the Eternal City against the slanders of the Protestants.[25]

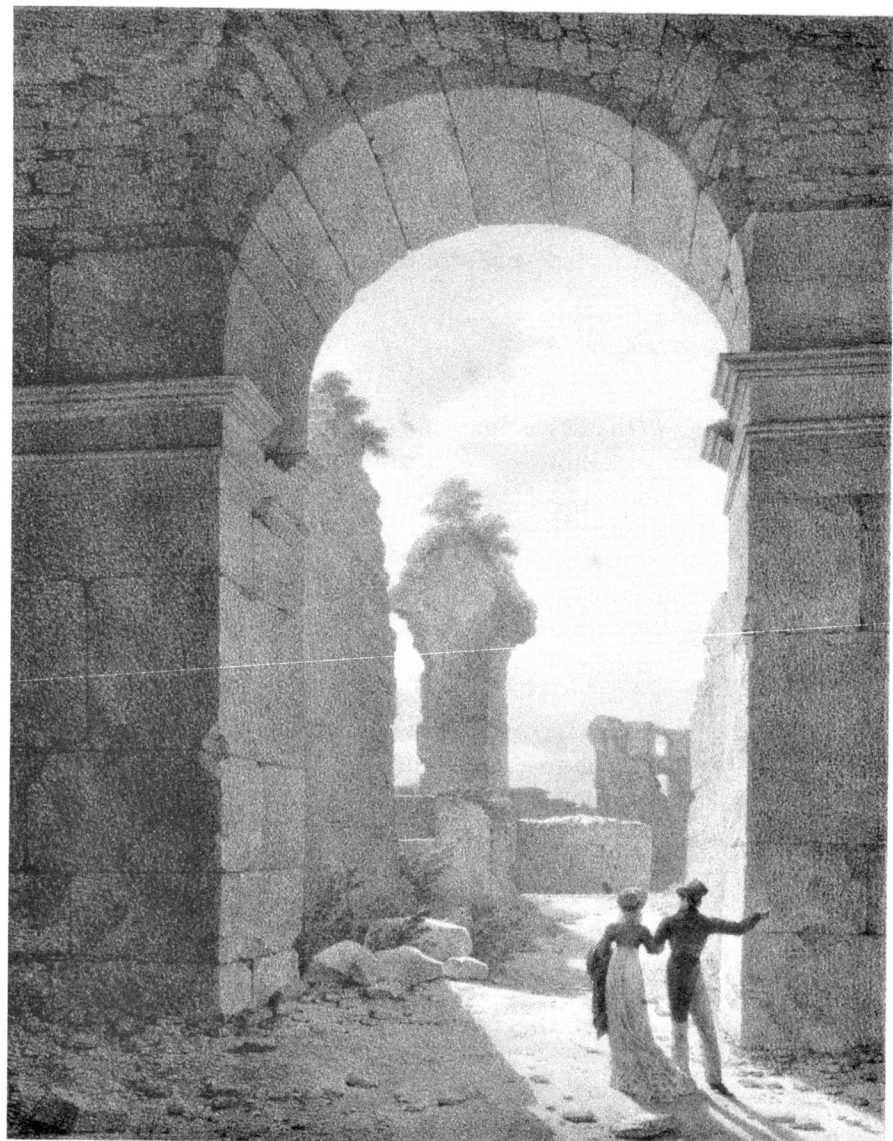

An early 18th-century image of tourists at the lower arches of the Colosseum in Rome. Jean Baptiste Isabey, *Voyage en Italie* (Paris: 1823), Plate 2, from ETH-Bibliothek Zürich, Rar 9742, https://doi.org/10.3931/e-rara-51063.

Still other Europeans of the era came to Rome on an artistic pilgrimage, since by the 15th century Rome had become the cultural capital of Catholic Europe. Rome boasted at least 267 "architects, sculptors, painters, plasterers, engravers, and silversmiths" in the 1600s, attracting connoisseurs from throughout Catholic Europe.[26] Rome was a city of music, too, as well as a hub of the literary world. As Eric MacPhail noted, Rome occupied a lynchpin role in the French Renaissance. "As the capital of Latin Literature and the headquarters of the Roman Empire," MacPhail contends, Rome represented the "power and creativity of the classical past."[27] As a result, France "sent some of its best minds to Rome" during the 16th century, some of whom studied at Rome's prestigious universities, including the Sapienza, the Collegio Romano, and various resident missionary colleges.[28]

Thanks to this influx of Catholic-world visitors, Rome's population became increasingly international in the 16th century. Southern Germans still frequented the streets of Rome, as did Corsicans, Albanians, Slavs, and Greeks. The French were more common still; indeed, a common saying of the age held that "in Rome, there are more French than red dogs (*chiens rouges*)."[29] When French Essayist Michel de Montagne visited Rome, he noted that Rome contained "such a large number of Frenchmen" that "almost every person he met on the streets" addressed him "in own tongue."[30]

Even more common than the French were the Spanish, whose community in Rome may have topped 30,000 by the end of the 16th century, or about 25 percent of Rome's total population.[31] These Spanish migrants followed in the train of a steady stream of Spanish money. During the Counter-Reformation period, Spanish kings enriched by American bullion lavished tremendous resources on Rome with an eye towards assuming the role of protector of Rome that the Germans had previously enjoyed. In the process, Dandalet argues, Spain played a "fundamental role in the transformation of Rome into what was arguably seventeenth-century Europe's most dramatic and impressive urban stage."[32] Ultimately, these gifts were self-serving: by tying its own fortunes to that of the *caput mundi*, the young Spanish kingdom was in effect asserting its own claim of pre-eminence over the entire Catholic world.[33]

The "Infectious Enthusiasms" of the Early Modern Era

As many of these unacclimated French, Spanish, and other Catholic visitors no doubt discovered, however, the Eternal City could still be a dangerous place for foreign visitors. According to the French writer Nicholas de Bralion, who visited Rome in the early 17th century, travelers knew "from common experience" that the air of Rome was "very offensive and unhealthy, especially to young strangers, who ought to behave in moderation if they want to return to their country."[34] Conventional wisdom of the time held that Rome's bad air arose from "marshy places of the nearby countryside" though Bralion himself suspected that the "exhalations" of Roman's ancient ruins were also at least partially to blame.[35]

In a similar vein, French geographer Pierre Duval lamented Italy's *mauvais air*, generated (he believed) by stagnant waters and humidity in the soil. This bad air was annoying to the local Romans, but downright deadly for visiting foreigners, whom Duval advised to "take medicine for seven days after they arrive there, avoid bad odors, work little, guard against long periods of hunger and cold, abstain from fruit and women, and always drink only fresh water."[36] It is not clear what "medicine" Duval is talking about here. He may perhaps have meant the South American anti-fever medicine cinchona, better known to Western audiences in 1639 as "Jesuit's Bark" since it was first described in print by the Jesuit Father Bernabé Cobo.[37] But probably not: it would be many years before chichona came into common use a febrifuge in Europe and even then the bark was an expensive luxury.

For travelers of this time period, Rome's atmosphere of artistic inspiration and its air of fever were inseparable phenomena, two sides of the same coin. As historian Simon Wrigley has pointed out in his article "Infectious Enthusiasms," Rome's air was considered to be simultaneously inspiring and sickening. Visitors to Rome in the early modern age generally assumed that Rome's very atmosphere was "suffused with some unique element" which "stimulated artists to great achievements" yet also caused the diseases that "so often assailed visitors to the Eternal, but sometimes fatal, City."[38] Visiting Rome could therefore be a harrowing experience for both body and mind. As a result, travelers to Rome experienced interlinked psychological and physical shocks: "the extreme emotions brought on by confrontation with the assembled great art [in Rome]," Wrigley contends, "were paralleled by—or confused with—the effects of disease."[39]

Based on my own analysis of mortality patterns amongst Catholic cardinals, visitors to Rome of this era did indeed have good reason to fear the Eternal City's *mauvais air*. As noted in Chapter 3 above, August–September deaths amongst cardinals over time can serve as a useful proxy measurement of Rome's malaria rate, and fluctuations in that percentage could indicate changing levels of malaria risk in Rome. If this is accepted, then the immediate aftermath of the Reformation Rome remained a dangerous place. Between 1500–1600, summer season mortality stood at 25.9 percent, 9.23 percent higher than the expected average for those two months (16.67 percent). This was better than the overall average for the period from 496 to 1600, when 27.6 percent of all cardinal deaths occurred in the August–September malaria season, but only marginally. The period from 1600 to 1700 was slightly healthier still, with the excess mortality falling to only 6.63 percent. These changes are clearly seen in the diagram below, which overlays summer-season mortality upon the rise of Rome's urban population.

Despite this record of improvement, both the 16th and 17th centuries look positively pestilential in contrast with the overall 1701–1850 period, during which Miranda's data shows no summertime spike in mortality at all. Rather, in the post-1700 era the mortality peak amongst Catholic cardinals in Rome occurred in January–February and is most likely attributable to wintertime respiratory diseases.[40] As we shall see below,

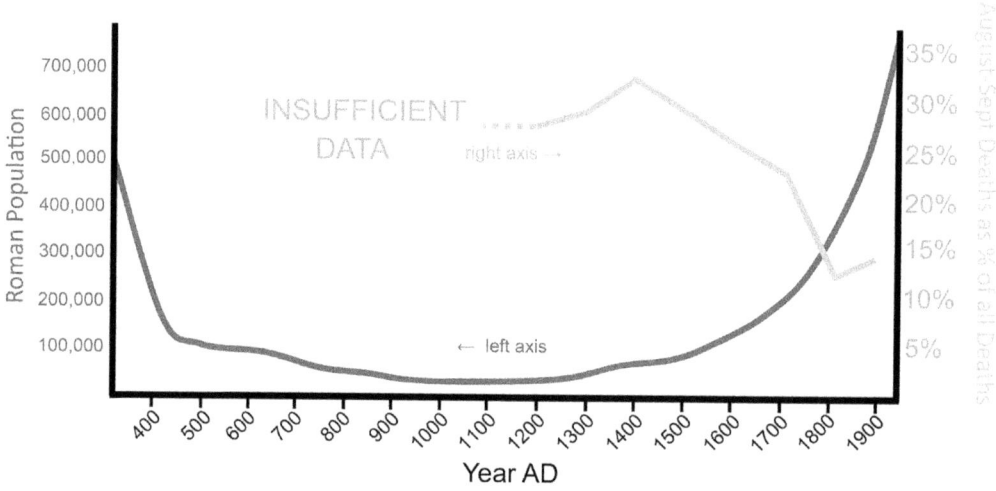

Population of Rome and % of August–September Deaths, 400–1900 CE. Benjamin James Reilly, "Cardinal Numbers: Changing Patterns of Malaria and Mortality in Rome, 494–1850," *Journal of Interdisciplinary History*, Vol. 49, no. 3 (2019), p. 414, © The Massachusetts Institute of Technology and The Journal of Interdisciplinary History, Inc.

this growing summer-season salubrity probably reflects a combination of urban growth, hydraulic engineering, and new medical treatment. But progress was slow, and for travelers in the first two centuries after the Protestant Reformation, Rome remained a deadly destination.

An objection could be raised: is comparing cardinals to Catholic travelers valid, or are we comparing apples to oranges? The cardinals in our list were after all generally full-year residents of Rome, living and dying in the vicinity of the Eternal City. In contrast, the Catholic artists, writers, craftsmen, and pilgrims of the Renaissance era were often just temporary visitors to Rome and could potentially have avoided the malarial season in Rome altogether. For it to be true that Roman Fever represented a risk to Catholic travelers to Rome, therefore, we must also establish that those travelers were actually in Rome during the dangerous summer season. If they were not, then the inadvertent religious quarantine of the Protestant Reformation would have exerted little impact on European history.

So *did* visiting Catholics remain in Rome through the summer during the 16th century? The existing literature has little to say on this subject. However, another study I carried out throws some light on exactly this issue. In fall of 2019, in an effort to determine the seasonality of transalpine European travel to Rome, I conducted a thorough reading of 271 pre–1750 travelogue documents, biographies, letter collections and the like, systematically recording where each author was on the 15th of each month. My initial goal was to determine whether Protestant and Catholic voyagers to Rome exhibited different seasonal travel patterns (they did, though not to the level of statistical significance). However, one unexpected finding of this study was that travel patterns to Rome changed quite dramatically over time. In the years from 1400 to 1750, foreign travelers were present in Rome throughout the calendar year, and while the number of foreign visitors in Rome did fall to an August–September low, the number of travelers in Rome during the lowest month (August) was only 47 percent lower than the number of travelers in Rome present during the highest traffic month (February). However, after 1750, travel to Rome became far more sharply seasonal. In these years, the drop-off between the busiest month (March, in this case) to the lowest month (September) rose to 77 percent, a three-quarters reduction in tourist volume. We will discuss the data on changing Italian travel patterns more thoroughly in the next chapter, which deals with the European Grand Tour. For now, suffice it to say that European travelers of the 16th century were in fact quite often in Rome during the dangerous summer season, especially in comparison with the centuries that followed.

All of these findings lead inevitably to one conclusion: that the 16th century, and to a lesser degree the 17th, was the time period in which the Protestant Reformation exerted the greatest selective pressure on European history. During this crossroads era, Protestant travel to Rome was sharply curtailed since such travel had become religiously inadvisable and politically problematic. However, due in part to an active campaign of encouragement by the Counter-Reformation church, Catholics continued to come to Rome—and perhaps in higher numbers than ever before. It may be that the French, Spanish, and other Catholic countries gained more than they lost through their connection to Rome in this period, at least in the political, intellectual, and perhaps scientific spheres. However, from the standpoint of demographics the lure of Rome must have exerted a sizable demographic drain on transalpine Europe's Catholic states, whose citizens were attracted by the siren's song of Rome's religious and cultural attractions only to fall prey to Rome's *mauvais air*. The 16th-17th centuries, therefore, was the time period in which the inadvertent quarantine of the Protestant Reformation mattered the most.

Malaria's Slow Decline

By the end of the 16th century Rome was already on its way to becoming a healthier destination for Catholics and Protestants alike due to long-term demographic growth and infrastructural improvement. The scale of Rome's demographic expansion in the early modern and modern era was both impressive and somewhat surprising, especially considering that Rome's population had fallen to just 10,000 after the Sack of Rome, merely 1 percent of its ancient era height. Some contemporary observers actually suspected that the Sack might prove to be a *coup de grace* from which Rome could never fully recover.[41] Writing just two decades after the Sack, William Thomas observed that, other than the populated Vatican Hill and the Borgo districts, most of the area within Rome's city walls consisted of little more than "rubble and old monstrous foundations" interspersed with "desert, pasture, and vineyards," much as it had been in the time of Romulus.[42]

Over the course of the next century, however, Rome's population began to soar, bolstered by an influx of Catholic visitors and by generous Spanish patronage. By the century's end Rome's population topped 100,000, the highest it had been in nearly 13 centuries. What was good news for the Romans however was bad news for their uninvited guests, *Anopheles* mosquitoes. As the area between Rome's ancient Aurelian walls began to fill, Rome's wastes, orchards, and gardens were progressively replaced by new construction.[43] In the process, *Anopheles* habitat gave way to paved roads, plazas, and housing, steadily reducing the fever risks, especially in the densely settled urban core.[44] Certain areas remained unhealthy, especially the Forum, the banks of the Tiber, the area around the Lateran, the lowest-lying areas in the Campus Martius, and the outskirts of the city in general. Nonetheless, by the end of the 16th century malaria was beginning to recede as a threat.

Rome's health was further improved by a series of much-needed hydraulic improvements put into place by the late Renaissance papacy. From the mid–16th century onwards a series of popes invested considerable time and money into restoring Rome's aqueducts, which had been in a state of severe disrepair since the dark days of the Lombard invasions. In part, these projects were a papal project to beautify the city. The Ottoman capital of Istanbul (the former Constantinople) had recently been decorated with a number of aqueduct-fed urban fountains, and in their jealous vanity the popes demanded similar adornments for the capital of Christendom.[45] However, urban health and sanitation were important papal goals as well. Indeed, the attention of the popes was first fixed upon the aqueducts by a fever epidemic in August of 1566 that was eventually traced to standing water and a broken aqueduct channel in the Campus Martius. For the pope at the time, Pius V, aqueduct reconstruction was part and parcel of a larger effort to rid Rome of "putrid water and to maintain salubrious air for the good of the public."[46]

In the years that followed, the popes carried out an ambitious program of urban hydraulic renewal in the Eternal City. By 1570, the papacy had restored the Acqua Vergine aqueduct, which supplied water to the Campus Martius, and fitted it with fountains whose jets and bubblers kept the water from becoming stagnant, and thus spoiled

14. Fork in the Road

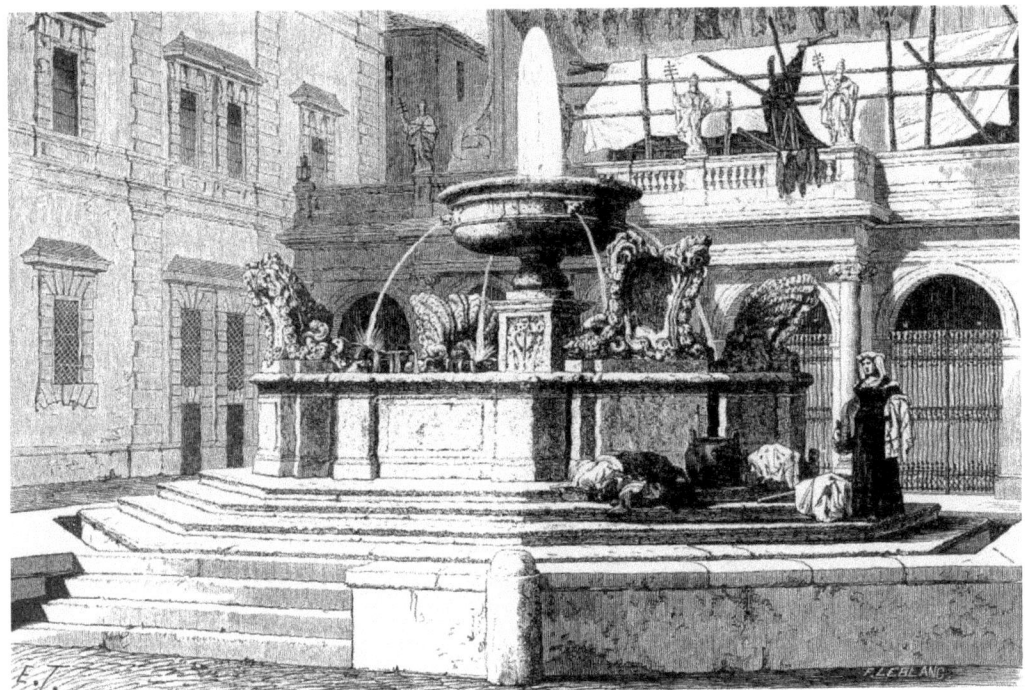

The Fountain in the Piazza Santa Maria in Trastevere, powered by the water of the Acqua Felice aqueduct. Note the gutter surrounding the octagonal fountain to catch runoff water, which the woman on the right side of the image seems to be re-using for her laundry. Jules Gourdault, *Rome et la Campagne Romaine* (Paris: Hachette, 1885), p. 189.

the breeding plans of *Anopheles* mosquitoes. In the 1580s the papacy bankrolled the restoration of another defunct Roman aqueduct, the Acqua Felice. Because this water arose high on the slopes of the Alban Hills, the Acqua Felice had a formidable flow pressure, allowing for the construction of more dramatic urban fountains. What is more, the Acqua Felice had enough pressure to reach the tops of Rome's abandoned hills; indeed, Rome's ingenious hydraulic engineers used airtight syphons to transfer the water up and down urban slopes, thus "engirdling Rome's hills with streams of Felice water."[47] Rome's hills, abandoned since the Lombards had cut the aqueducts in the 6th century, were now once again open to habitation. Later aqueducts followed, including the Acqua Paola, which sprang from the slopes of the Lake Bracciano volcano caldera and had such a powerful discharge volume that grain mills were later built along its course to harness the kinetic energy of its flow.[48]

One might imagine that this new influx of water into Rome would have rendered the city a more malarial place overall, but in fact the opposite occurred. In order to deal with the inevitable run-off from the urban fountains, Rome's hydraulic engineers constructed an elaborate set of sewers and drains. Water from the fountains was first collected and sold for secondary uses including drinking, laundering, manufacturing, and even flushing out the latrines.[49] Excess water was then shunted into an elaborate system of drains which emptied ultimately into the Tiber. Before these improvements were put in place, Rome had been crisscrossed with open-air drains full of trash, sewage, standing water, and swarms of mosquitoes.[50] Thanks to the new aqueducts, however, Rome's drains were now constantly flushed by water, keeping them relatively clean and preventing stagnant water from pooling up in the sewers. What is more, Rome's sewers were increasingly paved over to protect the drains from wheeled vehicles—and to protect the wheeled vehicles from the drains. In addition, increasing care was made to grade the streets, with an eye towards encouraging run-off and preventing puddles.[51] The sum result of these measures was a marked reduction in the amount of stagnant water in Rome, at least in comparison to preceding centuries, and a dramatic decrease in mosquito breeding habitat in the Eternal City.

Thanks to its growing population and hydraulic improvements, Rome was well on the way to becoming a healthier city. However, saying that Rome was *healthier* is not the same as saying it was *healthy*—the danger of Roman Fever was now less, but it was not negligible. Indeed, as we shall see in the following two chapters, malaria would continue to pose a threat to European travelers to the Eternal City for several centuries to come.

15

Homecoming

In October of 1786, novelist Johann Wolfgang von Goethe stood on the very threshold of Rome. The young German could barely contain his excitement. For as long as he could remember Goethe had felt an "irresistible need" to visit Rome, the "hub of the world." Those dreams were about to become a reality. "Tomorrow evening Rome! Even now I can hardly believe it. When this wish has been fulfilled," Goethe wrote, "what shall I wish for next?"[1]

Upon entering the city and seeing its marvels, however, Goethe found himself feeling, not just wonder, but familiarity, as if returning to a place he had visited once before. Even though Goethe hailed from a Protestant family, as a child he had been surrounded by images of Rome captured in "paintings, drawings, etchings, woodcuts, plaster casts and cork models." Now that he was in Rome itself, however, "all the dreams of my youth have come to life ... wherever I walk, I come upon familiar objects in an unfamiliar world; everything is just as I imagined it, yet everything is new."[2] Goethe was a stranger, but not in a strange land. He was home.

Goethe was by no means the only transalpine traveler of his era to feel a sense of unexpected familiarity in the Eternal City. As John Pemble has quipped, foreign visitors to the Eternal City tended not to "discover Rome" so much as they "recognize[d] a Rome they already knew, and for which they had already prepared a repertoire of responses."[3] In part, this is because young children of the age were steeped in the classics during their early education, which traditionally included a hefty serving of Roman history and Latin literature. As contemporary English traveler John Chetwode Eustice noted, "the name of Rome echoes in our ears from our infancy; our lisping tongues are tuned to her language; and our first and most delightful years are passed among her orators, poets, and historians." Small wonder, then, that English visitors to Rome "take a deep interest in her fortunes, and ... adopt her cause, as that of our own country, with spirit and with passion."[4]

For some travelers, however, the reality of Rome failed to match their overblown expectations. Like Goethe, the French traveler C.M.J.B. Dupaty could scarce believe he had finally reached Rome, the city of "centuries, emperors, nations," the seat of Caesar and the home of Horace.[5] Nonetheless Dupaty was deeply dismayed by the wretched appearance of the ruined city he found on the banks of the Tiber, which was "not Rome, but its corpse; the *campagna* is its tomb, and its teeming inhabitants are the worms that devour it."[6] But perhaps the disappointed Dupaty should have counted his blessings. Thanks to urban hygienic improvements, the decline of urban mosquito habitats, and increasing popular awareness of Rome's fever dangers, early modern Rome was considerably less likely to become the tomb of visiting Europeans than it had been for the

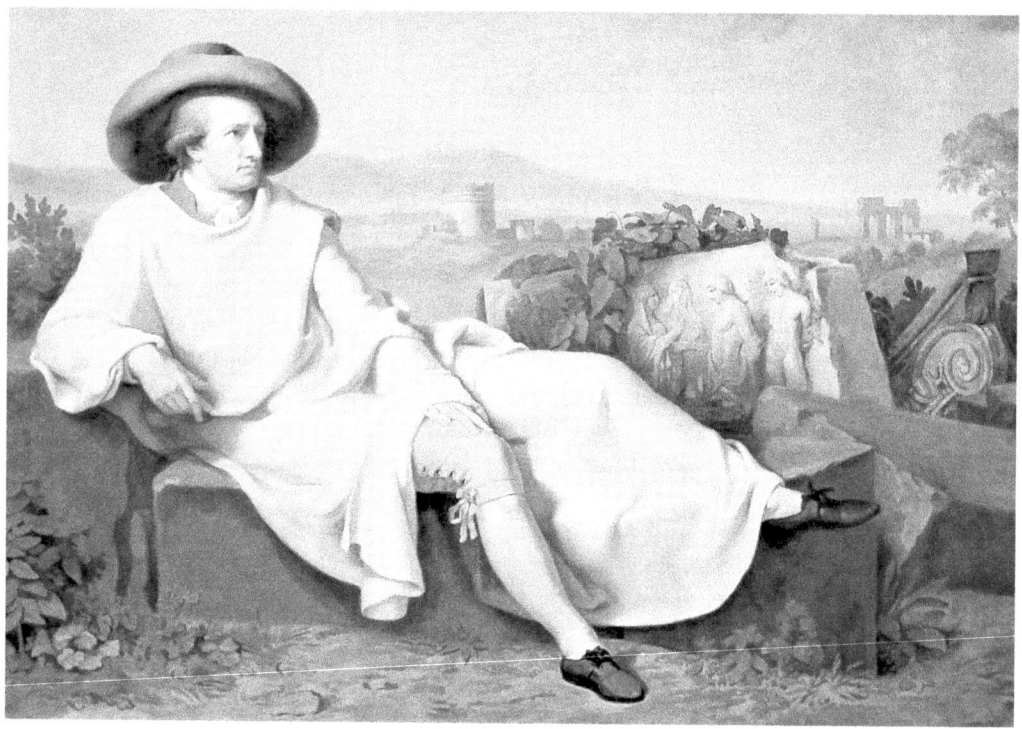

Portrait of Goethe reclining on ruins in the Roman *Campagna*, 1787, by Johann Heinrich Wilhelm Tischbein. CC By-SA 4.0, Städel Museum, Frankfurt am Main.

transalpine soldiers, appellants, pilgrims, and other visitors who had left their corpses the Eternal City during the Medieval era.

Rome and the Grand Tour

Though they came from different countries, and to different conclusions, Dupaty, Eustice and Goethe were all carried to Rome by the same cultural phenomenon: the "Grand Tour" tradition of the early modern era. Although the Grand Tour would later give its name to the modern concept of "tourism" it was originally imagined as an educational rather than recreational endeavor. Self-improvement, not entertainment, was the goal. Richard Lassels, an early popularizer of the Grand Tour, contended in a 1670 tract that the Grand Tour offered a plethora of benefits for young men. Travel teaches "wholesome hardship" and weans a young man from the effeminizing influence of "fondness of his mother." What is more, touring encourages humility, forces a pupil to practice his languages, and trains a young Englishman "for his country's service" by exposing him to foreign peoples and concepts. Lassels likens a young man who has returned from his tour to "a glorious Sun" who "shine[s] bright in the firmament of his country" [by which he means Parliament] and who "blesses his inferiors with the powerful influences of his knowing spirit."[7]

Although some of these benefits of travel could be obtained anywhere in Europe, Lassels believed that the ultimate goal of any Grand Tour should be Rome. In the *caput mundi*, Lassels wrote, "all languages are spoken, all sciences are taught, the ablest men of *Europe* meet, all the best *records* are found, all wits appear as upon their true theatre." Even the ruins themselves had stories to tell, since in Rome "every stone almost is a book; every statue a master; every inscription a lesson, every *Antechamber* an *Academy*." The Grand Tour, then, was a mobile finishing school for young men, and Rome was its capstone course.[8]

The roots of the Grand Tour go back to at least the 16th century. As historian Clare Howard points out, Renaissance-era parents believed foreign travel to be a "highly educating experience, by which one was made a complete man intellectually." What is more, the brilliance of the Italian Renaissance was a wake-up call of sorts for the Germans and English, who came to realize they were still "barbarians on the outskirts" of the more civilized Italian south.[9] In order to soak up this superior southern culture many Englishmen of this period set out to "do" Italy, touring its sights and enrolling in various Italian universities—and often having a good deal of fun in the process.[10] One such traveler was Edward de Vere, the Earl of Oxford, who may have spent as much as a year in Italy in the early 1570s.[11] Upon his return to England de Vere became a playwright and may in fact have been the real William Shakespeare. Whatever Shakespeare's true identity, the Immortal Bard was clearly an Italophile: no fewer than 11 of Shakespeare's plays are set in part or in their entirety within the Italian peninsula.

Almost as soon as this southward flow of Englishmen began, it was interrupted by the Protestant Reformation. As we saw in the last chapter, during and after the age of Henry VIII the number of Englishmen travelling to Italy and Rome dropped precipitously. English travel was further disrupted in the late 1660s by renewed war with France and then again by the War of Spanish Succession, a continent-wide conflict that raged from 1701 to 1714.[12]

Following the signing of the Peace of Utrecht in 1714, English travelers began to return in earnest to the continent, Rome included. But there was one last hiccup: five years later the Stuart Dynasty, which had been ejected from England in the Glorious Revolution of 1688, chose to make Rome their capital in exile. Nonetheless, the overall impact of the Stuarts on English Grand Tour patterns is unclear. For many would-be Grand Tourists and their families travel to Rome once again had a whiff of treason to it. However, pro–Stuart Englishmen—including some Protestants—flocked to the Stuart court in Rome, where their names were duly recorded by the local agent of the British Hanoverian dynasty, Baron von Stosch.[13] After 1746 the point became moot: Stuart hopes to re-take the English crown were shattered by the Hanoverian victory in the Battle of Culloden over the pro–Stuart Jacobites. Defanged by their defeat, the Stuart court declined to the status of a tourist attraction and no longer dissuaded any but the most die-hard Hanoverians from travel to Rome.[14]

So did the 17th-century revival of the Grand Tour mean that the Protestant Reformation's inadvertent religious quarantine had lost its potency and that transalpine Europeans were once more being exposed to Roman Fever? Yes and no. It is true that the Grand Tour did attract an annual flow of young elites to Rome and, potentially, its resident plasmodia species. Nonetheless, the nature of European travel to Rome had changed substantially since the Middle Ages. While tourism to Rome resumed other human currents, such as the stream of monks, bishops, priests, and other foreign European appellants that had once flooded the papal court, were not renewed. In addition, Rome continued to attract few pilgrims from the Protestant north, since Protestantism frowned upon pilgrimage, especially to Rome.[15] In one exceptional case that proves the rule Goethe encountered two Rome-bound Germans in full pilgrim regalia, including the traditional flowing cape, round hat, and scrip bag, while Goethe was in Venice, and his first reaction was surprise, since he had never seen this archaic outfit being worn by actual pilgrims. Goethe's main previous exposure to such antique regalia had been at Weimar's "fancy-dress balls" where similar get-ups had been worn by costumed masqueraders.[16]

As for the Jubilee, some Protestants did make a point of visiting Rome to watch the holy-year ceremonies, but they seem to have been motivated as much by sheer curiosity as by religious sentiment. One anonymous English tourist to Rome who was present at the 1700 Jubilee described the Catholic pilgrims of that year as

> … a continu'd Train of Sun-burnt, sad Weather-beaten Sinners of both Sexes, crawling along the High-ways…. Bishops in Coaches, Priests on Foot, Gentlemen on Horses, Beaus upon Mules, Pilgrims upon Asses, and thus they mov'd on higgle-de-piggle-de, like … they were running headlong to the Devil…. Had I not known the occasion that call'd them together in these numbers, instead of believing 'em to be Christians going to the *Jubilee*, I should have took 'em, by their Looks and Garbs, to have been *Infidel Indians*, moving towards *Grand Paw-Waw*.[17]

Other Grand Tourists were more appreciative of Catholic religiosity in Italy, which they increasingly saw as a charming theatrical performance rather than a threat to their immortal souls. English traveler John Moore quite enjoyed the pomp and spectacle he encountered in Rome during the 1775 Jubilee and even admitted in his letters that he had succumbed to temptation and "bowed the knee to Baal," kissing the pope's slippered toe during a private audience with the pontiff.[18] English tourist Anna Jameson attended a mass in Saint Peter's led by the pope himself in 1823 and later confided that "to see the high priest of an ancient and wide-spread superstition publicly officiate in his sacred character, in the grandest Temple in the universe, surrounded by all the trappings of his

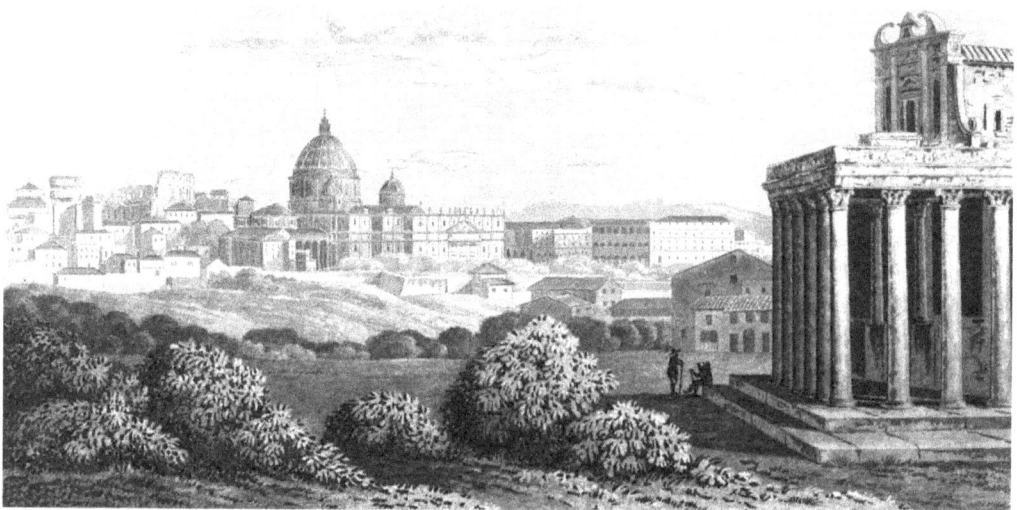

Idealized 19th-century engraving of a distant view of Rome, with Saint Peter's Basilica and the Vatican Palace in the foreground, and the Colosseum ruins behind. The artist has taken some liberties here, placing the viewer somewhere on the southern slopes of Monte Mario, though in reality from that angle the Colosseum should have been hidden behind Vatican Hill. Herman Friedlander, *Views in Italy* (London: Sir Richard Phillips and Co., 1821), p. 76.

spiritual and temporal authority, was an exhibition … to please and exalt a lively imagination." Indeed, Jameson admits that for half an hour she had almost wished herself Catholic.[19]

Some English of the period did indeed give in to this temptation and turned papist in Rome, but even those travelers who remained Protestant tended to schedule their trips to Rome with the spectacle and show of the Catholic holidays in mind. Like the majority of Rome-bound travelers since the Dark Ages, Grand Tourists tended to arrive in Rome in late November or December to ensure that they could celebrate Christmas in the city and then departed in March or April after the end of Holy Week. John Richard Digby Beste noted in April of 1824 that the English were present in the city in huge crowds "to witness the [Easter] ceremonies, which they ran after with the greatest eagerness." Once Easter was over, however, the English fled the city. By late April, Beste remarked that "scarcely an Englishman was to be found in Rome."[20] As for Beste himself, he soon followed the footsteps of other English travelers, abandoning the Eternal City in the first week of May.

Timing the Trip

In addition to arranging their trips according to the holiday cycle, visiting European tourists seem to have timed their itineraries to the weather, since Rome in the summer could be unpleasantly hot. The travelling tutor Monsieur de Blainville deeply regretted his choice to stay in Rome during the summer of 1707 where he suffered heat "never known in the memory of man" and lamented that he had "fifty times repented my shutting myself up with my companions in this cursed Place."[21] Goethe found a better way to survive the summer in Rome: he beat the heat by bribing a Vatican custodian to allow him daily access to the Sistine Chapel's cool interior. Goethe later claimed that "we even used to have meals there" beneath Michelangelo's masterpiece "and I remember that one day I was overcome by the heat and snatched a noon nap on the papal throne."[22]

Holidays and weather, however, only get us so far when trying to explain the observed patterns of European travel to Rome. Since the climate and the liturgical calendar are constants and are not subject to significant change over time, we might expect patterns of European travel to Rome to be similarly unchanging. But that was far from the case. As is clear from the radar chart below, which gives the findings of a 2019 study I conducted on transalpine travelers to Rome for the 1400–1850 time period, a significant change seems to have taken place in 1750 or so, at around the time that Grand Tour tradition reached its peak.[23] Before 1750, travel patterns to Rome were far more evenly distributed throughout the year, with a substantial number of travelers being present in Rome even in the summer. After 1750, however, the vast majority of travelers chose to visit Rome only during the December–April tourist season, which accounted for 64.9 percent of all months spent in Rome. During the same era, travel to Rome fell to a mere trickle during the July-through-September low season, which now accounted for only 13.7 percent of all travel.

Why did the European pattern of visiting Rome shift so dramatically after 1750? What had changed? I initially suspected that improvements in transportation were mainly the cause—as travel became faster and more dependable, I speculated, Europeans would have been able to fine-tune their trips to Rome to the preferred season. However, the evidence does not really bear this out. While there was some moderate improvements in the quality of roads in the modern period, including some Napoleonic-era road construction in the Alpine passes, it still took travelers at least three to four weeks to pass from London to Rome as late as the 1830s and 1840s.[24] This is somewhat faster than the six-week average for such trips in the high Middle Ages, but even during the Medieval era, a determined traveler willing to change horses could have made the trip in about 30 days, quite close to the best times set in the 1830s.[25] The real breakthrough in transportation speed would have to wait until the second half of the 19th century when railway and steamship replaced horse and sail, cutting the travel time between London and Rome to a mere 55 hours.[26] Transportation improvements, therefore, cannot explain the dramatic shift in travel patterns to Rome that occurred around 1750.

What about motives for travel? Did the post–1750 period attract a different sort of traveler than the pre–1750 era? To some degree, yes. When I compiled my list of 271 travelers for my 2019 study, I took note of what attracted each traveler to Italy and found that their motivations varied widely: 13 were involved in diplomatic service, 12 were pilgrims, 11 were ecclesiastics, and so on. The largest group by far however were tourists, whose primary or exclusive goal was to see the artistic and cultural sites of Italy. Such travelers were particularly common in the post–1750 period when they comprised 87 percent of the individuals on my list. Nonetheless, tourism was a major motivation for travel the pre–1750 period as well, when 63 percent of the travelers were tourists.[27] It seems reasonable therefore to infer that some of the difference between pre–1750 and post–1750 travel patterns can be ascribed to a greater degree of pure tourism over time. Still, given the magnitude of the seasonal shifts, other factors must have played a role as well.

Another possible explanation for the change in seasonal patterns was the dramatic increase in the number of convalescent travelers, men and women

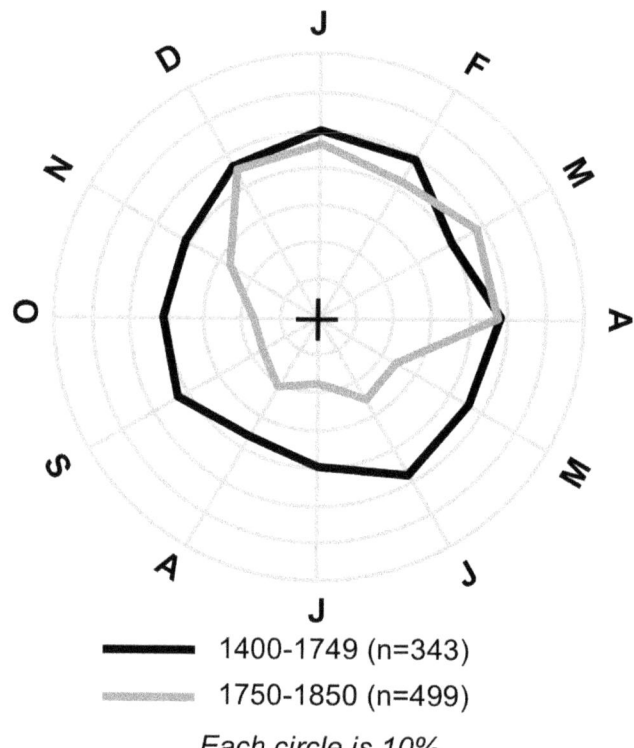

1400–1749 (n=343)
1750–1850 (n=499)

Each circle is 10%

European Visits to Rome as % of All Italian Travel. The dramatic change in European visiting patterns in Rome after 1750: while pre-1750 European visitors in Italy were in Rome throughout the calendar year, with only a slight tendency to avoid Rome in the summer malaria season, after 1750 the pattern of avoiding the Roman summer becomes far more pronounced. Benjamin Reilly, "Northern European Patterns of Visiting Rome, 1400–1850," *Journal of Tourism History*, Vol. 11, no. 2 (2019), p. 14.

who sought to remedy their ailments through a "change of the air." Such trips were by no means a new phenomenon. As early as the 1580s Michel de Montaigne visited the famous baths of Lucca in the foothills of the Apennines in hopes that its curative water would give him some relief from his chronic kidney stones.[28] What was new after 1750 was the number of European patients diagnosed with "consumption," now known as pulmonary tuberculosis, a progressive illness caused by a bacterial infection of the lungs. Such afflictions were becoming increasingly common in England with the advent of the industrial age, when urban overcrowding and lung-damaging air pollution favored the spread of the bacteria. Not understanding the true causes of the ailment, however, doctors suspected instead that consumption was a nervous disorder peculiar to middle and upper-class Englishmen caused by the "wear and tear of the living machine, mental and corporeal" due to exhaustion, "anxiety of mind" and "bad air."[29]

The antidote for bad air was of course good air, so "consumptives" were advised to leave the cold and damp of an English winter for the warmth of the Mediterranean south. Many consumptives therefore wintered in Rome, where humidity was lower and temperatures were on average 5–6 degrees Celsius higher than in London.[30] True, some consumptives were advised to avoid Rome even in the winter season due to the "sedative influence" of Rome's "malarious atmosphere," but even the sick were not immune to the many cultural attractions of the Eternal City.[31] As the 19th-century physician T.H. Burgess somewhat condescendingly noted, "no consumptive patient, who is able to drive to the spot, and to crawl over the walls," omits the traditional visit to the Colosseum by moonlight. "One might suppose that an individual in bad health would choose a more cheerful scene," Burgess noted, "at least, one less significant of his own condition; but it may be, perhaps, that ruins console each other."[32]

Managing the Threat: Grand Tourists and Malaria

The rise of tourism, including medical tourism, no doubt helps to explain why travelers abandoned Rome in the summer in the post–1750 period. However, I would argue that the most compelling explanation for the change in travel patterns is malaria—not necessarily the incidence of it, but *awareness* of it. This thesis gets strong support in my 2019 study, in which I searched each travelogue text both digitally and manually for references to malaria, bad air, miasma, *aria cattiva* (Italian for bad air) and *l'intempérance*, an idiosyncratic French term referring to seasonal fevers.[33] All told, I found that 91 of the 197 travelers on my list who spent time in Rome exhibited some knowledge of malaria in and around the Eternal City.[34]

For these authors, malaria was quintessentially a disease of place. The *campagna* was said to be particularly unhealthy, as was the marshy ground around Lake Bolsena north of Rome. Ostia and the mouths of the Tiber were reputedly feverish as well, just as they had been in the time of Belisarius over a millennium earlier. When Charlotte Anne Eaton visited ancient ruins and modern fortifications of Ostia in 1818, she found the town almost deserted. Curious, Eaton asked a local woman, "where are the people in town?" "Dead!" was the woman's laconic reply.[35]

Perhaps the most malarial landscape in Italy, however, was the Pontine Marshes, a vast coastal swamp south of Rome that had defied repeated drainage schemes since the time of Theodoric of the Ostrogoths. James Johnson described these fenlands as "neither fluid nor solid, but a hideous and heterogeneous composition of both" and declared them to be "more destructive of human life than the sword of war, or the tooth of famine."[36] According to French traveler Charles Coëtlosquet, the marsh's "rare inhabitants" were chronically "exhausted by malaria" especially "during the last two months of summer, and few people there escape them."[37] As a result, European visitors tended to avoid these marshes or else travel through them with great haste; Johnson's carriage for example "dashed" through the marsh "with little less velocity than that of an arrow from a bow," managing to cross the 28 miles of marshes in just two hours and forty minutes.[38]

As for Rome itself, visitors gave it mixed reviews, with some neighborhoods having better reputations for health than others. English traveler Alban Butler advised visitors to avoid the sparsely populated southern reaches of Rome near the Lateran Basilica since the air there was "extremely unhealthy, particularly to strangers."[39] Writing in 1828, French voyager M.R. Colomb wrote that the *aria cattiva* was bad in Rome's Saint-Pierre and Saint-Sebastian quarters, but the much frequented Champ-de-Mars [Campus Martius] area is now "covered with houses" and thus "no longer knows the effects of *mal'aria*." Colomb noted that Rome's *aria cattiva* usually set in around July 15, reaches its "highest peak towards the end of the August," and "finally ends with the first rains of October."[40] Most visitors to Rome followed the example of Marguerite Blessington, who left Rome on July 14, driven from the Eternal City "by the oppressive heat" with "'evil prophesies … of the malaria' ringing in her ears."[41] William Webb fled Rome even earlier in the summer, writing in June of 1822 that "whatever may be my sincere desire to stay and batten at Rome, I must yield as must all other strangers, since its summer is death. Such is the annual dread calamity of the Malaria."[42]

While nearly half of the authors who visited Rome made some reference to malaria in their texts, such knowledge was by no means equally distributed throughout the data sample. Instead, references to malaria increased steadily over time. While only four authors mentioned malaria or a similar term in the entire 1400–1674 period, 12 made note of malaria from 1675 to 1749, 21 between 1750 and 1799, and 34 between 1800 and 1824. What is more, this rising popular knowledge of malaria seems to have exerted a strong impact on the behavior of European travelers. As is clear from the diagram below, the number of months that visiting Europeans were willing to risk to the Roman summer declined as the knowledge of malaria rose. This relationship is epitomized by the 1800–1824 period. During these 25 years, textual mentions of malaria rose to 68.7 percent, the highest of any period, but willingness to travel to Rome during August and September bottomed out, reaching a low ebb of 6.5 percent. Fear of malaria therefore seems to have played an important role in dissuading European travelers from summer visits to the Eternal City.

The reverse was true as well: when fear of malaria subsided, European travelers became more willing to expose themselves to Rome's fever season. Rome actually saw a rebound in summertime travel in the post–1825 era and the experiences of English tourist Charles Terry help to explain why. Terry risked a visit to Rome in the mid-summer of 1846 and even decided to visit the catacombs of the church of S. Sebastiano despite their evil reputation for malarial fever. Notwithstanding the dangers, and despite the sickly appearance of the Capuchin monk that Terry hired as a guide, Terry willingly descended, candle in hand, into the very "bowels of the earth." There, he encountered inky darkness, but no human remains: there was "not a skeleton to be seen" in the catacombs,

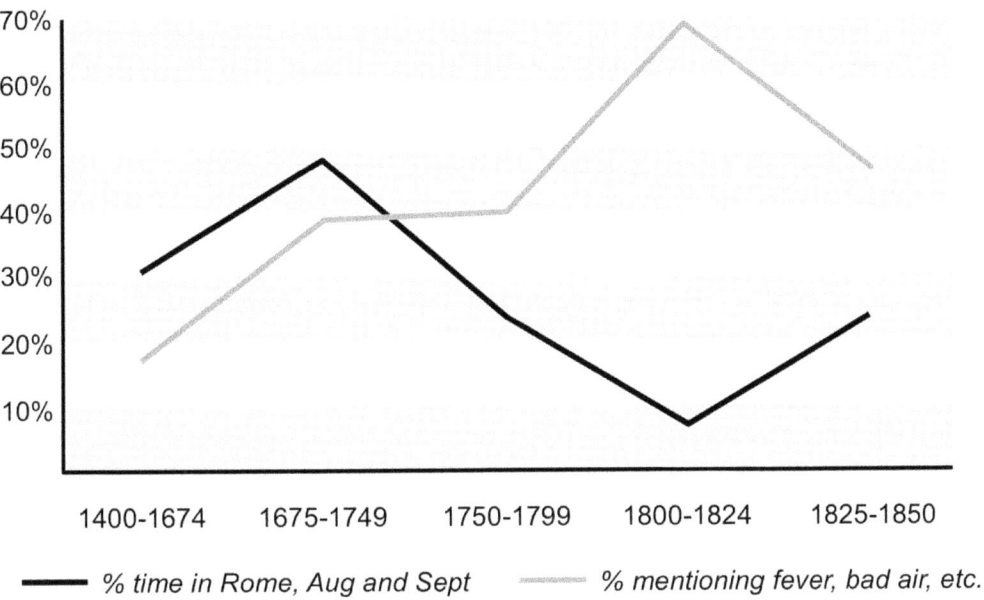

Knowledge of Malaria and Patterns of Visiting Rome, 1400–1850. Benjamin Reilly, "Seasons in Italy: Northern European Travelers, Rome, and Malaria," *Journal of Tourism and Cultural Change* (2020), p. 11.

Terry wrote, since "every bone had been taken away to serve as relics throughout the world."[43]

After seeing his fill of empty underground niches, Terry returned to the smothering heat and blinding light of the world above and paid the Capuchin the agreed-upon fee. In addition, taking pity on his guide's "pale, thin, worn, bony, eyeshrunk countenance," Terry "added a trifle for him to get some quinine to help sustain him."[44] Although Terry does not mention it—and his readers probably took it for granted—Terry was most likely following his own advice and taking regular doses of quinine as an antidote to Rome's famous fevers. If so, the treatment did not entirely work: when Terry left Rome in late August, he was glad to do so, as he felt "a touch of fever working in my veins."[45]

Quinine, which made it possible for visitors like Terry to risk a summer visit to the Eternal City, was by no means the first anti-malarial drug to be used by European travelers in Italy. Wealthy travelers had long used cinchona, the ground-up bark of a tree native to Peru, to ward off Roman Fever. In 1780, wealthy British expatriate Elizabeth Knight wrote that she had administered herself "an ounce of bark" when a malaria epidemic swept through her Corso neighborhood in Rome.[46] As late as the 1810s, cinchona was still the remedy of choice against malaria. When William Rose Stuart suffered a "short but sharp attack of the ague [acute fever]" in his summer quarters in Albano he took the bark to recover, though he complained that the cursed stuff "rendered me deaf and dizzy for four and twenty hours."[47] Cinchona was effective against malaria as it short-circuited the plasmodia's ability to dissolve hemoglobin, causing the invading plasmodia to poison themselves to death as their cellular bodies filled with toxic half-digested blood proteins.

The problem with cinchona, however, is that each parcel of the unrefined bark contains different amounts of the active anti-fever agent, making its effectiveness hit-or-miss. Treating malaria with cinchona is somewhat akin to treating your depression with St. John's Wort you have pulled from your own backyard.

Quinine is different. In 1820 two French pharmacists, Joseph Pelletier and Joseph Caventou, discovered a way to extract an alkaloid from cinchona bark and marketed it under the brand name of "Essence of Cinchona." By whatever name, quinine was a huge improvement over "the bark" since it was now possible to give the medication in precisely controlled dosages with much less chance of vomiting or other side effects.[48] What is more, quinine was water soluble and thus could be administered by means of a beverage—typically wine—to conceal the bitter taste. True, quinine (like cinchona itself) had some nasty side effects, including sweating, nausea, diarrhea, abdominal pain, tinnitus, and even temporary blindness. However, these disadvantages were well worth it since quinine is remarkably effective both as a preventive and a curative agent. In the words of 19th-century health expert Gabriele Taussig, when quinine is "given in proper times and doses" it is "as prompt as it is efficacious," often altering the "entire aspect of the disease, leaving only a simple malady, instead of one by which previously the life of the patient was threatened."[49] With the advent of quinine, malaria had met its match.

As a result, by the second half of the 19th century, quinine had transformed malaria from a deadly scourge of Rome's unacclimated visitors into a mere local curiosity. This change is most clearly visible in Henry James' popular novella *Daisy Miller*, the story of a failed romance between the socially naïve American girl Daisy and Winterborne, a buttoned-down English Grand Tourist. In the climactic scene, Winterborne catches Daisy viewing the Colosseum ruins by moonlight with an Italian paramour and berates her for putting herself at such a risk—and with such a man! Winterborne then pleads with Daisy to take her "pills," but the despondent Daisy, who has been unable to gain the acceptance she craves from Continental high society, petulantly declares that "I don't care whether I have Roman Fever or not." Daisy's foreshadowing soon proved deadly: the young American girl fell ill within a few days of visiting the Colosseum ruins and perished a week later from a "terrible case of the fever."[50] However, the reader knows that she died of a broken heart, not malaria: her refusal of the quinine which could have saved her was tantamount to suicide.

Indeed, by the time *Daisy Miller* was written in the 1880s, many European visitors from across the Alps must have seen malaria as just another one of Rome's antiquities—a vestige of the past with increasingly little relevance to the present. As Rome's population grew, mosquito habitat shrunk, banishing malaria to the margins of the town. Population growth probably triggered a beneficial autocatalytic cycle, with urban construction reducing malaria frequency and reduced malaria frequency helping to further drive urban development. What is more, transalpine Europeans became increasingly savvy to the danger they faced in Rome and timed their trips to avoid the summer malaria season accordingly. The advent of quinine after 1820 further reduced the malaria threat. For most Europeans who visited Rome after 1825, malaria was no longer worth mentioning—except, perhaps, as a plot point in a novel.

Nonetheless, the dance between visiting Europeans and Roman fever was not quite finished. True, Rome's malaria was no longer a major threat to most European travelers, who either left Rome before the fever season or used quinine to mitigate the ravages of malaria. Nonetheless, during the 19th and 20th centuries, the winds of war would propel new pulses of European soldiers over the Alps to Rome. They came as an occupying force—but as we shall see, malaria was happy to occupy the occupiers, leading to yet another wave of deadly fevers amongst transalpine visitors to the Eternal City.

16

Last Gasps

In most respects, the Grand Tour experience of John Morritt of Rokeby was entirely typical. The scion of a wealthy Yorkshire family, Morritt set out on his finishing-school adventure circa 1793 at the age of 22 immediately after his graduation from St. John's College in Oxford. After "doing" Vienna, Istanbul, Athens, and Naples, Morritt arrived in the Eternal City just before the start of the Easter season, as was customary for English traveler to Rome. Like many of his countrymen Morritt found the Catholic Holy Week ceremonies fascinating, an "inexhaustible scene of curiosity and wonder." He took the expected tour of Saint Peter's Basilica, which he compared favorably to Saint Paul's cathedral in London—though he did note that Rome lacked the "thick hazy smoke of London" that made Saint Paul's dome look higher in comparison. What is more, like other Grand Tourists of the age, Morritt fretted about Rome's miasmic air, or "*malaria*, as it is called," which made parts of Rome "scarce[ly] inhabitable" during the summer months.[1] Fear of fever, however, did not dissuade Morritt from the customary moonlight visit to the Colosseum ruins, which he described as "broken into beauty by time." "I have seen scarce any scene," Morritt wrote to his aunt, "that ever struck me more."[2]

Morritt's run-of-the-mill Grand Tour, however, was about to go off the rails. Like many Grand Tourists Morritt had intended to spend nearly a month in the art galleries of Florence after making the rounds in Rome, but his plans were interrupted by French general Napoléon Bonaparte's string of stunning victories in North Italy. "The Austrians have lost in killed and prisoners about 18,000 men, and have evacuated all their posts as far as Mantua," Morritt reported to his relatives. Worse yet, Morritt had heard that the northwest Italian state of Piedmont had already surrendered most of its fortresses to the French, effectively giving Napoléon "the keys of Italy."[3] Morritt ultimately slunk back to England by a roundabout route, taking a boat up the Adriatic Sea to Trieste from which he fled through the Alps to the relative safety of Vienna.[4] Although Morritt didn't know it at the time, he was witnessing the end of one era and the start of another. The golden age of the Grand Tour was now over, and a new age of French imperial domination of Italy had begun.

Napoléon I, Rome, and aria cattiva

French hegemony over Rome during the Napoléonic era unfolded in two acts. At first, the French ruled Rome indirectly through a puppet state, dubbed the "Ridiculous Republic" by the Romans. A few local Roman revolutionaries celebrated its creation by planting a tree of liberty in the ruin-strewn soil of the Forum. In the meantime, French officials systematically liberated Rome of its artistic treasures, seizing as many paintings, statues, and other works as they could. "This Babylon," a French commissioner said, "gorged with the spoils of the universe, must feed us and pay our debts."[5] As Susan Nicassio has quipped, the loot that France could seize from the Eternal City was "limited only by their ability to ship it."[6] The Romans had seen nothing like this since the Sack of 1527. When the populace was finally provoked into rebellion by French greed they were slaughtered in the streets and their ringleaders publicly executed. No one mourned when the Ridiculous Republic was crushed under the boots of an allied army in 1799 while Napoléon was distracted by his doomed Egyptian campaign.

The French would return to power in Rome following Napoléon's brilliant victory over the Austrians at Marengo in 1800. Bonaparte allowed the pope to maintain his sovereignty in Rome, but only under the watchful eye of the French embassy and through the new French cardinals foisted upon the pope, including Napoléon's own uncle Joseph Fesch. He even forced the pope to play a part in his most famous act of political theater, the imperial coronation ceremony in Notre Dame on 2 December 1804. To the dismay of the pope, Napoléon tore up the script mid-event and placed the imperial diadem on his own head, symbolizing he had earned the crown by his own merits and through the acclaim of the French people rather than by grace of the papacy. Five months later, he re-established the Kingdom of Italy and awarded himself another crown, the Iron Crown of the Lombards, in an elaborate ceremony celebrated in Monza Cathedral in Milan. Through these coronations, Napoléon sent clear signal to all of Europe that France was usurping Germany's old claim to Roman imperial authority. Napoléon also inherited the German Empire's old pretentions of superiority over clerical authorities. "I am Charlemagne, the sword of the Church" Napoléon wrote to his cardinal uncle. "I notify the pope of my wishes. If the pope does not accept, I shall reduce him to the situation in which was before Charlemagne."[7]

In 1808, Napoléon made good on these threats. Frustrated like the German emperors before him by the pope's unwillingness to support his imperial objectives, Napoléon seized Rome in 1808. At first, the French agreed to leave the pope in place as Rome's puppet ruler, but in 1809 Napoléon formally declared Rome to be a free imperial city under direct French authority. The pope responded by excommunicating him, who then retaliated by arresting Pius VII and imprisoning him in France. Napoléon was now sovereign of Rome, though he theoretically ceded that sovereignty to his first-born son, who was duly declared "King of Rome" in 1811. In the future, Napoléon decreed, all emperors of the Bonaparte dynasty would be crowned first in France and then in Rome, the "second city" of the French Empire, just as it had been during the Carolingian age.[8]

Although theoretical sovereignty over Rome was held by Napoléon and his kin, real authority lay in the hands of a French-appointed bureaucrat whose power grew out of the gun barrels of a substantial French military garrison. The man in question, at least from 1810 onwards, was the young prefect Camille de Tournon, whose excellent and systematic study of Rome and the surrounding area is one of our best sources for the period. De Tournon had never been to Rome before being appointed to rule it; for de Tournon, as for most men of the period, Rome was the land of "dreams and epic poetry and opera and nursery stories, not a place where real life people lived."[9] And like many others European visitors before him, de Tournon found that the actual city of Rome did not match up to his sky-high expectations. Upon reaching the city's "sacred soil," he wrote to his mother that the "appearance of its ruins and the desert [the *campagna*] which surrounds it fills the soul with a singular melancholy." Perhaps, de Tournon hoped, he might play a role in "plant[ing] some seeds of prosperity in this soil which is so poetic, but so wretched."[10]

Despite these first impressions, de Tournon soon discovered that the impoverished appearance of Rome's *campagna* was not due to the laziness of the inhabitants but rather the region's "*aria cattiva*," or bad air. There was nothing new about this—any well-read Grand Tourist could have told him as much. What set de Tournon apart was his systematic and scientific approach to the problem. Indeed, for de Tournon, cracking the code of *aria cattiva* was literally a matter of life or death, since thousands of French soldiers were under his care and he knew from history that foreign troops stationed in Rome traditionally paid "a terrible tribute to death."[11]

While de Tournon does not provide the reader with systematic mortality records for French troops in Rome during the imperial occupation, the anecdotes he does provide suggest the French suffered horribly from fever. One regiment of 80 men stationed at the Piazza del Popolo the northern edge of Rome suffered 30 malaria cases in just three summer weeks, and 27 of the afflicted died.[12] In the same year, de Tournon found that 170 out of 265 customs officers guarding Rome's coastline fell ill; 22 of these men died and another 45 had to be reassigned.[13] France had to defeat malaria, or at least understand it, before malaria defeated France.

To this end de Tournon made a careful study of the problem, mapping out the physical and temporal parameters of Roman Fever much more systematically than anyone before him. Much of de Tournon's findings confirmed what German emperors and English Grand Tourists already knew—that the high malaria season was from August to September and that Lake Bolsena, the *campagna*, the vicinity of ancient Ostia, and the Maremma plain of Tuscany were all hotbeds of fever.[14] De Tournon also found that as a general rule the malarial zone ended heights of 120 to 150 meters above the *campagna* plain. Borrowing native Italian terminology, de Tournon argued that places below that elevation had *pessima* [worst], *cattiva* [bad], or *sospetta* [suspect] air, while above that elevation the air was *buona* [good], *fina* [fine], or *ottima* [excellent]. Thus Monte Mario, "raised 130 meters above the level of the plain," was in the *aria buona* range, and thus was "inhabitable year-round," a fact that retroactively explains both why this hilltop was the preferred camping-ground of the German emperors and why it later became a preferred country residence of the exiled English royal dynasty, the Stuarts. At 180 meters, Tivoli's air was even better, in the "*ottima*" range, as was the air of Frascati, Albano, and Velletri in the Alban hills.[15] On the other end of the spectrum was the Pontine Marshes, cursed with the most *pessima* air in Italy. These marshes were all but abandoned as a consequence: "the virgin forests of America," de Tournon observed, "do not offer a more savage aspect."[16]

Interestingly, although de Tournon regarded the Pontine Marshes as the very epitome of a malarial landscape, he did not believe that malaria was caused by mere proximity to marshy land. "The closeness or distance from stagnant water has little influence on the state of health," de Tournon noted, for "some high and perfectly dry areas of plain between Rome and Tivoli, and Rome and Frascati, are nearly as unhealthy as the edges of the marshes at Ostia." On this point de Tournon was perfectly correct. Although *Anopheles* mosquitoes need stagnant water to breed, once they are born they can travel up to five kilometers across flat terrain in search of blood meals.[17] This observation was a breakthrough of sorts as it challenged the old paradigm that malaria was caused by the foul stench of rotting vegetation, a theory still embraced by influential geologist and malaria authority John MacCullough as late as the 1820s.[18]

Nonetheless, de Tournon never ended the threat that Roman Fever posed to the Napoleonic occupying army. In fact, it is likely that the French presence in Rome was itself a factor in making the problem worse. Napoléon's occupation of the Eternal City discouraged Grand Tourists and pilgrims from visiting Rome, much to the dismay of the guides, art sellers, innkeepers, prostitutes, souvenir mongers, and restaurateurs who depended upon their business.[19] What is more, the new Babylonian captivity of the pope after 1809 must have greatly reduced the flow of appellants, newly-elected bishops, and other such ecclesiastical visitors to Rome. As a result, Rome's population fell sharply during the Napoleonic years, from nearly 135,000 in 1809 to 123,000 just two years later, and perhaps a low of 118,000 by 1813.[20] Since malaria rates rise as population density declines—a phenomenon that de Tournon himself noted—the stage was set for a temporary resurgence of malarial fevers in the *caput mundi*.[21]

And indeed, the travel accounts of the few travelers who did brave the roads to Rome in this period make it clear that malaria was on the rise during and immediately after the Napoleonic era. Prussian traveler John Bramsen recounted in 1814 that "*malaria is found yearly to spread so widely*" that that it was "making increasing advances upon Rome itself," threatening to turn the city into "little better than a splendid wilderness … at certain seasons many parts of Rome, especially those in the vicinity of the river, are almost deserted."[22] Two years later Marie-Henri Beyle, who is better known by his pen name Stendahl, found that "the *aria cattiva* advances yearly [in Rome]. Places which were reputedly the most healthy for the last thirty years are being attacked."[23]

By 1817, Napoléon was in exile and the pope was once again enthroned in Rome, but the malaria situation did not immediately improve. The perceptive French traveler Louis Simond, who visited Rome in the winter of 1817–1818, found that most of Rome was "uninhabited and uninhabitable due to the risk of acquiring a violent tertian fever, which by its long duration often became mortal." What is more, Simond correctly diagnosed the link between malaria and population density, noting that "the *mal'aria* affects the diverse quarters of Rome in proportion inverse to their population." As a result, Rome's outlying districts were becoming "each day more deserted, because they are unhealthy, and more unhealthy because they are deserted."[24] Jean-Pierre Giegler's 1818 travel guide on Italy makes much the same points. Because of the recent population decline, Giegler argues, "bad air" now "circles Rome from all direction" and has "insensibly conquered … the ancient capital of the world … convert[ing] to solitude many quarters that were once well peopled" and threatening to reduce Rome to a "frightful desert."[25]

By Giegler and Simond's time, however, Rome's population was beginning to tick upwards once again as foreign visitors took advantage of the post–Napoléonic peace to return to the Eternal City. During Holy Week of 1818, Simond noted, Rome attracted a "crowd of strangers from the extremities of Europe, especially England."[26] Just two years later, English traveler Thomas Pennington found Rome so thick with visitors in late March that the Sistine Chapel could not accommodate the throng of humanity attracted by the Maundy Thursday mass. In the end, women and VIPS were given priority seating, but all others were "left to mob it as they could," leading to a virtual scrum in which handkerchiefs were lost and coats were torn.[27] Three days later, during Easter mass in Saint Peter's, Pennington observed "there were so many English in the church, that we almost forgot for the time that we were out of England."[28] Clearly, Rome was on the road to recovery.

Imperial Redux: French Bodies, Roman Parasites and Napoléon III

A generation later, however, European travel to Rome was disrupted by yet another Napoleonic occupation. The architect of invasion this time was Louis Napoléon, nephew of the great Bonaparte, who rose in popularity by catering to conservative Catholic sentiment in France: his election manifesto was 1848 was "religion, family, property, the eternal basis of all social order."[29] Thanks to these conservative ideals, not to mention his famous name, he managed to secure election as president of France following the Revolution of 1848. Once in power, however, he borrowed a page from his uncle's authoritarian playbook, abolishing the elected assembly and declaring himself emperor of France.

He also followed his uncle's example of sending troops to Rome, though for different reasons than his illustrious predecessor. In late 1848, the papacy begged the French for assistance against the Italian nationalists who took advantage of the 1848 revolutions to seize power in Rome. To placate conservative Catholics in France, who saw these revolutionaries as an impious rabble, Napoléon III sent 10,000 men to the Roman Coast. However, the French force proved to be far too weak to take the city, whose defenses had been stiffened by the arrival of Italian revolutionary general Giuseppe Garibaldi. As a result, the French were forced to hunker down and await reinforcement, and by start of June *P. vivax* was beginning to debilitate the French force. According to a French newspaper correspondent accompanying the expedition, "one hundred men swollen with malaria fever came in here yesterday" and he predicted that "in another week the hospitals will not contain the number of sick who will claim admittance."[30] The French either needed to retreat, or attack. Spending the summer in the malarial Roman *campagna* was not an option.

Napoléon III decided to attack, and despite heroic resistance by Garibaldi's soldiers and other revolutionary fighters Rome fell to French forces on July 3, right at the cusp of Rome's *P. falciparum* season. If the French had hoped to be safe from malaria once they were within the walls of the Eternal city, however, they were rudely disappointed. By high summer the hastily-established military hospitals were overflowing with the sick and nearly every bed was occupied by a fever patient. At the apex of the epidemic the hospital dedicated to fevers, Santo Spirito, received a hundred new fever patients a day and fully 12 percent of the French force was incapacitated.[31] All told, 781 French troops would die in fever hospitals in the first year of the French occupation of Rome, almost four times as many as were killed during the military siege. As is typical of *P. Falcparum* infections, the French death rate peaked in August and September before declining with the temperatures of late autumn.[32]

As in the day of de Tournon, the leaders of the 1849–1870 occupational force wanted to solve the malaria problem, not just describe it. To this end French medical official Felix Jacquot conducted a close and detailed study about the relative health different sites in hopes that future military expeditions to Rome would "no longer recklessly post their soldiers in places where death and malady must devour them."[33] Jacquot found that troops

16. Last Gasps 173

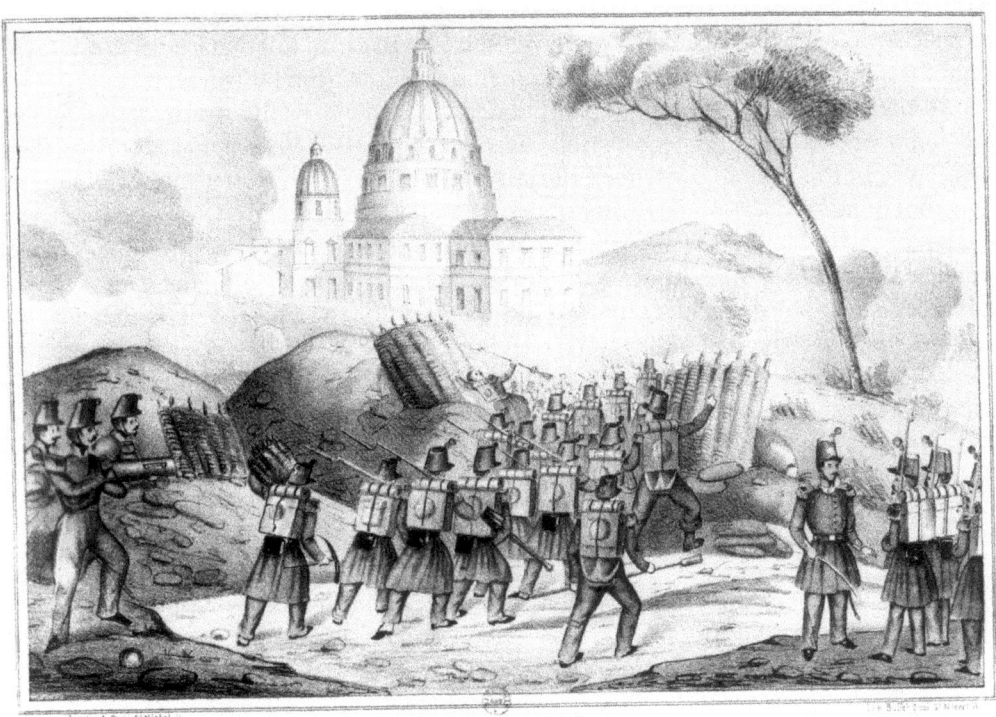

SIÈGE & PRISE DE ROME, 1849.

The 1849 French siege of Rome. Photo 12/Alamy Stock Photo.

posted near the well-populated center of town suffered low rates of malarial infection. So too did the troops garrisoned in the Alban hills and, to a lesser degree, the papal *villeggiatura* town of Viterbo. On the other hand, soldiers encamped in the "vacant, uninhabited peripheral zone, which makes up two-thirds of the city," suffered far higher morbidity and death rates.[34] French troops stationed near the Forum, the lair of Saint Sylvester's dragon and the site of the Lacus Curtius, suffered from particularly high rates of malaria. So did the artillery regiment stationed near the Piazza de Popolo where once grew the haunted nut-tree that had sprung from the grave of Nero.[35] In many ways, Rome's landscape of fever had changed little since the Middle Ages.

Nonetheless, the French occupation of Rome was different from its Medieval counterparts in one crucial way: unlike their German imperial predecessors, the French had quinine. True, there was not yet any clear consensus on how this drug was to be used. As Jacquot points out, despite France's north Africa experiences "the greatest anarchy reign[ed] amongst medical doctors as to the treatment of endo-epidemic summer-autumn fevers." Doctors were in "complete disagreement as to doses of sulfate of quinine, as to the timing and dosage of evacuants, as to the necessity or utility of anti-inflammatory and anti-spasmodic medications, etc."[36] Some doctors tried to treat their malarial patients with vomatives or with arsenic combined with laxatives.[37] When French doctors did prescribe quinine, they often gave it in insufficient doses: in general, French troops showing malarial symptoms were given a single gram of quinine, while two grams is the recommended daily dosage for quinine today.[38] Trial and error, however, proved to be an invaluable teacher, and French doctors began to make progress treating malarial infections. The second year of the occupation, in fact, witnessed a huge spike once again of August–September fevers, but the overall death toll that year was only 113.[39] If not for quinine, French losses would have undoubtedly been far worse.

In the end, the French military would occupy Rome for a full twenty years, leaving only in the aftermath of France's terrible defeat in the Franco-Prussian war. During those twenty years, the French presence in Rome had been a thorn in the side of the Italian Kingdom of Sardinia, a modernizing state based in Northwest Italy, whose goal was unification of the Italian peninsula. When that thorn was finally removed in 1870 by French military disaster, Sardinian King Victor Emmanuel and his prime minister Count Cavour moved quickly to annex papal territories in Italy despite the protests of the papacy. Not even the Vatican remained under papal control—the popes would not regain sovereignty over the Vatican City until 1929, when Mussolini re-gifted it to the Catholic Church in return for formal papal acceptance of the reality of Italian unification.

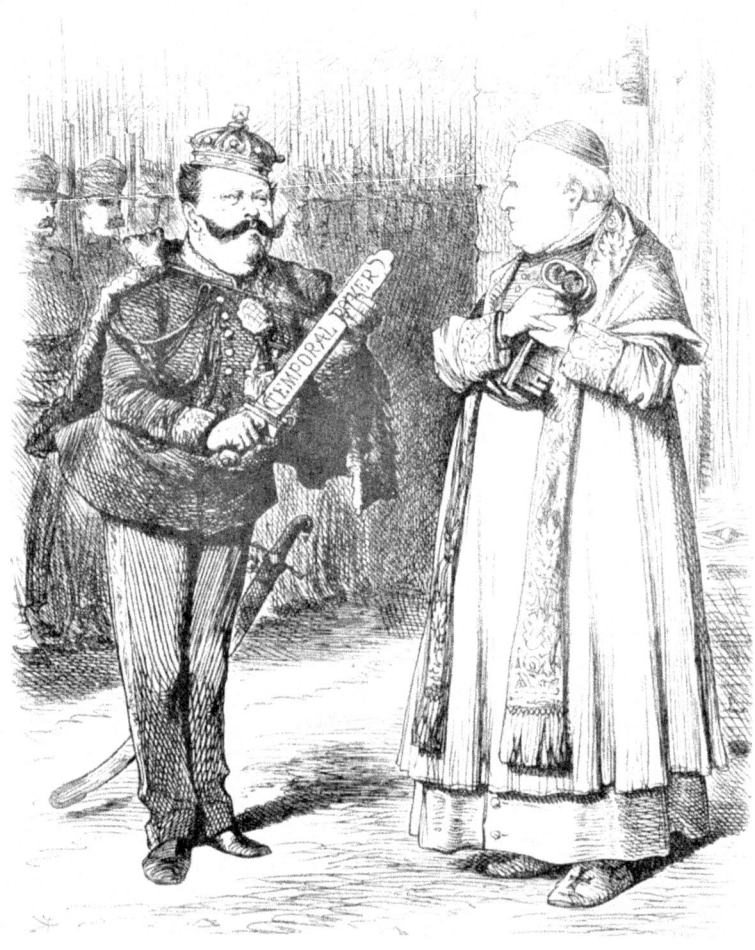

A cartoon from *Punch* depicting Victor Emmanuel (holding a sword marked TEMPORAL POWER) compelling the Pope Pius IX to surrender control over Rome. The original caption read, "I must needs surrender the *sword*, my son: but *I keep the keys!*" Eleanor McNees, "'Punch' and the Pope: Three Decades of Anti-Catholic Caricature," *Victorian Periodicals Review*, Vol. 37, No. 1 (Spring 2004), p. 38.

Independent Italy and Malaria

Italy was now unified for the first time since the age of the Roman Empire. Nonetheless, a cloud of *aria cattiva* continued to hang over the young Italian state. Count Cavour himself would die of malaria, probably contracted from a mosquito born in the rice paddies of his own northwest Italian estate. Victor Emmanuel, the "father of the fatherland," died from malaria as well.[40] Some Italians even argued against making Rome the capital of the new Italian state for fear of malaria; *caput mundi* Rome may be, but the city remained synonymous with fever.[41] These fears seemed confirmed in 1879 when a "true malarial pandemy raged" in Rome, triggered by exceptionally high spring rainfall. In all, Rome's hospitals received 34,217 fever cases, an increase of 80 percent over the previous year.[42] Thankfully, quinine was there to mitigate the mortality.

After 1880, the malaria rate in Rome began to drop as rapid population growth filled in the Eternal City's empty spaces, but the situation in the countryside seemed to be getting worse.[43] In the post-unification period, a number of new rail lines were built to knit the young country together. Unfortunately, these railways became new hotbeds of malaria infection. Track construction led to the damming up of many small streams and the creation of new quarries and ditches, creating prime *Anopheles* habitat. What is more, Italy's railroad builders had an inexhaustible appetite for wooden ties, leading to large-scale deforestation, erosion of upland soils, and the creation of new malarial lowland marshes.[44] According to Italian senator and health expert Luigi Torelli, the cost of quinine distribution to railway workers alone was 1.5 million lira per year in the late 1870s, "a true tribute," Torelli wrote, "to *Dea Febbre*."[45] If you factored in the cost of fever hospitals, the price of the quinine consumed by the general public, the work hours lost to malarial languor, and the neglect of productive but malarial land, Torelli argued, the true financial cost of malaria was far higher.

In addition to this tribute in coin, the malaria continued to demand a high payment of human lives from the inhabitants of the Italian peninsula. According to Torelli, 43,000 Italian soldiers had been treated for malarial fevers in military hospitals in the second half of the 1870s alone.[46] As late as 1898, Italian civilian hospitals were still admitting approximately two million malaria patients each year.[47] Hospital statistics suggested that about 186,000 Italians lost their lives to malaria between 1887 and 1898, but health department officials suspected that the true malaria death toll may have topped 100,000 annually.[48] In some areas of Italy, the malaria infection rate could be as high as 40–90 percent, though it varied with rainfall and temperature from year to year.[49] As always, the malarial Minotaur preferred to take its tribute in children. Boys and girls under five years of age accounted for 50 percent of the annual victims.[50] Demographers found that the life expectancy for farm workers in highly malarial parts of Italy was only 22.3 years, more than 13 years fewer than in the healthier towns of the mountains and the Italian north.[51]

As for transalpine Europeans, they now looked upon Italy's fevers with continued curiosity but with considerably less fear. Quinine might have been too expensive for many poor Italian *paisanos* but was easily affordable for European tourists from beyond the Alps, especially after the price of quinine dropped from $100 per kilo in 1880 to only $7 in 1893.[52] What is more, the railway and the steamship vastly improved transportation time and reliability, making it ever easier to time vacations to a preferred month, week, or even day. By the century's end, Roman Fever expert W. North claimed, "vast majority" of travelers were arriving in Rome "between November and April" and thus ran "practically run no risk at all" of malaria infection. Despite the safety of the season, many such travelers never strayed far from their quinine which "may without exaggeration be said to form a not inconsiderable portion of the dietary of such mere sight-seers."[53] In the age of Daisy Miller, death by malaria was a mental failing rather than a physical one—the result of poor planning, ignorance, neglectfulness, or perhaps willing self-destruction.

Thanks to the quinine and the steam engine, the number of European travelers to Rome exploded in the century after 1850. Already by 1886, the number of foreign visitors to Rome may have reached 18–25,000 annually, and many of these were from Northern European countries like Britain and Germany, though Americans made up an increasingly large share of the tourists. By 1913, however, Italy was receiving 90,000 travelers annually from Britain alone.[54] Nearly all of these visitors departed Italy in the summer months or else left Rome for popular *villeggiatura* spots in the Apennines or the cooler north, where they girded themselves against the rigors of summer with ample doses of quinine. As a result, in the judgment of historian John Pemble, by the turn of the 20th century, "death from malaria among visitors to the large Mediterranean cities was extremely rare."[55]

Fighting the Fever

For Europeans living north of the Alps, malaria was largely forgotten, but it was not yet gone, as the Italians still living in malarial districts knew all too well. Italian mothers of the 19th and early 20th century were still burying their babes during the summer heats, just like the mothers of Lugnano had done nearly a millennium and a half before. No one in Italy disagreed with Torelli that the scourge of malaria had to be stopped. But how? To eradicate a disease, you must eliminate its cause. But what caused malaria? By this time, most experts accepted that the malaria was not an exclusively Italian disease, but was in fact the same disease that seasonally afflicted the fishermen of the English Fens, the coast-dwellers of Holland, and even the Brahmins of India.[56] That realization, however, made malaria an even more perplexing riddle, since researchers were forced to look for commonalities connecting disparate sites with varying latitudes, altitudes, soils chemistries, rainfall patterns, and temperature profiles. The question remained, why was "Roman Fever" so much more deadly than the otherwise similar tertian fevers that prevailed elsewhere in Europe?[57]

The experts of the time had many opinions, but no real answers. Echoing a common definition, Torelli defined "malaria" as "air which contains suspended elements that are harmful to man when breathed" and believed that these airborne toxins usually but not always arose from stagnant water.[58] Malaria expert Francesco Puccinotti, on the other hand, discounted the miasma theory of aerial particles and argued instead that malaria was produced by some sort of "terrestrial radiation" that was strongest in flat and uncultivated land.[59] As late as the 1890s influential malariologist W. North was still clueless about the causal agent of malaria. North argued that waterlogging of the subsoil seemed to play a role, but so did "sudden and excessive change[s] of temperature" such as the transition from dawn to day and evening to night.[60] Ironically, North believed that mosquito nets were protective against malaria—not by blocking mosquitoes, but because they "hinder[ed] radiation," much like the fishing nets used by some English gardeners to protect their plants from harmful frost.[61]

Just a year after North had published this nonsense, the shroud of ignorance over malaria was finally lifted. While stationed in India, British medical doctor Dr. Ronald Ross established that malaria parasites were transmitted by bites of the *Anopheles* mosquito. Almost simultaneously, Italian malariologist Giovanni Grassi came to the same independent conclusion. Grassi also demonstrated that malaria had several distinct types, including *P. vivax* and *P. falciparum*, which in turn solved the mystery as to why "Roman Fever" was uniquely deadly.

Grassi and Ross's findings were the tools the Italians needed to attack malaria at its source. As the 19th century gave way to the 20th, the Italian government inaugurated what malaria scholar Frank Snowden has called a program of "eradication … through chemotherapy." Anti-malaria workers used larvicides to control *Anopheles* breeding in malarial hotspots within Italy while quinine was distributed *en masse* in hopes of expunging the parasites from the collective Italian blood stream. These efforts were further supported by an educational campaign designed to combat popular misconceptions about the disease and extoll the virtues of quinine, which for many Italian peasants was quite literally a bitter pill to swallow.[62] As a consequence of these efforts the overall death rate from malaria in Italy fell from over 20,000 a year in the late 19th century to less than 4,000 in 1910.[63] The anti-malaria campaign proved particularly successful in the Roman *campagna*, where malaria rates fell from 32 percent to only 4 percent from 1900 to 1906, laying the groundwork for resettlement and agricultural development of this long-neglected plain.[64]

Although Italian anti-malarial measures had subdued the beast, they by no means killed it. Eradication through quinine, the Italian health authorities were eventually forced to acknowledge, was an impossible dream. Even high doses of quinine could not eradicate malaria parasites that were hiding dormant in the liver, a fact that greatly complicated the task of eradication. What is more, many Italians refused to take their quinine consistently, using it only in the acute stages of a fever crisis. Other Italians were unable to stomach quinine or were unwilling to tolerate the mediation's numerous side-effects.[65] Malaria therefore persisted and even staged a brief comeback tour during World War I when it ran riot in the bodies of soldiers who had been drafted from fever-free parts of Italy and then marched into malarial zones for their military service.[66]

In the years following World War I, therefore, the Italians adopted a new anti-malarial strategy. Benito Mussolini and his violently nationalistic Fascist party had by then seized power in Italy, capitalizing on Italian disillusionment with the post-war settlement and fear of Communist revolution. In 1928, Mussolini decided to resume the anti-malarial offensive, but this time with a distinctive Fascist spin. Rather than relying on chemical eradication, Mussolini focused on large-scale drainage works and set his sights in particular on the Pontine Marshes, which had been synonymous with malarial fever since the time of the ancient Romans. At Mussolini's direction Italian engineers dug an elaborate network of canals through the marshes, ensuring that spring-season floods would now be diverted out to sea. What is more, in keeping with the Fascist vision that the Italian farmer was the backbone of the state, Mussolini re-settled nearly 60,000 war veterans into the 5,000 farms and two new towns he founded in the reclaimed Latina province. Settlers were protected from malaria not only by the drainage works but through quinine distribution, modern housing with screened windows, and the liberal use of a new larvicide, Paris green.[67]

Mussolini's anti-malarial campaign was, according to Snowden, a "dramatic but qualified success." The construction of the drainage works, popularly dubbed "Mussolini canals," was performed by manual laborers in atrocious conditions and many of these diggers and dredgers no doubt succumbed to fever. What is more, progress was achieved by diverting anti-malarial resources from other areas, particularly the highly malarial far south. Furthermore, academic life stagnated in Italy during the Fascist era, costing Italy its lead at the forefront of anti-malarial science.[68] Nonetheless, the Latina province project itself was a glittering propaganda triumph, allowing Mussolini to brag that he and the Fascist party had at long last "liberated Rome from the toxic fields that encircled it."[69]

The Latina scheme also had a strategic angle to it: Mussolini hoped that the lessons learned in the *bonificazione* of Italy would be applicable to the malarial regions of

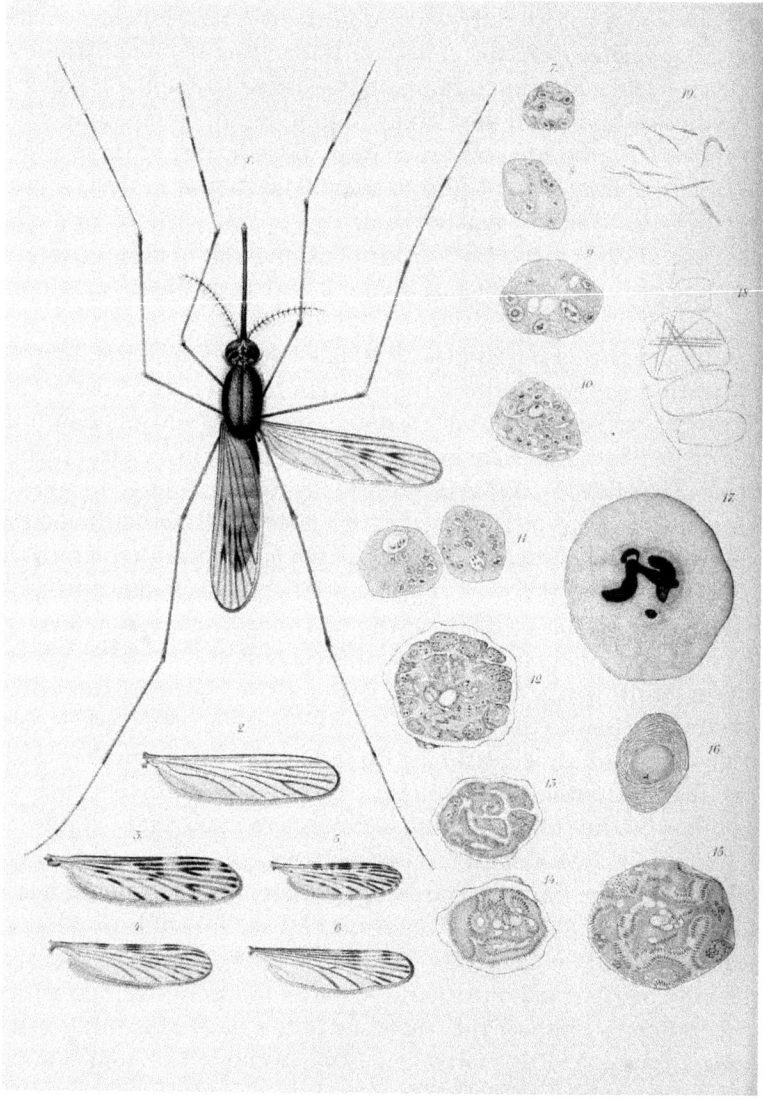

An illustration by Giovanni Grassi of *Anopheles* mosquito variants and various stages of parasite development within the blood cells. Giovanni Battista Grassi, *Studi di Zoologo Sulla Malaria*, 2nd ed. (Rome: R. Accademia dei Lincei, 1901), Plate 5.

Africa. Not content to rule Italy alone, Mussolini dreamed of presiding over a vast new Roman Empire, larger than the original, that would "join the two shores of the Mediterranean and of the Indian Ocean into a single Italian territory."[70] Mussolini moved a step in this direction in 1935–1936 when his modern army overwhelmed the African state of Ethiopia and added it to Italy's existing holdings on the Horn of Africa. Future expansion in Africa and Asia, however, was blocked by the existing colonial holdings of the English and French, who occupied the lion's share of the territory that Mussolini needed to achieve his imperial vision.

As a result, Mussolini allied himself with the rising power of Germany and Japan and in June of 1940 declared war on Britain and France. It soon became clear, however, that Mussolini's grandiose imperial dreams far exceeded Italy's modest military capabilities. Italy was able to conquer Greece and the Balkans during World War II, but only with considerable German help. What is more, Italy was even less successful in North Africa, where his Libyan-based invasion of British Egypt turned into a rout after the British victory at El Alamein, and both Libya and Tunisia were lost to a British counterattack. A year later, the United States and Britain took the war to Italian territory, invading the strategically important island of Sicily.

Defeated on the battlefield and by this time wildly unpopular at home, Mussolini was removed from power and arrested by King Victor Emmanuel III on July 25, 1943. The new government publicly resolved to keep fighting the war, but privately opened negotiations with the Allied powers and eventually signed an armistice on September 3. Unwilling to allow Italy to become a back-door invasion route to Germany, however, the Nazis rushed into Italy to fill the void, and occupied the peninsula as far south as Naples.

1944: The Last Epidemic

The stage was now set for one final encounter between malaria and an invading foreign army, though this time with several new twists. For once, malaria was not a problem for the occupying Germans, who were well-advised by their own malaria specialists and who benefited from the *bonificazione* work accomplished by previous Italian governments. However, the Germans seem to have been intent on making malaria a problem for the advancing Allied forces, perhaps in hopes of re-creating the malarial epidemic disasters that had befallen previous foreign invaders into Italy. Knowing that the Latina province and the Roman *campagna* would soon become a war zone, the Germans destroyed the water pumps and dynamited sea walls and drainage ditches that Mussolini had built. The Germans even deliberately introduced seawater into the restored Pontine Marshes, perhaps in hopes of creating salinity conditions favorable to anthropophilic *Anopheles labranchiae* mosquitoes. As a result, according to Edward Snowden, "not only were mosquitoes immensely more numerous in 1944 than ever before, but also that nearly all of the mosquitoes present were *Anopheles labranchiae* rather than their harmless competitors."[71] Germany's actions, Snowden contends, were designed to "slow Allied northward progress" by knowingly "creating a medical emergency" in Lazio province. As such, they constitute a "deliberate act of biological warfare," a war crime according to the terms of the 1925 Geneva Protocol on biological and chemical weapons.[72]

These are bombshell accusations, and they have not gone unchallenged. In 2010 medical researcher Erhard Geissler and security expert Jeanne Guillemin attacked

Snowden's "biological warfare" claims, arguing that Germany's primary goal was to render the area impassible to the tanks and heavy equipment of the allied forces, not to foster malaria infections amongst Italian civilians. What Snowden failed to understand, these authors contend, is the important legal distinction between "a battlefield tactic that results in grievous harm to civilians and the active promulgation of biological warfare."[73] I suspect that the truth lies somewhere in between the Snowden and the Geissler/Guillemin positions. Based on the weight of evidence Snowden presents, it seems likely that the Germans knew that their actions would foster malaria infections, but as Geissler and Guillemin point out, the advancing allies rather than Italian civilians were the intended target of the Germans.

If so, the German tactic misfired. As it turned out, the Allies brought with them two powerful talismans against malarial infection: DDT, a miracle insecticide, and atabrine, a synthetic substitute for quinine. Thanks to their protection, the invading British and Americans suffered relatively few malaria cases. The same, however, could not be said for the Italians of Latina province, who had lost most of their hard-won acquired immunity following the successful Italian anti-malarial programs of the early 20th century. The result was a dramatic spike in malaria cases, 110,000 of which were recorded in hospitals between 1944 and 1946, a twenty-fold increase over the previous five years. What is more, given the inadequacy of wartime record keeping, these statistics probably understate the scale of the problem—one Italian health expert suspected that Latina province suffered 100,000 malaria cases in 1944 alone, and that many of these were of the dangerous *P. falciparum* variety.[74] Ironically, a foreign invasion of Italy had led to a malaria epidemic, but this time around it was the Italians and not the invaders who suffered the consequences.

Thankfully for the long-suffering Italian people, the 1944–46 outbreak of malaria proved to be its parting shot. Almost as soon as the war ended, Italian medical professionals partnered with U.N. health agencies and the American Rockefeller Foundation to eliminate malaria from Italy once and for all by using DDT to destroy malaria's *Anopheles* vectors. Following aggressive residential spraying campaigns, malaria was eradicated in mainland Italy by the late 1940s and Sicily followed close behind in the 1950s. Finally, in November 1970, the WHO delighted both Italians and transalpine Europeans alike when it declared that Italy was officially malaria free.[75] At long last, Roman Fever was no more.

Conclusion

In early September of 2017, a young Italian girl named Sofia Zago showed signs of fever, so her parents hurried her to the local hospital in their home town of Trento. Doctors initially believed that Sofia's ailment was nothing worse than a bad sore throat. To their astonishment, however, Sofia's blood work came back positive for *P. falciparum* malaria, a disease that her doctors had initially ruled out since Sofia had never been to a malarial area. Poor Sofia was immediately packed into an ambulance and rushed to a hospital in Brescia with more experience with tropical diseases. Despite the move, Sofia fell into a cerebral malarial coma shortly after her diagnosis, never regained consciousness, and died in the early morning hours of September 4.[1]

Sofia's shocking death attracted a lot of attention at the time and, not surprisingly in this partisan day and age, different groups gave it a different spin based on their pre-conceived notions. For some environmentalists, the return of a deadly tropical disease to an area where it had been abolished could only be the result of global warming. Right-wing Italian nationalists, on the other hand, ascribed Sofia's death to uncontrolled illegal immigration from disease-ridden Africa.

In actuality, neither of these scenarios hold water. While global warming is a real phenomenon and is likely to prove problematic in many other ways, rising temperatures alone are unlikely to lead to a return of malaria in places where it has been eliminated. As we have seen, malaria requires several preconditions to develop, namely the existence of an *Anopheles* vector, an existing reservoir of infected humans, and sufficiently high temperatures to foster its development within the mosquito. Just raising the temperature alone will not automatically raise the malaria rate: to return to the dance analogy, global warming might add new square footage to the dance floor, but malaria cannot jitterbug there unless someone invites it to the ball. So long as Italy remains a first-world country with a stable government and well-developed medical sector, endemic malaria is unlikely to return to its shores.[2]

The illegal immigration hypothesis, although a bit closer to the mark, is not quite right either. Sofia's malaria was eventually traced back to a hospital in Trento which Sofia visited regularly to treat her childhood-onset diabetes. While Sofia was there, the hospital also hosted two young African girls being treated for *P. falciparum* they had brought back with them as a ghoulish souvenir of a recent trip to Burkina Faso. Although investigators are not entirely sure how Sofia was infected, an analysis revealed that Sofia's strain of malaria was identical to that of the Burkina Faso girls. In all likelihood, then, Sofia was infected through a hospital error, perhaps from a blood-work mix-up or by the re-use of a contaminated medical instrument. What is certain is that immigration into Italy, whether legal or illegal, cannot by itself re-introduce malaria on a large scale without an efficient insect vector, and the home range of anthropophilic mosquitoes in Italy is much smaller today than it was before the 20th-century eradication campaigns.[3]

The main take-away from Sofia Zago's tragic death, then, is that malaria is no longer native to Italy. All reported 21st-century cases have been introduced cases, irruptions from the outside. However, as we have seen throughout this book, the exact opposite situation prevailed throughout most of recorded European history. For much of the past two millennia, Italy has been synonymous with fever, and foreign travelers into Italy, far from introducing malaria plasmodia into Italy, were the ones who generally suffered the most from its deadly effects.

Had Italy been a backwater, attracting only the occasional traveler, Italy's fevers would not have been a problem. But the opposite was the case: Rome was the *caput mundi*, the threshold of the apostles, the wonderland of art, the Holy City of the Holy Church, and the fountainhead of imperial legitimacy. As a result, the Eternal City received an uncountable stream of European pilgrims, appellants, soldiers, kings, emperors, artists, invalids, spies, churchmen, and tourists over the last 15 centuries. Most of these roamers eventually made their way back home, but not all—since Europeans living north of the Alps generally lacked acquired immunity to malaria, especially Rome's endemic *P. falciparum* infections, a fraction of these visitors left their bodies in Italy. Exactly how many is impossible to say. What we do know is that non–Italians were about three times more likely than native Italians to die in Rome during the August–September fever season, suggesting that the loss of life might have been considerable indeed.

Of course, visiting Europeans were by no means helpless against the threat of Roman Fever. From the 17th century onwards, cinchona and quinine were available to mitigate the malaria risk of Rome. Before then, the best medicine available to travelers from the unacclimated north was their own two feet: from at least the time of Alcuin, visiting Europeans were advised to flee Rome and the Italian south before the pestilential summer season, when bad air haunted the streets of the Eternal City. As we have seen throughout this book, Alcuin's advice was generally followed, not only by English pilgrims but also by German imperial commanders and early modern Grand Tourists, all of whom tried to time their itineraries to avoid the August–September peak fever season. Nonetheless, while the flow of transalpine humanity fell to a trickle in the summer, it did not stop entirely. Nearly every year, some visiting Europeans seem to have stayed in Rome through the summer due to business concerns, ongoing litigation, travel delays, political considerations, or perhaps sheer personal idiosyncrasy. What is more, in a few years this trickle of summertime visitors rose to a flood, especially during the Jubilees and during the various German and French European military campaigns into the Eternal City.

So how did the interplay between European travelers and Roman plasmodia impact European history? Based on what we have seen, it is clear that Rome exerted a steady demographic drain on Europe for at least a millennium and a half. In most of those years, however, I suspect the drain was so small that it served as little more than background noise for the more significant events of the time. Nonetheless, there are two periods in which I think the fatal attraction of Rome helped to shape European history: the Medieval struggle between the German Empire and the papacy, and the Protestant Reformation.

When he accepted the imperial crown in Rome in 800, Charlemagne signaled to all of Europe that the German people had emerged from the cold northern forests and had inherited the imperial glory of the Roman Caesars. Politically, the coronation was a triumph. Biologically, however, it proved to be a disaster. Charlemagne's crown yoked Germany, where malaria was fairly weak and episodic, together with Italy, where the prevalence of malaria may have been an order of magnitude higher than north of the Alps and where deadly *P. falciparum* reigned during the season of the Dog Star. Charlemagne's coronation ensured that a steady stream of future German emperors-elect would seek their own crowns amidst the feverish ruins of Rome. As a result, a half-million men would clamber up a steep disease gradient over the next five centuries and repeated malaria epidemics were the inevitable consequence.

Worse yet, fear of fever meant that the German presence in Italy tended to be weak and ephemeral, preventing the creation of lasting imperial structures in Italy. As a result, each successive emperor had to start from scratch in their quest to realize their imperial dreams. The short campaign seasons that malaria imposed upon the emperors compounded the problem, predisposing the Germans towards violent shock-and-awe tactics that alienated the very Italians they sought to incorporate into the imperial polity. From the standpoint of biology, then, the Germanic Empire was indeed a monstrosity, a fundamentally unstable entity that harmed Germans and Italians alike.

While the establishment of the German Empire hindered the growth of transalpine Europe by tying its fortunes to Roman Fever, the Protestant Reformation may have had the opposite effect. I am not the first author to argue that the Protestant reformation may have played an indirect role in the relative rise of Protestant Europe. Back in 1905, Max Weber argued in his influential *The Protestant Ethic and the "Spirit" of Capitalism* that the religious ideals of the Protestant Reformers predisposed Protestant northerners to hard work, thrift, and capital accumulation, ultimately paving the way for the industrial revolution.[4] The problem with Weber's thesis is that "ethics" and "spirits" are difficult to quantify, making the notion almost impossible to demonstrate empirically.

In contrast with Weber's Protestant work ethic thesis, my own argument—that the Reformation served as an inadvertent but beneficial quarantine against Roman Fever—rests on more solid evidentiary ground. For the hypothesis to be plausible, a number of propositions must be proven true: (1) that Rome was a hotbed of malarial fever throughout the period under study, (2) that unacclimated transalpine travelers were disproportionately vulnerable to Rome's fevers, (3) that Rome attracted a large number of visitors from throughout Europe, (4) that some such travelers remained in Rome through the dangerous summer season, and (5) that travel to Rome from the Protestant north declined in the immediate aftermath of the Reformation. As we have seen in the previous chapters, all of these propositions are strongly grounded in fact. The Protestant Reformation must therefore have reduced a long-standing demographic drain on parts of northern Europe, thought the exact magnitude of that drain is impossible now to determine.

That being said, the beneficial effect of the Protestant Reformation religious quarantine was limited in both space and time. Ironically, although Germany was the cradle of the Reformation, it probably gained the least in a demographic sense as any benefits it received from breaking ties with Rome were counterbalanced by the horrific death toll wreaked by the resulting religious warfare, in particular the Thirty Years' War, which slew as many as eight million Germans through battlefield deaths, famine, and disease. Nonetheless, the inadvertent quarantine may have had a more positive impact on other Protestant states, most notably England and the Netherlands, both of which begin to rise as European powers during precisely this period. Of course, other factors also contributed to the development of these northwestern European states. Of particular importance was what historian Kenneth Pomeranz has dubbed the "ghost acreage" of the newly-discovered Americas, which allowed maritime countries like England and the Netherlands to overcome the environmental and resource limits imposed on them by European geography.[5] Nonetheless, the cessation of a long-standing demographic drain exerted by the fevers of the Eternal City was an unexpected benefit to these countries and must have played a significant though heretofore unappreciated role as well. This is not to say that the rise of Europe's northern states was solely or even largely due to unintended biological consequences of the Protestant Reformation. Nonetheless, I would repeat the sensible words of pioneer interdisciplinary scholar W.H.S. Jones: Rome's endemic malaria may not have played a determinative role in shaping European history but was nonetheless "one out of many causes, a single component of a most complex whole."[6]

That being said, the window of time during which the Protestant Reformation would have bolstered the fortunes of the Protestant Europe in comparison to Catholic Europe was fairly narrow. Based on the weight of the evidence, I would suggest that the 16th and early 17th centuries was the period when the Protestant Reformation exerted its greatest demographic effect. During that era, malaria infections were frequent, in part because Rome still hosted high levels of plasmodia and mosquito habitat, and in part because some visitors of that period still tended to remain in Rome through the August–September high fever season. Indeed, during these crossroad years the French, Spanish, and other Catholic peoples flocked to Rome and its fevers in greater numbers than ever before, attracted by a deliberate Counter-Reformation program of glorifying the Eternal City. While Protestant Europeans did occasionally venture into Rome during this era, such visits were rare and Rome seems to have attracted outliers rather than mainstream representatives of Protestant European society. The English King Henry VIII's self-serving embrace of Protestantism, therefore, ended up serving his subjects well, greatly reducing what could have been a significant demographic drain on the English people. The 16th century and early 17th century, therefore, is when the Protestant Revolution exerted its greatest beneficial effect on northern European development, at least from the standpoint of biology and demography.

Protestant northern Europeans returned *en masse* to the *caput mundi* in the later 17th century, but by that time, the worst of the Roman Fever threat had passed into history. Growing knowledge of Rome's fever risk, increasingly seasonal patterns of travel to Italy, and the wider availability of *cinchona* and (later) quinine medical remedies rendered Italy a progressively less dangerous destination for foreign travelers. Transalpine Europeans would still die of malaria in the age of Daisy Miller, but aside from the deaths associated with the Napoléonic French expeditions to Rome of the 19th century, these deaths were remarkable mainly for their rarity. The threat that Roman Fever posed to foreign visitors was finally over—though not before leaving an indelible mark upon the history of Europe.

Chapter Notes

Preface

1. Benjamin Reilly, *Disaster and Human History: Case Studies in Nature, Society, and Catastrophe* (Jefferson, NC: McFarland & Company, 2009), p. 332.
2. See Benjamin Reilly, "Malaria, Protestants, and Google." *Environmental History*, Vol. 16 (April, 2011), pp. 312–321; Reilly, "Cardinal Numbers: Changing Patterns of Malaria and Mortality in Rome, 494–1850." *Journal of Interdisciplinary History*, Vol. 49, Vol. 3 (2019), pp. 397–417; Reilly, "Northern European Patterns of Visiting Rome, 1400–1850." *Journal of Tourism History*, 2019. DOI: 10.1080/1755182X.2019.1607571; and Reilly, "Seasons in Italy: Northern European Travelers, Rome, and Malaria." *Journal of Tourism and Cultural Change* (2020). DOI: 10.1080/14766825.2019.1693582.

Introduction

1. Jean-Pierre Giegler, *Manuel du voyageur en Italie, ou Nouvelle description de tout ce que ce pays offer* (Milan, 1818), p. 448. My translation
2. Reilly, *Disaster and Human History*, pp. 349–350.

Chapter 1

1. David Soren, *Malaria, Witchcraft, Infant Cemeteries, and the Fall of Rome*. San Diego State: Gail A. Burnett Lectures in Classics, 2002, p. 9. See also Soren, "Can Archeologists Excavate Evidence of Malaria?" *World Archeology*, Vol. 35, No. 2 (2003), pp. 193–209; and L. L. Lane, "Malaria, Medicine, and Magic in the Roman World." David Soren and Noelle Soren eds., *A Roman Villa and a Late Roman Infant Cemetery*. Rome: L'Erma di Bretschneider, 1998, pp. 633–651.
2. Sonia Shah, *The Fever: How Malaria has Ruled Humankind for 500,000 Years* (New York: Farrar, Straus and Giroux, 2010), p. 20. This section of text also draws information from James L. A. Webb, *Humanity's Burden: A Global History of Malaria* (New York: Cambridge University Press, 2009) and Randall Packard, *The Making of a Tropical Disease: A Short History of Malaria* (Baltimore: Johns Hopkins University Press, 2007).
3. Benjamin Reilly, *Slavery, Agriculture, and Malaria in the Arabian Peninsula* (Athens: Ohio University Press, 2015), p. 105.
4. See Michael T. White, George Shireff, Stephan Karl, Arza C. Ghani, and Ivo Mueller, "Variation in Relapse Frequency and the Transmission Potential of Plasmodium *vivax* malaria." *Proceedings of the Royal Society B*, Vol. 283 (2016).
5. Webb, p. 26.
6. See Emanuele Angelluci, Nigel Burrows, Stefano Losi, Chris Bartiromo, and X. Henry Hu. "Beta-thalassemia (BT) Prevalence and Treatment Patterns in Italy: A Survey of Treating Physicians." *Blood*, Vol. 128 (2016). doi.org/10.1182/blood.V128.22.3533.3533.
7. D. Maffi et al., "Glucose-6-phosphate dehydrogenase deficiency in Italian blood donors: prevalence and molecular defect characterization." *Vox Sang*, Vol. 106, No. 3 (2014), pp. 227–233.
8. Technically gorilla falciparum is *P. preaefalciparum*, meaning "pre-falciparum," a distinct but closely related species of the plasmodia. On the evolution of *P. vivax* and *P. falciparum*, see Dorothy E. Loy et al., "Out of Africa: Origins and Evolution of the Human Malaria Parasites *Plasmodium falciparum* and *Plasmodium vivax*." *International Journal of Parasitology*, Vol. 47 (2017), pp. 87–97.
9. There is some scholarly disagreement over this issue. According to Randall M. Packard, *falciparum* was probably unable to find a permanent foothold in humans before the dawn of agriculture in Africa. James Webb, on the other hand, believes that the "paracultivation" of yams by hunter-gatherers may have allowed for both high enough populations for *falciparum* infections and micro-environments suitable for falciparum's *Anopheles* mosquito vectors. However, Both scholars agree that falciparum infections rose over time as humans established large, permanent agricultural settlements in rainforest environments. See Packard, p. 23; Webb, pp. 32–35.
10. See Timothy C. Winegard, *The Mosquito* (New York: Dutton, 2019), p. 32.
11. Richard Carter and Kamini N. Mendis. "Evolutionary and Historical Aspects of the Burden of Malaria." *Clinical Microbiology Reviews*, Vol. 15, No. 4 (2002), p. 568; Isaac Oludare Oluwayemi, "Cerebral Malaria." *Malar Chemoth Cont Elimination*, Vol. 3, No. 116. doi:10.4172/2090-2778.1000116.
12. Robert Sallares, *Malaria and Rome: A History*

of Malaria in Ancient Italy (New York: Oxford University Press, 2002), p. 102.
   13. L. W. Hackett, *Malaria in Europe: An Ecological Study* (London: Oxford University Press, 1937), p. 278.

Chapter 2

   1. Charles de Brosses, *Lettres Familières, Écrites d'Italie en 1739 & 1740*, Vol. 1. (Paris: Librarie Académique, 1869), p. 305. My translation.
   2. Charles de Brosses, Vol. 1, pp. 308–309. My translation. De Brosses was not alone in his negative assessment of Rome's location; German writer Goethe wrote that "the seven hills are not hills at all; it is only in relation to ancient river bed of the Tiber, which later became the Campus Martius, that they appear to be heights… I am convinced that no inhabited site among the peoples of old was as badly placed a Rome." See Johan Wolfgang von Goethe, *Italian Journey* (New York: Penguin, 1962), pp. 165–166.
   3. De Brosses, Vol. 1, p. 312.
   4. Gregory S. Aldrete, *Floods of the Tiber in Ancient Rome* (Baltimore: Johns Hopkins University Press, 2007), pp. 11–12.
   5. See W. H. S. Jones, *Malaria: A Neglected Factor in the History of Greece and Rome* (London: Macmillan, 1907), pp. 64–65.
   6. Winegard, p. 65.
   7. *Ibid.*, p. 66.
   8. Joël Le Gall, *Le Tibre: Fleuve de Rome dans L'Antiquité* (Paris: Presses Universitaires de France, 1953), pp. 40–41.
   9. See E. Rodriguez Almeida, *Il Monte Testaccio, ambiente, storia, material* (Rome: Quasar, 1984).
   10. For a good discussion of Rome's aqueducts, see P. Bono and C. Boni, "Water Supply of Rome in Antiquity and Today." *Environmental Geology*, Vol. 27, No. 2 (1996), pp. 126–134.
   11. Aldrete, pp. 205–208.
   12. Aldrete notes that by the early imperial period the *insulae* apartments favored by the poor tended to be built on low-lying, flood-prone terrain, while private homes (*domus*) were overwhelmingly built on hills and outside the flood zone. See Aldrete, pp. 213–215.
   13. Aldrete, p. 55.
   14. *Ibid.*, pp. 16–17.
   15. *Ibid.*, p. 26.
   16. *Ibid.*, p. 27.
   17. Michelle Ziegler, "Malarial Landscapes in Late Antique Rome and the Tiber Valley." *Landscapes*, Vol. 17, No. 2 (2016), p. 148.
   18. See Jean-Marie André, "La notion de "Pestilentia" à Rome: du tabou religieux à l'interprétation préscientifique." *Latomus*, Vol. 39, No. 1 (1980), pp. 9–10.
   19. See Aldrete, p. 148–149.
   20. John Hopkins, "The 'Sacred Sewer': Tradition and Religion in the Cloaca Maxima." In Mark Bradley ed., *Rome, Pollution, and Propriety* (New York: Cambridge University Press, 2012), pp. 81–102.
   21. Aldrete, p. 175.
   22. Sallares, pp. 112–113.
   23. Donald Hughes, *Environmental Problems of the Greeks and Romans: Ecology in the Ancient Mediterranean* (Baltimore: Johns Hopkins University Press, 2014), p. 155, 234.
   24. *Ibid.*, p. 103.
   25. Horace, *The Complete Odes and Epodes*. David West Trans. (New York: Oxford University Press, 1997), p. 32. See also Verner J. Warner, "Epithets of the Tiber in the Roman Poets." *The Classical Weekly*, Vol. 11, No. 7 (1917), pp. 52–54.
   26. *Ibid.*, p. 70.
   27. See Lara O'Sullivan, Andrew Jardine, Angus Cook, and Philip Weinstein, "Deforestation, Mosquitoes, and Ancient Rome: Lessons for Today." *BioScience*, Vol. 58, No. 8 (Sept., 2008), pp. 756–758.
   28. Franco Bonelli, "La malaria nella storia demografica ed economica dell'Italia: Prima lineamenti di una ricerca." *Studi Storici*, Vol. 7, No. 4 (Oct.-Dec., 1966), pp. 679–680.
   29. G. De Matthaeis, *Sul Culto Reso dagli Antichi Romani alla Dea Febbre* (Roma: Stamperia de Romanis, 1814), p. 30.
   30. *Ibid.*, p. 36.
   31. See François Retief and Louis Cilliers, "Malaria in Graeco-Roman Times." *Acta Classica*, Vol. 47 (2004), pp. 127–137.
   32. Jones, p. 85.
   33. For a good summary of the historiography surrounding the Jones thesis, see Christopher Baron and Christopher Hamlin. "Malaria and the Decline of Ancient Greece: Revisiting the Jones Hypothesis in an Era of Interdisciplinarity." *Minerva*, Vol. 53 (2015), pp. 327–358.
   34. Sallares, p. 39.
   35. Hackett, p. xi.

Chapter 3

   1. For a good discussion of pre-modern beliefs about disease, see Christopher Hamlin, *More than Hot: A Short History of Fever* (Baltimore: Johns Hopkins University Press, 2014).
   2. Timothy P. Newfield, "Malaria and malaria-like disease in the early Middle Ages." *Early Medieval Europe*, Vol. 25, No. 3 (2017), pp. 269–270.
   3. *Ibid.*, p. 294.
   4. *Ibid.*, p. 295.
   5. See Paolo Squatriti, "The Floods of 589 and Climate Change at the Beginning of the Middle Ages: An Italian Microhistory." *Speculum*, Vol. 85 (2010), pp. 779–826.
   6. For an excellent survey of references to fevers, including the semi-tertian fevers that are probably cases of *P. falciparum* infection, see Retief and Cilliers. "Malaria in Graeco-Roman Times." *Acta Classica*, Vol. 47 (2004), pp. 127–137. On the historical prevalence of malaria in Italy see also Sallares, pp. 34–42; and Robert Sallares, Abigail Bouwman, and Cecilia Anderung. "The Spread of Malaria to Southern Europe in Antiquity: New Approaches to

Old Problems." *Medical History*, Vol. 48 (2004), pp. 311–328.

7. Sallares et al., p. 318. Sallares, Bouwman, and Anderung ascribe the spread of malaria into the region to colonization of the delta by highly anthropogenic *A. Sacherovi* mosquitos, which are endemic in the nearby Balkan Peninsula.

8. *Ibid.*, p. 327.

9. Angelo Celli, *Malaria, According to the New Researches* (New York: Longmans, Green, 1900), p. 149.

10. *Ibid.*, p. 156

11. Leonard Jan Bruce-Chwatt and Julian de Zulueta, *The Rise and Fall of Malaria in Europe: A Historico-Epidemiological Study* (New York: Oxford University Press, 1980), p. 84, 96. Bruce-Chwatt and de Zulueta give only raw numbers of malaria deaths for the period 1887 to 1901, so I was obliged to infer a 12% infection rate for 1887 by comparing multiplying the death rate for 1877 (21,033) by the average ratio of cases per death that Bruce-Chwatt and de Zulueta provide for the period after 1902.

12. *Ibid.*, p 80.

13. Félix Jacquot, *Lettres Médicales sur L'Italie, Comprenant L'Histoire Médicale du Corps d'Occupation des États Romains* (Paris: Librairie de Victor Masson, 1857), p. 85. Jacquot actually uses the term "*fièvres paludéennes*," or "swamp fevers," a common French term for malaria.

14. For historical data on typhoid in Europe, see William T. Sedgewick and Charles-Edward A. Winslow, "Statistical Studies on the Seasonal Prevalence of Typhoid Fever in Various Countries and Its Relation to Seasonable Temperature." *Memoirs of the American Academy of Arts and Sciences*, Vol. 12, No. 5 (Aug. 1902), pp. 467, 469–470, 521–571. A modern study by Neil J. Saad et al. came to much the same conclusion: that typhoid in Europe largely tracks with temperature, and thus peaks in August and September. Unlike malaria however, though the bell curve is fairly shallow, and a significant number of cases continue to occur throughout the winter. See Neil J. Saad, Victoria D. Lynch, Marina Antillón, Chongguang Yang, John A. Crump and Virginia E. Pitzer, "Seasonal Dynamics of Typhoid and Paratyphoid Fever." *Scientific Reports*, Vol. 8 (2018). On-line at https://www.nature.com/articles/s41598-018-25234-w/.

15. Jacquot, p. 83.

16. Jacquot, pp. 382–383. Malaria killed roughly 10% of the Corsican army garrison every year in the first half of the 19th century; see Bruce-Chwatt and Zulueta, p. 79.

17. Brent D. Shaw, "Seasons of Death: Aspects of Mortality in Imperial Rome." *The Journal of Roman Studies*, Vol. 86 (1996), p. 120; Walter Scheidel, "Libitina's Bitter Gains: Seasonal Mortality and Endemic Disease in the Ancient City of Rome." *Ancient Society*, Vol. 25 (1994), p. 167.

18. Scheidel, "Libitina's Bitter Gains," p. 159.

19. Shaw, p. 127.

20. Scheidel, "Libitina's Bitter Gains," p. 160.

21. Walter Scheidel, "Death and the City: Ancient Rome and Beyond." R. Smith and E. A. Wrigley (eds.), *publication of the conference on the fiftieth anniversary of the Cambridge Group for the History of Population and Social Structure*. Cambridge, 2014.

22. Salvador Miranda's Cardinals of the Holy Roman Church is online at http://www2.fiu.edu/mirandas/cardinals.htm. For a longer discussion of this archival resource, see Alessio Fornasin, Marco Breschi, and Matteo Manfredini, "Mortality Patterns of Cardinals (Sixteenth-Twentieth Centuries)," *Institut National d'Études Démographiques*, LXV (2010), 631–652.

23. In his study of early modern Florentine ideas on disease, Carlo M. Cipolla noted that Florentine doctors imagined disease as a sliding scale, in which one disease could morph into another if environmental conditions improved or worsened. By this logic, "plague" was not a specific *type* of disease, but an *intensity* of disease, on the severe end of the spectrum. As a corollary, Cipola and other disease historians suspect that frequency of bubonic plague in history has been seriously over diagnosed, while other diseases, such as malaria, have probably been undercounted. See Carlo M. Cipolla, *Miasmas and Disease: Public Health and the Environment in the pre-industrial Age* (London: Yale University Press, 1992), pp. 67, 76.

24. See Reilly, "Cardinal Numbers."

25. Reilly, "Cardinal Numbers," p. 413.

Chapter 4

1. Kyle Harper, *The Fate of Rome: Climate, Disease and the End of an Empire* (Princeton, NJ: Princeton University Press, 2017), p. 151.

2. Livy, *The History of Rome*. Canon Roberts trans. London: Everyman's Library, 1905, Book 5, Section 48.

3. Julius Caesar, *The Commentaries of Caesar on His Wars in Gaul* (Dublin: John Cumming, 1844), pp. 98–99.

4. Tacitus, *The Agricola and Germania*, R. B. Townshend trans. (London: Methuen, 1894), p. 57

5. Harper, p. 192.

6. Thomas Hodgkin, *Italy and Her Invaders*, Vol 1, Part 1 (Oxford: Clarendon Press, 1892), p. 75. Although dated, Hodgkin's work on Rome and invaders from the north shows much greater sensitivity to the role played by malaria than that of most recent historians, perhaps in part because malaria was still very much an ongoing concern for foreign visitors to Rome in Hodgkin's own lifetime.

7. Henry Wace and Philip Schaff, *Nicene and Post-Nicene Fathers of the Christian Church* (New York: Scribner's, 1912), pp. 499–500.

8. Hodgkin, Vol. 1, Part 2, p. 387. See also Eric Faure, "The death of Alaric I (c. 370–410AD), the vanquisher of Rome: Additional arguments strengthening the possible involvement of malaria." *European Journal of Internal Medicine*, Vol. 37 (Jan., 2017), pp. e14-e15, doi: 10.1016/j.ejim.2016.06.021

9. Hodgkin, Vol. 2, p. 156.
10. See Harper, p. 196.
11. See Jordanes, *The Origin and Deeds of the Goths*, Charles C. Mierow trans (Princeton, 1908), p. 222.
12. Sallares et al., p. 318.
13. Hodgkin, Vol 5, p. 231.
14. Gregory of Tours, *History of the Franks*, Ernest Brehaut ed. (New York: Columbia University Press, 1916), p. 69.
15. New research now suggests that the impact of Justinian's plague on late Roman population has been greatly exaggerated, though it is still likely the outbreak of this contagion distracted the Byzantines from their war effort against the Ostrogoths. See Lee Mordechai et al., "The Justinianic Plague: An inconsequential pandemic"? *Proceedings of the national Academy of Science USA*, Vol. 116, No. 51 (Dec, 2019), pp. 22546–25554. doi: 10.1073/pnas.1903797116
16. Procopius, *History of the Wars*, Vol. IV. H. B. Dewing trans (Cambridge, MA: Harvard University Press, 1919), p. 297. The *Liber Pontificalis*, or book of popes, clarifies Procopius's remark, declaring that during Totila's siege the famine in Rome was so bad that "people ate their own children." See *Liber Pontificalis*, Louise Ropes Loomis trans. (New York: Columbia University Press, 1916), p. 158.
17. *Ibid.*, p. 323.
18. Hodgkin, Vol. 5, p. 492.
19. On Ostrogoth/Lombard settlement patterns in Italy, see John Moorhead, "Ostrogothic Italy and the Lombard Invasions." In Paul Fouracre ed., *The New Cambridge Medieval History: I* (Cambridge, UK: Cambridge University Press, 2005, pp. 150–161).
20. Hodgkin, Vol. 6, p. 316.
21. Chris Wickham, *The Inheritance of Rome: Illuminating the Dark Ages, 400-1000* (New York: Penguin Books, 2009), p. 78.
22. See Christopher Hibbert, *Rome: the Biography of a City* (New York: Penguin Books, 1985), p. 74; Hodgkin, Vol. 5, p. 316.
23. Hibbert, *Rome*, p. 74.

Chapter 5

1. Parks, p. 32.
2. Requoted from George B. Parks, *The English Traveler to Italy* (Stanford, CA: Stanford University Press, 1954), p. 72.
3. According to Alfonso Corradi's index of epidemic disease in Italy, after a peninsula-wide outbreak of the epidemic in 599, there were no documented outbreaks of bubonic plague afterwards except in 652 (in Alghero) and in 746–48 (in Calabria and Sicily). See Corradi, *Annali delle Epidemie Occorse in Italia dalle Prime Memorie Fino al 1850*, Vol. VII (Bologna: Tipi Gamberini e Parmeggiani, 1865), p. 222.
4. John Theilmann and Frances Cate, "A Plague of Plagues: The Problem of Plague Diagnosis in Medieval England." *Journal of Interdisciplinary History*, Vol. 37, No. 3 (Winter, 2007), p. 390. The term "plague" was particularly associated with fevers; Hamlin, p. 61.
5. Matthew 16: 18–19, King James Version.
6. Roger Collins, *Keepers of the Keys of Heaven: A History of the Papacy* (New York: Basic Books, 2009), p. 14.
7. See John Vidmar, *The Catholic Church Through the Ages: A History* (New York: Paulist Press, 2014), pp. 31–33.
8. Collins, p. 35–36.
9. Brett Edward Whalen, *The Medieval Papacy* (New York: Palgrave Macmillan, 2014), p. 49.
10. Ferdinand Gregorovius, *History of the City of Rome in the Middle Ages*, Vol. 2. Mrs. Gustavus W. Hamilton Trans. (New York: Ithaca Press, 2000), p. 42. Gregorovius' work, like that of Thomas Hodgkins, is somewhat dated in its style, but has the great advantage of being highly sensitive to malaria, which was still very much on the minds of transalpine visitors to Rome during the later 19th century when Gregorovius composed his text. See footnote 34 in chapter 7 below for a case study example of Gregorovius' value to the study of malaria in Rome compared with the insensitivity of more recent historians to disease concerns.
11. Norwich, John Julius. *Absolute Monarchs: A History of the Papacy* (New York: Random House, 2011), p. 41.
12. Ziegler, p. 141.
13. Shortly before his death, Gregory confided in a letter that, in addition to stomach pain, "I also suffer from a constant succession of slow fevers." See Fernand Mourret, *The History of the Catholic Church*, Vol. 3 (London: B. Herder, 1946), p. 71.
14. Sallares, p. 211.
15. Parks, p. 28.
16. *Ibid.*, p. 30.
17. Judith Champ, *The English Pilgrimage to Rome: A Dwelling for the Soul* (Leominster, UK: Gracewing, 2000), p. 16.
18. Bede, p. 203.
19. See Corradi, Vol. 1, pp. 70–71.
20. Parks, p. 55.
21. *Ibid.*, p. 80. Alcuin himself visited Rome at least twice, the first time as the "youthful companion" of a pilgrim and traveler named Aelberht, the second time to "collect the pallium for his friend Eanbald, the new Archbishop of York." It was during the second voyage that Alcuin met Charlemagne and was summoned into his service as a scholar of the court; see Douglas Dales, *Alcuin: His Life and Legacy* (Cambridge, UK: James Clark and Co., 2012), p. 109.
22. *Ibid.*, p. 13.
23. Bede, *A History of the English Church and People*. Leo Sherley-Price trans (New York: Dorset Press, 1968), pp. 246, 307, 336–337.109.
24. C. R. Dodwell, *Anglo-Saxon Art: A New Perspective* (Ithaca, NY: Cornell University Press, 1985), p. 179.
25. Bede, p. 312.

26. *Ibid.*, p. 68.
27. *Ibid.*, p. 59.
28. Edward Kylie ed., *The English Correspondence of Saint Boniface* (London: Chatto and Windus, 1911), pp. 99–100.
29. W. J. Moore, "The Saxon Pilgrims to Rome and the Schola Saxonum." Ph.D. Diss., University of Fribourg, 1937, p. 91.
30. *Ibid.*
31. Peter Llewellyn, *Rome in the Dark Ages* (London: Faber and Faber Ltd., 1971), p. 179.
32. See Anselo M. Tommasini, *Irish Saints in Italy*, J. F. Scanlan trans. (London: Sands and Company, 1937), p. 99.
33. Llewellyn, p. 175–177.
34. Jonathan Sumption, *The Age of Pilgrimage: the Medieval Journey to God* (Mahwah, NJ: Hidden Spring, 2003), p. 312.
35. "Dedication of a Church and an Altar" *International Committee on English in the Liturgy*, 1978, p. 17.
36. *Ibid.*, p. 32
37. Gregorovius, Vol 3, p. 74.
38. Nancy Lenkeith, *Dante and the Legend of Rome* (London: Warburg Institute, 1952), p. 10.
39. *The Marvels of Rome*, p. 29. On the influx of relics from the holy land to Rome, see Brian Barefoot, *The English Road to Rome* (Reading, UK: Images Publishing, 1993), p. 18.
40. Hibbert, *Rome*, p. 76.
41. See for example Arsenio Frugoni, *Il Giubileo di Bonifacio VIII* (Rome: Editori Laterza, 1999), p. 86.

Chapter 6

1. Thomas Wright ed., *Gesta Romanorum; or Entertaining Stories*, Vol. 2. (London: John Camden Hotten, 1871), pp. 87–90.
2. Arturo Graf, *Roma nella Memoria e nelle Immaginazioni del Medio Evo* (Turin: Giovanni Chiantore, 1923), p. 142. My Translation
3. Graf, p. 144.
4. These "Emperors" are an odd mix of real Roman Emperors (Caesar, Vespasian, Diocletian, etc.), German Holy Roman Emperors (Henry II, Otto, Frederick, etc.), people who were rulers but not actual Roman Emperors (Alexander, Pompey, etc.) and random names pulled from the pages of history, including the historian Pliny and the North African theologian Fulgentius.
5. Wright, Vol. 2, pp. 97–100.
6. Henry A. Myers, ed. *The Book of Emperors: A Translation of the Middle High German Kaiserchronik* (Morgantown, WV: West Virginia University Press, 2013), pp. 77–79.
7. *The Marvels of Rome*, Francis Morgan Nichols trans. (NY: Ithaca Press, 1986), p. 18.
8. *Ibid.*, p. 4.
9. *Ibid.*, p. 21, p. 28.
10. Wright, Vol. 1, pp. 145–146.
11. Richard Lassels, *The Voyage of Italy, Or a Compleat Journey through Italy* (London: John Starkey, 1670), pp. 129–130.
12. https://www.livius.org/articles/place/rome/rome-photos/rome-forum-romanum/lacus-curtius/
13. *The Marvels of Rome*, p. 41.
14. Raymond Keaveney, *Views of Rome* (Scala Books, 1988), p. 146.
15. William Caxton, *The Golden Legend; or Lives of the Saints*, Vol. 2 (London: J. M. Dent and Co., 1900), pp. 203–204.
16. Myers, pp. 252–253.
17. Peregrine Horden, "Disease, Dragons, and Saints: the Management of Epidemics in the Dark Ages." In Terence Ranger and Paul Slack eds., *Epidemics and Ideas* (London: Cambridge University Press, 1992), p. 70.
18. *Ibid.*, p. 59–60.
19. Caxton, Vol. 2, p. 127.
20. See Mirko Grmek, *Diseases in the Ancient Greek World* (Baltimore, MD: Johns Hopkins University Press, 1991), p. 272.

Chapter 7

1. On Pepin's negotiations with Pope Zacharias, see Pierre Riché, *The Carolingians: A Family Who Forged Europe* (Philadelphia: University of Pennsylvania Press, 1993), pp. 66–73.
2. Einhard, *The Life of Charlemagne* (Ann Arbor, MI: University of Michigan Press, 1960), p. 23.
3. Collins, p. 132. The quote on the Lombards is by Pope Stephen III, who held the papacy from 786–772.
4. On papal/Lombard relations, see Paolo Delogu, "Lombard and Carolingian Italy." In Rosamond McKitterick ed., *The New Cambridge Medieval History: II* (Cambridge, UK: Cambridge University Press, 2008), pp. 290–319.
5. Gregorovius, Vol. 2, p. 323.
6. On Franco-Papal relations in this period, see Thomas F. X. Noble, "The Papacy in the Eighth and Ninth Centuries." In Rosamond McKitterick ed., *The New Cambridge Medieval History: II* (Cambridge, UK: Cambridge University Press, 2008), pp. 563–586, and Delogu, pp. 290–319.
7. For a more detailed discussion of series of events that led up to Charlemagne's coronation, as well as description of the event itself, see Matthias Becher, *Charlemagne* (New Haven, CT: Yale University Press, 2003), pp. 7–17.
8. Gregorovius, Vol 1, p. 4. On the importance of Roman coronation to the political legitimacy of the Germanic Emperors, who styled themselves *imperator augustus* from 996 onwards, see also Timothy Reuter, *Germany in the Early Middle Ages, 800–1056* (New York: Longman, 1991), pp. 274–275; and Peter H. Wilson, *Heart of Europe: A History of the Holy Roman Empire* (Cambridge, MA: Belknap Press of Harvard University Press, 2016), pp. 309–311.
9. For a more fine-detailed accounting of Europe's historical malaria intensity than this map

allows, see Hackett's somewhat dated but highly comprehensive *Malaria in Europe*.

10. For a good discussion of the former, see Daniel Defoe, *Tour through the Eastern Counties of England in 1722* (London: Cassell and Company, 1888). As is typical of a malarial zone, Defoe notes that young men seasoned to the feverish climate of the place "did pretty well with it," but their brides from the surrounding "uplands" typically "changed their complexion, got an ague [acute fever] or two, and seldom held it above half a year, or a year at most." (p. 30).

11. See Martin R. Howard, "Walcheren 1809: A Medical Catastrophe." *BMJ*, Vol 310, No. 7225 (Dec 18, 1999), pp. 1642–1645.

12. William McNeill, *Plagues and Peoples* (New York: Anchor Books, 1976), p. 102.

13. Llewellyn, p. 184.

14. In the process, the Arabs and their African slaves may have introduced or augmented the S Hemoglobin trait in Sicily, which is today a hotbed of sickle-cell disease; see Giovanna Russo-Mancuso, Maria Antonietta Romea, Vincenzo Guardabasso, and Gino Schiliro. "Survey of Sickle-Cell Disease in Italy." *Haematologica*, Vol. 83 (1998), p. 875.

15. Gregorovius, Vol. 3, p. 179.

16. Collins, p. 142.

17. Robert Comyn, *History of the Western Empire from its Restoration by Charlemagne to the Accession of Charles V*, Vol. 1 (London: William Allen, 1851), Vol. 1, p. 54.

18. Roger Collins, *Early Medieval Europe, 300–1000* (London: Macmillan, 1991), p. 309.

19. *The Chronicle of Regno of Prüm and Adalbert of Magdeburg*, p. 128.

20. Sallares et al., p. 318. The notion that Pepin and his army suffered from malaria has been floated by other scholars; see for example R. S. Bray, *Armies of Pestilence: The Impact of Disease on History* (Cambridge, UK: James Clarke and Co., 1996), p. 100. If Pepin did succumb to malaria, it was likely of the *P. vivax* or *P. malariae* variety, as Venice is outside of *P. falciparum*'s normal range.

21. Riché, p. 161.

22. For more on the complex politics of this era, see Eric J. Goldberg, *Struggle for Empire: Kingship and Conflict under Louis the German, 817–876* (London: Cornell University Press, 2006).

23. *The Chronicle of Regno of Prüm and Adalbert of Magdeburg*, p. 155.

24. Ibid.

25. Ibid., p. 143.

26. Ibid., p. 160.

27. Comyn, Vol. 1, p. 90.

28. Wilson, p. 48.

29. Liutprand of Cremona, *The Complete Works of Liutprand of Cremona*. Paulo Squatriti trans. (Washington, DC: Catholic University of America Press, 2007), p. 236.

30. Ibid., p. 225.

31. *History and Politics in Late Carolingian and Ottonian Europe: The Chronicle of Regno of Prüm and Adalbert of Magdeburg*, Simon MacLean trans. (New York: Manchester University Press, 2009), p. 266.

32. See G. A. Loud, "Southern Italy in the Tenth Century." In Timothy Reuter ed., *The New Cambridge Medieval History*, Vol. 3 (Cambridge, UK: Cambridge University Press, 1999), p. 629.

33. Gregorovius, Vol. 3, p. 479.

34. Gerd Althoff, *Otto III*. Phyllis G. Jestice trans (University Park, PA: Pennsylvania State University Press, 2003), p. 83.

35. Eckhard Müller-Mertens, "The Ottonians as Kings and Emperors." In Timothy Reuter ed., *The New Cambridge Medieval History*, Vol 3 (Cambridge, UK: Cambridge University Press, 1999), p. 258.

36. Gregorovius, Vol. III, p. 489. Gregorovius' sensitivity to malaria and fever during the reign of Otto III stands in sharp contrast to the disregard of later historians, who have not seen not malaria as relevant to the study of Otto's reign. Gerd Althoff's influential biography of Otto III, for instance, fails to locate Otto's Roman palace on the healthy Aventine hill (see footnote 31 above), ignores Otto's complaints to the pope about the unhealthiness of the Italian climate, and ascribes Otto's death to some "unknown, perhaps epidemic illness," not even entertaining the possibility it may have been malaria. This is despite the fact that contemporary sources ascribe Otto's death to "morbus Italicus," meaning "the Italian disease." See Althoff, p. 129.

37. Althoff, p. 105; Levi Roach, "Emperor Otto III and the End of Time." *Transactions of the Royal Historical Society*, Vol. 23 (2013), p. 92.

38. Roach, p. 91.

39. Ibid., p. 129.

40. Müller-Mertens, p. 260.

41. Ibid., p. 3, 7. On scholarly opinions of Otto III's Italian dreams, see also David A. Warner, "Ideals and Action in the Reign of Otto III." *Journal of Medieval History*, Vol. 25, No. 1 (1999), pp. 1–2.

42. Althoff, p. 13.

43. James Bryce, *The Holy Roman Empire* (London: Macmillan, 1871), p. 135.

Chapter 8

1. Müller-Mertens, p. 261.

2. Comyn, Vol. 1, p. 132. Disease historian R. S. Bray suspects that Henry II's army was undone by malaria; see Bray, p. 100.

3. Ibid., Vol. 1, p. 139.

4. La Due, p. 90.

5. Whalen, p. 81.

6. See Richard Krautheimer, *Rome: Profile of a City, 312–1308* (Princeton, NJ: Princeton University Press, 2000), p. 310.

7. La Due, p. 82.

8. See Chris Wickham, *Medieval Rome: Stability and Crisis of a City, 900–1150* (Oxford, UK: Oxford University Press, 2015), p. 196.

9. Gregorovius, Vol. 3, p. 224.

10. See Norwich, *The Popes*. p. 89; Gregorovius, Vol. 4, Part 1, p. 47.

11. Geoffrey Barraclough, *The Medieval Papacy* (New York: W. W. Norton, 1968), p. 94.
12. Walter Ullmann, *A Short History of the Papacy in the Middle Ages* (New York: Routledge, 2003), p. 128.
13. Gregorovius, Vol. 4, Part 2, p. 610.
14. See Wilson, *Heart of Europe*, pp. 85–92, 329–330.
15. I. S. Robinson, "Innocent II and the Empire." in John Doran and Damien Smith eds., *Pope Innocent II: The World vs. the City* (New York: Routledge, 2016), p. 35.
16. On the demographics of the Norman migration into south Italy, see Jean-Marie Martin, *Italies Normandes: XIe-XIIe siècles* (Paris: Hachette, 1994), pp. 31–48.
17. Gordon S. Brown, *The Norman Conquest of Southern Italy and Sicily* (London: McFarland, 2003), pp. 93–94.
18. Robinson, *Henry IV of Germany*, p. 161.
19. Gregorovius, Vol. 4, Part 1, p. 236.
20. Robinson, "Innocent II and the Empire," p. 31.
21. Wilson, p. 62. This specific piece of symbolism had its origins in the Donation of Constantine, in which Constantine performs the same service for Sylvester I; see Robinson, "Innocent II and the Empire," p. 55.
22. Robinson, "Innocent II and the Empire," p. 51.
23. Gregorovius, Vol. 4, Part 2, p. 439.
24. Dante Aligheri, *The De Monarchia of Dante Alighieri*, Aurelia Henry trans. (New York: Houghton Mifflin, 1904), pp. 40.
25. C. C. Bayley, "Petrarch, Charles IV, and the 'Renovatio Imperii.'" *Speculum*, Vol. 17, No. 3 (Jul., 1942), pp. 388.
26. Aligheri, *De Monarchia*, pp. 59, 60, 187.
27. *Ibid.*, p. 176, 177, 156, 206.
28. See Paul J Alexander, "The Medieval Legend of the Last Roman Emperor and Its Messianic Origin." *Journal of the Warburg and Courtauld Institutes*, Vol. 41 (1978), pp. 1–15.
29. Wilson, p. 39; Roach, p. 78.
30. Roach, p. 85.
31. Ullmann, p. 192.
32. Peter Munz, *Frederick Barbarossa: A Study in Medieval Politics* (Ithaca, NY: Cornell University Press, 1969), p. 31.
33. *Ibid.*, pp. 72–73.
34. *Barbarossa in Italy*, Thomas Carson ed. and trans. (New York: Italica Press, 1994), p. 30. *P. falciparum* malaria often manifests as diarrhea amongst patients with no previous exposure to the disease; see Ram Naresh Prasad, and Kamal Jeet Virk, "Malaria as a cause of diarrhoea—a review." *PNG*, Vol. 36 (1993), pp. 337–341.
35. Munz, p. 221.
36. Otto of Freising, *The Deeds of Frederick Barbarossa*, Charles Christopher Mierow trans. (New York: Columbia University Press, 2004), pp. 337–338.
37. In the modern era, the Dog Star (Sirius) no longer rises in the sky during the summer malaria season due to changes in the earth's tilt; see Shah, p. 70.
38. John Freed, *Frederick Barbarossa: The Prince and the Myth* (New Haven, CT: Yale University Press, 2016), pp. 343–344.
39. See Munz, pp. 249–250.
40. *Ibid.*, p. 298.
41. Comyn, Vol. 1, p. 271. Malaria infection in any case can cause diarrheal symptoms, especially in the unacclimated; see Prasad (1993).
42. J. A. Watt, "The Papacy." In David Abulafia ed., *The New Cambridge Medieval History*, Vol. V (Cambridge, UK: Cambridge University Press, 1999), p. 130.
43. David Abulafia, *Frederick II: A Medieval Emperor* (New York: Oxford University Press, 1988), pp. 81–82. See also Richard F. Cassady, *The Emperor and the Saint: Frederick II of Hohenstaufen, Francis of Assisi, and Journeys to Medieval Places* (DeKalb, Illinois: Northern Illinois University Press, 2011), p. 16.
44. See Comyn, Vol. 1, p. 274. Other sources blame his death on "a cold caught while hunting" or on a "typhus-like fever"; see Cassady, p. 27; Horst Furmann, *Germany in the High Middle Ages, c. 1050–1200* (Cambridge, UK: Cambridge University Press, 1986), p. 186.
45. Constance's death was foreshadowed by the demise of many Spanish knights who had been sent to Sicily from Aragon as part of her dowry. Frederick had hoped to use them to consolidate his control over Italy, but before they could see combat, "disease struck and the survivors, demoralized, returned home to Aragon." See Abulafia, *Frederick II*, p. 106.
46. Comyn, Vol. 1, p. 294.
47. See Abulafia, *Frederick II*, p. 165; Cassidy, p. 239.
48. In his 18th century travels into Southern Italy, the English author J. R. Forster noted that Brindisi is "unhealthy all the year round, but in summer it is the worst in Italy; and the garrison [of the Kingdom of Naples], which is changed once in three years, always leaves half of its men behind." See Forster, *Travels through Sicily and that Part of Italy Formerly Called Magna Graecia* (London: Edward and Charles Dilly, 1773), p. 199.
49. Gregorovius, Vol. 5, part 1, p. 253; Marcel Brion, *Frédéric II de Hohenstaufen* (Paris: Librarie Jules Tallandier, 1978), p. 238.
50. *Ibid.*, p. 211.
51. *Ibid.*, p. 216.
52. Gregorovius, Vol V, Part 2, p. 410.

Chapter 9

1. See Peter Herde, "From Adolf of Nassau to Lewis of Bavaria, 1292–1347." In Michael Jones ed., *The New Cambridge Medieval History*, Vol. VI (Cambridge, UK: Cambridge University Press, 2015), p. 230.
2. Abulafia, David. "The Italian South." In

Michael Jones ed., *The New Cambridge Medieval History*, Vol. VI. (Cambridge, UK: Cambridge University Press, 2015), p. 500.

3. David Gilmour, *The Pursuit of Italy: A History of a Land, Its Regions, and their Peoples* (New York: Farrar, Straus and Giroux, 2011), p. 70; William M. Bowsky, *Henry VII in Italy: The Conflict of Empire and City-State, 1310–1313* (Lincoln, NE: University of Nebraska Press, 1960), p. 116.

4. Bowsky, p. 119. If so, the culprit was likely *P. vivax*, as Brescia is outside of the normal range of *P. falciparum*.

5. Gregorovius, Vol. V, part 2, p. 658–659.

6. Gregorovius, Vol. VI, part 1, p. 47.

7. Abulafia, "The Italian South," pp. 489–490.

8. Theitmar of Merseberg for example wrote in the early 11th century that "there are many conspiracies in the regions of Rome and Lombardy. For all visitors there is scant affection and everything that a guest requires must be bought, treachery being part of the deal. Many here also die from poisoning." See Thietmar of Merseburg, *Ottonian Germany: The Chronicon of Thietmar of Merseburg*. David A. Warner trans. (New York: Manchester University Press, 2001), p. 309. On Italians as poisoners, see also Antoni Mączak, *Travel in Early Modern Europe* (Cambridge, UK: Polity Press, 1995), p. 249.

9. Corrado Tommasi-Crudeli, *The Climate of Rome and the Roman Malaria* (London: J. & A. Churchill, 1892), p. 57.

10. Herde, p. 536. The Maremma coastal plain was dangerous even to native Italians, as demonstrated by the malaria deaths of three members of the Medici family of Florence within three weeks of each other after a late summer excursion into the Maremma plain in 1562. Their deaths were blamed on "severe malaria" by contemporaries, and this diagnosis has recently been confirmed by a chemical analysis of their skeletal remains, which tested positive for *P. falciparum* antigens. See Gino Fornaciari et al., "*Plasmodium falciparum* Immunodection in Bone Remains of Members of the Renaissance Medici Family." *Transactions of the Royal Society of Tropical Medicine and Hygiene*, Vol. 104 (2010), pp. 583–587.

11. Gregorovius, Vol VI, Part 2, p. 381. Gregorovius is re-quoting Matteo Villani.

12. Gregorovius, Vol VI, Part 2, p. 381; Ivan Hlaváček, "The Luxemburgs and Rupert of the Palatinate, 1347–1410." In Michael Jones ed., *The New Cambridge Medieval History*, Vol. VI (Cambridge, UK: Cambridge University Press, 2015), p. 553.

13. See Peter H. Wilson, *The Holy Roman Empire 1495–1806* (New York: Palgrave, 2011), pp. 3–5; Wilson, *Heart of Europe*, pp. 1–3.

14. *Ibid.*, p. 3.

15. Horst Fuhrmann, "*Quis teutonicos constituit iudices nationum?* The Trouble with Henry." *Speculum*, Vol. 69, No. 2 (Apr. 1994), pp. 348.

16. Tyler, pp. 39–40, 41.

17. Gregorovius, Vol. VI, part 1, p. 28.

18. *The Deeds of Frederick Barbarossa*, p. 201.

19. Gregorovius, Vol. IV, part 2, p. 329.

20. See Otto Kestner, "Alpenpässe und Römische Malaria in der mittelalterlichen Kaiserzeit." *Historische Vierteljahrsschift*, Vol. 30 (1935), pp. 686–719.

21. See Munz, p. 72.

22. By "probable malaria case," I mean a premature death or large-scale disease outbreak occurring in a malarial zone and during the summer malaria season, particularly the months of August and September, which is not obviously the result of a non-malarial disease pathogen. See Chapter 3 above for a fuller explanation of why I am opposed to more restricted methods of determining probable malarial infections, which I believe can lead us to misleading false negative results.

23. Or perhaps Frederick II was just lucky. Some scholars hold that malaria resistance can be lost in as little as six months if an individual is no longer exposed to constant re-infection, so Frederick's acquired immunity to malaria could have been partially or wholly lost during his time in Germany. See Carter and Mendis, p. 567.

24. Wilson, *Heart of Europe*, p. 51.

25. William McNeill, *The Pursuit of Power* (Chicago, IL: University of Chicago Press, 1982), p. 3.

Chapter 10

1. Christopher Cheney, *Pope Innocent III and England* (Stuttgart: Anton Hiersemann, 1976), p. 25.

2. Barefoot, p. 35.

3. Julia Bolton Holloway, *The Pilgrim and the Book: A Study of Dante, Langland, and Chaucer* (New York: Peter Lang, 1992), p. 2.

4. *Ibid.*, p. 16.

5. Alan Kendall, *Medieval Pilgrims* (London: Wayland Publishers, 1970), p. 11.

6. Debra J. Birch, *Pilgrimage to Rome in the Middle Ages: Continuity and Change* (Rochester, NY: Boydell Press, 1998), pp. 136, 151–154. See also Joyce Hill, "From Rome to Jerusalem: An Icelandic Itinerary of the Mid-Twelfth Century." *Harvard Theological Review*, Vol. 76, No. 2 (1983), pp. 175–203; Francis Peabody Magoun, "The Rome of Two Northern Pilgrims: Archbishop Sigeric of Canterbury and Abbot Nikolás of Munkathverá." *Harvard Theological Review*, Vol. 33, No. 4 (Oct. 1940), pp. 267–289.

7. Kendall, p. 36.

8. *Ibid.*, p. 146.

9. See Barefoot, p. 38. According to Liutprand of Cremona, Berengar, the King of Italy, sent a spy to Rome in the guise of a poor pilgrim; see Liutprand of Cremona, p. 182.

10. See Michael Keevak, *The Pretended Asian: George Psalmanazar's Eighteenth-Century Formosan Hoax* (Detroit: Wayne State University Press, 2004).

11. Katherine L. Jansen, Joanna Dell, and Frances Andrew. *Medieval Italy: Texts in Translation* (Philadelphia: University of Pennsylvania Press, 2009), p. pp. 293–294.

12. Sumption, p. 147.
13. Étienne Van Cauwenbergh, *Les Pèlerinages Expiatoires et Judiciaires dans le Droit Communal de la Belgique au Moyen Âge* (Louvain: Bureaux du Recueil, 1922), p. 39.
14. Ibid., p. 165.
15. Tyler, p. 27.
16. Albert d'Haenens, "Aller à Rome au Moyen Age." *Institut Historique Belge de Rome*, Vol. 50 (1980), p. 104.
17. Dante Alighieri, *The Inferno*. John Ciardi trans. (New York: Penguin, 1982), pp. 27–32.
18. Norbert Ohler, *The Medieval Traveller*, Caroline Hillier trans. (Woodbridge, UK: Boydell Press, 1989), p. 196.
19. Edmond René Labande, "Recherches sur les pèlerins dans l'Europe des Xie et XIIe siècles." *Cahiers de Civilisation Médiévale*, Vol. 1, no. 3 (1958), p. 341.
20. Geoffrey Chaucer, *The Canterbury Tales*, Michael Murphy trans. On-line at <http://academic.brooklyn.cuny.edu/webcore/murphy/canterbury/2genpro.pdf>.
21. Holloway, p. 234.
22. Ibid., p. 174.
23. Webb, p. 22.
24. Champ, p. 31.
25. Birch, p. 199.
26. Herbert Thurston, *The Holy Year of Jubilee: An Account of the History and Ceremonial of the Roman Jubilee* (London: Sands and Co., 1900), p. 12.
27. Dante *The Inferno*, p. 159.
28. Ibid., pp. 18, 26.
29. Frugoni, p. 102; Giovanni Villani, *Selections from the First Nine Books of the Chroniche Fiorentine of Giovanni Villani*, Rose E. Selfe trans. (Westminster, UK: Archibald Constable, p. 1896), p. 320.
30. Thurston, p. 19
31. Ibid., p. 23.
32. Webb, p. 64; Holloway, p. 157.
33. Frugoni, p. 42.
34. Thurston, p. 14.
35. Furgoni, p. 106. On Sardinia's malaria, see Marcus Hall, "Environmental Imperialism in Sardinia: Pesticides and Politics in the Struggle against Malaria." In Marco Armiero and Marcus Hall eds., *Nature and History in Modern Italy* (Athens, OH: Ohio University Press, 2010), pp. 70–86.
36. Thurston, p. 26.
37. Sumption, pp. 330, 338.
38. Thurston, p. 56.
39. Ibid., p. 57.
40. Ibid., p. 58.
41. Furgoni, p. 124.
42. Fiorenza Cilli, *Giubilei: Breve Storia Degli Anni Santi* (Rome: Olmata, 2016), pp. 32–33.
43. Thurston, p. 64.
44. Ibid., p. 65.
45. Ibid., p. 68.
46. Ibid. Paulo notes that "Many people died... more particularly, of the pilgrims."
47. Celli, p. 59. My translation.
48. Arnold von Harff, *The Pilgrimage of Arnold Von Harff*, Malcolm Tetts trans. (London: Hakluyt Society, 1949), p. 39.
49. Ibid., pp. 20–34.
50. Ibid., p. 35. The same story appears in the 15th-century pilgrim guide of William Brewyn, who clarifies that these demons were causing a "horrible and terrible plague" which "kill[ed] by suffocation all who passed through the Flaminian gate." See William Brewyn, *A XVth Century Guide-Book to the Principal Churches of Rome* (London: Marshall Press, 1933), pp. 40–41.
51. Parks, p. 354.
52. See Champ, p. 43, and Rudyard Kipling, *Debits and Credits* (New York: Scribner's, 1926), p. 152.

Chapter 11

1. Thomas of Marlborough, *History of the Abbey of Evesham* (Oxford, UK: Clarendon Press, 2003), pp. 193–194.
2. Ibid., p. 229.
3. On the well-documented Evesham case, see Collins, *Keeper of the Keys*, pp. 245–250; Parks, pp. 241–242.
4. Cheney, p. 109.
5. Bettenson ed., p. 105.
6. Noble, p. 585.
7. Robinson, "Reform and the Church: 1073–1122." In David Luscombe and Jonathan Riley-Smith eds., *The New Cambridge Medieval History*, Vol. IV, Part 1 (Cambridge, UK: Cambridge University Press, 1999), p. 316.
8. La Due, p. 100.
9. Robinson, "The Papacy, 1122–1198." In David Luscombe and Jonathan Riley-Smith eds., *The New Cambridge Medieval History*, Vol. 4 (Cambridge, UK: Cambridge University Press, 2004), p. 325.
10. Barraclough, p. 104.
11. Robinson, "The Institutions of the Church, 1073–1216." In David Luscombe and Jonathan Riley-Smith eds., *The New Cambridge Medieval History*, Vol 4, Part 1. (Cambridge, UK: Cambridge University Press, 1999), p. 383. See also Z. N. Brooke, *The English Church and the Papacy: From the Conquest to the Reign of John* (Cambridge: Cambridge University Press, 1931), pp. 28–29.
12. R. W. Southern, *Western Society and the Church of the Middle Ages* (New York: Viking Penguin, 1992), p. 115–177. Re-quoted from La Due, p. 110.
13. La Due, p. 119.
14. Robinson, "The Institutions of the Church," p. 438.
15. John of Salisbury, *The Historia Pontificalis*, Marjorie Chinball trans (New York: Thomas Nelson and Sons, 1962), p. 81.
16. John of Salisbury, p. 76.
17. Robinson, "Reform and the Church," p. 324.
18. William E. Lunt, *Financial relations of the Papacy with England to 1327* (Cambridge, MA: The Mediaeval Academy of America, 1939), p. 483.
19. See Cheney, p. 44–45.

20. Parks, p. 117.
21. *Ibid.*, p. 99.
22. *Ibid.*, p. 97.
23. *Ibid.*, p. 82.
24. *Ibid.*, p. 127.
25. *Ibid.*, p. 187.
26. *Ibid.*, pp. 227–228.
27. Parks, p. 126.
28. Brenda Bolton, "Papal Italy." In David Abulafia ed., *Italy in the Central Middle Ages* (New York: Oxford University Press, 2004), p. 96.
29. See de Camille de Tournon-Simiane, *Études Statistiques sur Rome*, Vol. 1 (Paris: Librarie de Firmin Didot Frères, 1855), p. 105.
30. Matthaeis, G. de. *Sul Culto Reso dagli Antichi Romani alla Dea Febbre* (Roma: Stamperia de Romanis, 1814), p. 28.
31. Bolton, p. 96.
32. *Ibid.*, p. 98.
33. Parks, p. 129–130, 200–201.
34. Cheney, p. 109.
35. Lunt, p. 181.
36. *Ibid.*, p. 182.
37. Bernard de Clairvaux, *On Consideration*, George Lewis trans. (Oxford: Clarendon Press, 1908), p. 20.
38. *Ibid.*, p. 77.

Chapter 12

1. Gregorovius, Vol. V, Part 2, p. 570.
2. Norwich, p. 191.
3. Gregorovius, Vol. V, Part 2, p. 576.
4. Philip H. Wicksteed, ed. *Villani's Chronicle* (London: Archibald Constable and Co., 1906), p. 347.
5. Gregorovius, Vol. V, Part 2, p. 595.
6. Gregorovius, Vol. V, part 2, p. 599.
7. Ullmann, p. 279.
8. Norwich, p. 203.
9. *Ibid.*, p. 197.
10. *Ibid.*, pp. 203–204.
11. *The Essential Petrarch*. Peter Hainsworth trans. (Cambridge, UK: Hackett Publishing, 2010), p. 60.
12. *Ibid.*
13. Unn Falkeid, *The Avignon Papacy Contested: An Intellectual History from Dante to Catherine of Siena* (London, UK: Harvard University Press, 2017), pp. 101–102.
14. Gregorovius, Vol. VI, part 2, pp. 436–437.
15. Michel Grenon, *Charles d'Anjou: Frère Conquérant de Saint Louis* (Paris: L'Harmattan, 2012), p. 163.
16. *Ibid.*, p. 198.
17. On the reign of Joanna, see Georges Jehel, *Les Angevins de Naples: Un Dynastie Européenne, 1246–1266–1442* (Paris: Ellipses, 2014).
18. Contemporary accounts of Louis of Anjou's 1383 campaign note that there was already illness in the army in June, but that the "plague intensified with the warm weather." See William Caferro, *John Hawkwood: An English Mercenary in Fourteenth-Century Italy* (Baltimore: Johns Hopkins University Press, 2006), p. 240.
19. See William Urban, *Medieval Mercenaries: The Business of War* (London: Greenhill Books, 2006), pp. 229–231.
20. Caferro, p. 63.
21. *Ibid.*, pp. 65, 256
22. *Ibid.*, p. 256.
23. *Ibid.*, p. 209.
24. Norwich, p. 219.
25. Norwich, p. 239.
26. Collins, p. 319. Judith Hook estimated that as many as 3% of Roman's 55,000-odd citizens got their living from prostitution by the early 16th century; see Judith Hook, *The Sack of Rome* (London: Macmillan, 1972), p. 66.
27. La Due, p. 175.
28. Parks, pp. 337–341.
29. La Due, p. 176.
30. *Ibid.*
31. Norwich, p. 234.
32. Norwich, p. 262.
33. Nicolo Machiavelli, *The Prince*, W. K. Marriott trans. On-line at http://www.gutenberg.org/files/1232/1232-h/1232-h.htm.
34. Norwich, p. 255.
35. Michael Mallet and Christine Shaw, *The Italian Wars, 1494–1559* (New York: Routledge, 2012), p. 24.
36. Hibbert, *Rome*, p. 135.
37. Christopher Hibbert, *The Borgias* (London: Constable, 2009), p. 119.
38. Mallett and Shaw, pp. 33–34.
39. Luigi Guicciardini, *The Sack of Rome*, James H. McGregor Trans (New York: Italica Press, 1993), p. 62.
40. *Ibid.*, pp. 245–246. The pope was apparently already ill in July, when he complained of a "slight dysentery." Nor was he alone: in July of 1503, fever (probably *P. falciparum*) swept through Rome, inflicting high casualties.
41. La Due, p. 183.
42. Norwich, pp. 282–283.
43. *Ibid.*, p. 285.
44. Wendy J. Reardon, *The Deaths of the Popes: Comprehensive Accounts, Including Funerals, Burial Places, and Epitaphs* (London: McFarland, 2004), p. 180.
45. While there is considerable overlap between cardinals and popes, some popes were elevated to the office without becoming cardinals first, though this became increasingly rare over time. Note that these statistics exclude popes who abdicated, died by violence, or passed away outside of Rome.
46. Hook, p. 144.
47. *Ibid.*, p. 162.
48. Guicciardini, p. 93.
49. Norwich, p. 294.
50. Guicciardini, p. 107.
51. *Ibid.*, p. 111.
52. *Ibid.*, p. 98.
53. Guicciardini, pp. 114.

54. *Ibid.*, pp. 111–112.
55. Hook, p. 190.
56. Hibbert, *Rome*, p. 160. Judith Hook makes a similar argument (see Hook, p.190).
57. See Corradi, Vol. VIII, p. 121.
58. Hook, p. 206.
59. *Ibid.*, pp. 214–215. See also Mallet and Shaw, p. 163.
60. William Henry Smyth, *The Mediterranean: A Memoir* (London: John W. Parker, 1854), p. 228. George Cowan suggests that these forces were destroyed by typhus rather than malaria, but without any substantiating evidence; see George Cowan, *The Most Fatal Distemper: Typhus in History* (Diadem Books: Scotland, UK, 2016), p. 13.
61. *Ibid.*, p. 237.
62. Henry VII, *Assertio Septem Sacramentorum, or Defense of the Seven Sacraments* (New York: Benziger Brothers, 1908), p. 462.

Chapter 13

1. Martin Luther, *The Life of Luther Written by Himself*, William Hazlitt trans. (London: George Bell and Sons, 1904), p. 15. On Luther in Rome, see also Robert H. Bainton, *Here I Stand: A Life of Martin Luther* (Peabody, MA: Hendrickson, 1950), pp. 29–32.
2. *Ibid.*
3. *Ibid.*
4. *Ibid.*, p. 16.
5. *Ibid.*, p. 17.
6. Martin Luther, "An Open Letter to the Christian Nobility of the German Nation Concerning the Reform of the Christian Estate." C. M. Jacobs ed. (1520), pp. 58, 83, 80.
7. *Ibid.*, p. 80.
8. *Ibid.*, p. 95.
9. Mark Greengrass, *Christendom Destroyed: Europe 1517–1648* (New York: Viking, 2014), p. 309.
10. *Ibid.*, p. 81.
11. *Ibid.*, p. 84.
12. *Ibid.*, p. 88..
13. Greengrass, p. 335.
14. Stephen J. Vicchio, *The Legend of the Anti-Christ: A History* (Eugene, Oregon: Wipf and Stock, 2009), p. 198.
15. Martin Luther, *Against the Roman Papacy: An Institution of the Devil*. Requoted from Helmet Lehmann ed., *Luther's Works, American Edition*, Vol. 41 (Philadelphia: Fortress Press, 1957–1981), pp. 356–358.
16. Guicciardini, p. 110.
17. *Ibid.*, p. 109.
18. Hook, p. 174.
19. Helmet Lehmann ed., *Luther's Works, American Edition*, Vol. 49 (Philadelphia: Fortress Press, 1972), p. 169.
20. Greengrass, p. 277.
21. Vidmar, p. 213.
22. Luther, "Letter to the Christian Nobility," p. 114.
23. *Ibid.*, p. 115.
24. Gilles Bertrand, *Le Grand Tour Revisité: Pour Une Archéologie du Tourism: Le Voyage des Français en Italie*. (Rome: École Français de Rome, 2008), p. 74. My translation.
25. Reilly, "Malaria, Protestants, and Google," pp. 312–321.
26. A symbol of this change is the "Quadruple Alliance" of 1815, signed by Anglican Britain, Lutheran Prussia, Catholic Austria, and Orthodox Russia for mutual assistance against the French revolutionary threat.
27. *Ibid.*, p. 320.

Chapter 14

1. Logan Pearsall Smith, *The Life and Letters of Sir Henry Wotton*, Vol 1. (Oxford: Clarendon Press, 1907), pp. 19–21.
2. Anthony Munday, *The English Romayne Lyfe* (Plaistow, UK: Curwen Press, 1925), p. 1.
3. Fynes Moryson, *The Itinerary of Fynes Moryson*. Vol. 1 (London: J. Beale, 1617), p. 303.
4. Edward Webbe, *His Trauailes* (London: Bloomsbury, 1590), p. 31.
5. Barefoot, p. 71.
6. William Lithgow, *Travels and Voyages through Europe, Asia, and Africa* (Edinburgh: J. Murray and J. Cochran, 1770), pp. 21–22.
7. J. A. Symonds, *Sir Philip Sidney* (London: Macmillan, 1906), p. 29.
8. M. L. Clarke, "British Travellers to Rome in Tudor and Stuart Times." *History Today*, Vol. 28, No. 1 (Nov. 1978), p. 747.
9. *Ibid.*, 746.
10. Barefoot, p. 67.
11. Jeremy Black, *Italy and the Grand Tour* (London: Yale University Press, 2003), p. 2.
12. Clarke, p. 746.
13. Gerrit Verhoeven, "Calvinist Pilgrimages and Popish Encounters: Religious Identity and Sacred Space on the Dutch Grand Tour (1598–1685)." *Journal of Social History*, Vol. 43, No. 3 (2010), p. 623, 618.
14. *Ibid.*, p. 627.
15. Barefoot, p. 67.
16. Jean Delumeau, *Rome au XVIe Siècle* (London: Hachette, 1975), pp. 35, 39.
17. Norwich, p. 313.
18. *Ibid.*, p. 47.
19. Thurston, p. 93.
20. Delumeau, p. 43.
21. *Ibid.*, p. 44
22. *Ibid.*, p. 40.
23. Hook, p. 28.
24. Delemeau, p. 41.
25. François Brizay, "L'image de l'Italie dans les guides et les relations de voyage publiés en France au XVIIe siècle (1595–1713): sa construction et son évolution." Ph.D. Thesis, University of Tours, 1996, p. 230–231.
26. *Ibid.*, p. 47.

27. Eric MacPhail, *The Voyage to Rome in French Renaissance Literature* (Saratoga, CA: ANMA Libri and Co., 1990), p. 3.
28. *Ibid.*, p. 2; Burke, Peter. "Rome as a Center of Information and Communication for the Catholic World, 1550–1650." In H. Jones and Thomas Worcester eds., *From Rome to Eternity: Catholicism and the Arts in Italy, ca. 1550–1650*. (Boston: Brill, 2002), p. 260.
29. MacPhail, pp. 51–52.
30. Michel de Montagne, *The Journal of Montaigne's Travel in Italy by Way of Switzerland and Germany in 1580 and 1581*, Vol 2. (London: John Murray, 1903), p. 74.
31. Thomas James Dandelet, *Spanish Rome, 1500–1700* (New Haven: Yale University Press, 2001), p. 120.
32. Dandalet, p. 59.
33. *Ibid.*, p. 8.
34. Brisay, p. 345. My translation.
35. *Ibid.*, p. 345.
36. *Ibid.*
37. Fiammetta Rocco, *Quinine: Malaria and the Quest for a Cure That Changed the World* (New York: HarperCollins, 2003), p. 77.
38. Richard Wrigley, "Infectious Enthusiasms: Influence, Contagion, and the Experience of Rome." In Chloe Chard and Helen Langdon eds., *Transports: Travel, Pleasure, and Imaginative Geography, 1600–1830* (London: Paul Mellon Center for Studies in British Art, 1996), p. 77.
39. *Ibid.*
40. See Reilly, "Cardinal Numbers," p. 411. See also Brent D. Shaw, "Seasons of Death: Aspects of Mortality in Imperial Rome." *The Journal of Roman Studies*, Vol. 86 (1996), pp. 119–121.
41. Hibbert, *Rome*, p. 161.
42. William Thomas, *The History of Italy*, George B Parks ed. (Ithaca, NY: Cornell University Press, 1963), p. 27.
43. Delumeau, p. 72.
44. On the connection between urban density and malaria intensity, see Salares, p. 211; Reilly, "Cardinal Numbers," p. 413–414.
45. Katherine Rinne, *The Waters of Rome: Aqueducts, Fountains, and the Birth of the Baroque City* (London: Yale University Press, 2010), p. 41.
46. Katherine Rinne, "Urban Ablutions: Cleansing Counter-Reformation Rome." In Mark Bradley ed., *Rome, Pollution, and Propriety* (New York: Cambridge University Press, 2012), p. 197.
47. Rinne, *The Waters of Rome*, p. 136.
48. *Ibid.*, p. 146.
49. *Ibid.*, p. 156.
50. *Ibid.*, p. 198.
51. *Ibid.*, p. 211.

Chapter 15

1. Johan Wolfgang von Goethe, *Italian Journey* (New York: Penguin, 1962), pp. 127–128.
2. *Ibid.*, p. 129.

3. John Pemble, *The Rome We Have Lost* (Oxford, UK: Oxford University Press, 2017), p. 13.
4. John Chetwode Eustace, *A Classical Tour through Italy*, Vol. 1 (London: J. Mawman, 1815), p. 342.
5. C. M. J. B. Dupaty, *Lettres sur l'Italie en 1785* (Paris: Depélafol, 1822), Vol. 2, pp. 178–179.
6. *Ibid.*, p. 178. My translation.
7. Richard Lassels, *The Voyage of Italy, Or a Compleat Journey through Italy* (London: John Starkey, 1670), preface. I've modernized the text and corrected some of Lassel's typos. See also Rosemary Sweet, *Cities and the Grand Tour: The British in Italy, 1690–1820* (Cambridge, UK: Cambridge University Press, 2012), pp. 23–24.
8. Lassels, p. 257.
9. Clare Howard, *English Travellers of the Renaissance* (London: John Lane, 1914), p. 22.
10. Thomas, pp. xv–xvi. See also Lewis Einstein, *The Italian Renaissance in England* (New York: Colombia University Press, 1903), pp. 115–130.
11. Clare, p. 64.
12. Barefoot, pp. 95–96.
13. Edward Corp, *The Stuarts in Italy, 1917–1766: A Royal Court in Permanent Exile* (New York: Cambridge University Press, 2011), pp. 2–4.
14. Sweet, p. 150. Note that Grand Tourists also hailed from other parts of the Protestant north, especially Germany (Goethe being a notable example). However, scholarly sources on such travelers are extremely meager.
15. On the "depleted" pilgrimage tradition following the Protestant Reformation, see Champ, pp. 83–84.
16. Goethe, p. 75.
17. Anonymous, *Travels of an English Gentleman from London to Rome* (London: A. Bettesworth, 1718), pp. 118–119.
18. John Moore, *A View of Society and Manners in Italy*, Vol. 2 (London: W. Strahan and T. Cadell, 1781), pp. 48–49.
19. Anna Jameson, *Diary of an Ennuyée* (London: Henry Colburn, 1826), p. 198.
20. John Richard Digby Beste, *Transalpine Memoirs* (Bath: Richard Cruttwell, 1826), Vol. 1, p. 128.
21. Monsieur de Blainville, *Travels through Holland, Germany, Switzerland, but Especially Italy*, Vol. 2 (London: John Noon, 1757), pp. 415–416.
22. Goethe, p. 380.
23. See Reilly, "Seasons in Italy: Northern European Travelers, Rome, and Malaria" and Reilly, "Northern European Patterns of Visiting Rome, 1400–1850."
24. See John Pemble, *The Mediterranean Passion: Victorians and Edwardians in the South* (London: Faber and Faber, 2009), p. 18; Tyler, p. 26.
25. Barefoot, p. 33; Albert C. Leighton, *Transport and Communication in early Medieval Europe, AD 500–1100* (Newton Abbot, UK: David and Charles, 1972), p. 177.
26. Pemble, *The Mediterranean Passion*, p. 27.
27. Reilly, "Northern European Patterns of Visiting Rome," p. 15.

28. See Montaigne, Vol. 3.
29. Christopher Hoolihan, "Health and Travel in Nineteenth-Century Rome." *The Journal of the History of Medicine and Allied Sciences*, Vol. 44 (1989), pp. 466–467.
30. *Ibid.*, p. 465.
31. T. H. Burgess, *The Climate of Italy in Relation to Pulmonary Consumption* (London: Longman, Brown, Green and Longmans, 1852), p. 168. R. E. Scoresby-Jackson also argued that Rome's climate was not advantageous enough for invalids to "warrant the physician putting his patient to the expense and inconvenience of so long a journey." See R. E. Scoresby-Jackson, *Medical Climatology: or, A Topographical and Meteorological Description of the Localities Resorted to in Winter and Summer by Invalids* (London: John Churchill, 1862), p. 406.
32. Burgess, p. 176.
33. Montesquieu, for example, defined *l'intempérance*—literally meaning overindulgence—as "an illness which reigns during the summer at Rome, around Rome and in the Kingdom of Naples," which "begins with an imperceptible fever, which afterwards rises. After which, one almost always dies." He also notes that it was particularly common in the *Campagna* of Rome, and that it was associated with stagnant water. Given these symptoms, the location, and timings, he seems to be talking about *P. falciparum* malaria. See Albert de Montesquieu, *Voyages de Montesquieu*, Vol. 1 (Paris: Alphonse Picard & Fils, 1895), p. 196.
34. For a more thorough accounting of the relationship between growing European understanding of the threat of Roman Fever and the seasonality of Roman travel, see Reilly, "Seasons in Italy."
35. Charlotte Anne Eaton, *Rome, in the Nineteenth Century*. Vol. 3 (Edinburgh: Archibald Constable and Co., 1822), p. 414.
36. James Johnson, *Change of Air, or the Philosophy of Travelling* (New York: Samuel Wood and Sons, 1831), p. 219.
37. Charles Pau Coëtlosquet, *Souvenirs de Voyages* (Paris: Chez Waille, 1843), p. 122. My translation. For a longer discussion on Northern perceptions of malaria in Rome, the *campagna*, and the Pontine marshes, see Robert Casillo, *The Empire of Stereotypes: Germaine de Stael and the Idea of Italy* (New York: Palgrave Macmillan, 2006), pp. 166–179.
38. Johnson, p. 217.
39. Alban Butler, *Travels through France and Italy... During the Years 1745 and 1746* (Edinburgh: John Moir, 1803), p. 210.
40. M. R. Colomb, *Journal d'un Voyage en Italie et en Suisse* (Paris: Verdière, 1833), pp. 271–274, 278.
41. Marguerite Blessington, *The Idler in Italy*. Vol. 2 (London: Henry Colburn, 1839), p. 107.
42. William Webb, *Minutes of Remarks... Made in a Course along the Rhine, and During a Residence in Swisserland and Italy*, Vol. 2 (London: Baldwin, Cradock, and Joy, 1827), p. 122.
43. Charles Terry, *Scenes and Thoughts in Foreign Lands* (London: William Pickering, 1848), pp. 141, 143–144.
44. *Ibid.*, p. 145.
45. *Ibid.*, p. 149.
46. Elizabeth Knight, *Lady Knight's Letters from France and Italy, 1776–1795* (London: Arthur L. Humphreys, 1905), p. 95.
47. William Stuart Rose, *Letters from the North of Italy*, Vol. 1 (London: John Murray, 1819), p. 103.
48. Bruce-Chwatt and Zulueta, p. 71.
49. Gabriele Taussig, *The Roman Climate: Its Influence on Healthy and Disease, Serving as a Hygienical Guide* (Rome: Roman Typography, 1870), p. 88.
50. Henry James, *Daisy Miller* (London: Martin Secker, 1878), pp. 111–114.

Chapter 16

1. G. E. Marindin, ed., *The Letters of John B. S. Morritt of Rokeby* (London: John Murray, 1914), pp. 296, 300.
2. *Ibid.*, p. 297.
3. *Ibid.*, p. 303.
4. *Ibid.*, p. 292.
5. Desmond Gregory, *Napoleon's Italy* (Teaneck, NJ: Fairleigh Dickinson University Press, 2001), p. 51.
6. Susan Vandiver Nicassio, *Imperial City: Rome Under Napoleon* (London: University of Chicago Press, 2005), pp. 20–21. *Ibid.*, p. 22.
7. *Ibid.*, p. 84.
8. *Ibid.*, p. 89.
9. Nicassio, p. 31.
10. *Ibid.*, p. 188.
11. De Tournon, p. 232. My translation.
12. French Doctor J. B. Michel gives more details about this incident, noting that these troops suffered from "intermittent and pernicious intermittent fevers," "jaundice," "sweating." In addition, some of these troops suffered "comas," meaning they probably suffered cerebral malaria, a symptom of *P. falciparum*. According to Michel, the barracks outside the Porto de Popolo were judged to be uninhabitable from June 20 to the 30th of October. See J. B. Michel, *Recherches Médico-Topographiques sur Rome et L'Agro Romano* (Rome: L'Imprimerie de Deromanis, 1811), p. 145.
13. De de Tournon-Simiane, Vol. 1, pp. 232–233.
14. *Ibid.*, pp. 234, 230.
15. *Ibid.*, pp. 239, 107, 133.
16. *Ibid.*, p. 139. My translation.
17. Angelo Celli, *Malaria, According to the New Researches* (New York: Longmans, Green, 1900), p. 83.
18. John Macculloch, *Malaria: an Essay* (London: Longman, Rees, Orme, Brown, and Green, 1827), p. 37.
19. Gregor, p. 154.
20. Nicassio, p. 57; Taussig, p. 40.
21. See de Tournon, p. 232.
22. John Bramsen, *Letters of a Prussian Traveller*, Vol 2 (London: Henry Colburn, 1818), pp. 246–247. His italics.

23. Marie-Henri Beyle [Stendhal], *Rome, Naples et Florence*, Vol. 3 (Paris: Delaunay, 1826), p. 43. My translation.
24. Louis Simond, *Voyage en Italie et en Sicile*, Vol. 1 and 2 (Paris: A. Sautelet and Company, 1828), pp. 39, 43.
25. Giegler, p. 565. My translation.
26. *Ibid.*, p. 69.
27. Thomas Pennington, *A Journey into Various Parts of Europe*, Vol. 2 (London: George B. Whittaker, 1825), pp. 74–75.
28. *Ibid.*, p. 85.
29. Philippe Séguin, *Louis Napoléon Le Grand* (Paris: Bernard Grasset, 1990), p. 125.
30. See David I. Kertzer, *The Pope Who Would Be King* (New York: Random House, 2018), p. 207.
31. Jacquot, pp. 75–76.
32. *Ibid.* p. 74.
33. *Ibid.* p. 3.
34. *Ibid.*, p. 151.
35. *Ibid.*, pp. 82–83.
36. *Ibid.*, pp. 386.
37. *Ibid.*, p. 341–350.
38. *Ibid.*, p. 166.
39. *Ibid.*, p. 144.
40. Gilmour, pp. 203, 227.
41. Tommasi-Crudeli, p. 53.
42. W. North, *Roman Fever* (London: Sampson Low, Marston and Co., 1896), pp. 145–146.
43. See Celli, pp. 148–149. Overall, the number of malaria cases in Roman hospitals declined from 5,528 in 1864 to 4,390 in 1898, which represents a much higher *per capita* decline, as Rome's population probably doubled during the same period.
44. Luigi Torelli, *La Malaria D'Italia* (Rome: Stabilimento Tipografico Italiano, 1883), pp. 54–59. Modern research has borne out Torelli's observations; see for example Piero Bevilacqua, "The Distinctive Character of Italian Environmental History," In Marco Armiero and Marcus Hall eds., *Nature and History in Modern Italy* (Athens, OH: Ohio University Press, 2010), pp. 17–21.
45. *Ibid.*, p. 34.
46. *Ibid.*, p. 22.
47. Celli, p. 19.
48. See Celli, p. 18; Frank M. Snowden, "From Triumph to Disaster: Fascism and Malaria in the Pontine Marshes, 1928–1946." In John Kickie, Jonn Foot, and Frank M. Snowden eds., *Disastro: Disasters in Italy since 1860: Culture, Politics, Society* (New York: Palgrave, 2002), p. 115.
49. Bonelli, p. 663.
50. Frank M. Snowden, "'Fields of Death': Malaria in Italy, 1861–1962" *Modern Italy*, Vol. 4, No. 1 (1999), p. 27.
51. *Ibid.*, p. 31.
52. Bruce-Chwatt and Zulueta, p. 109.
53. North, p. 385.
54. Pemble, pp. 39–40.
55. *Ibid.*, p. 243.
56. See Richard Wrigley, "Pathological Topographies and Cultural Itineraries: mapping 'mal'aria' in 18th- and 19th-century Rome." In Richard Wrigley and George Revill eds., *Pathologies of Travel* (Rodopi Bv Editions, 2000), p. 213.
57. See Taussig, pp. 212–213.
58. Torelli, p. 9. This is essentially the same definition as the one proposed by Gabrielle Taussig's influential *On the Roman Climate*; see Taussig, p. 90.
59. Francesco Puccinotti, *Storia delle Febbri Intermittenti Perniciose di Roma*, Vol. 2 (Napoli: Puzziello, 1838), p. 136.
60. North, p. vii. On the original text the page number is printed as "iiv," which of course makes no sense.
61. *Ibid.*, p. 378.
62. Snowden, "Fields of Death," pp. 40–41. On peasant folk beliefs on malaria and resistance to the Italian government's quinine campaign, see also Paola Corti, "La Malaria nel Mezzogiorno tra Otto e Novecento." In F. Della Peruta ed., *Storia d'Italia*, Vol. 7 (Einaudi, 1984), pp. 635–678.
63. Bonelli, p. 684.
64. W. O. Blanchard, "Malaria as a Factor in the Italian Environment." *The Scientific Monthly*, Vol. 27, No. 2 (Aug. 1928), p. 174.
65. Snowden, "Fields of Death," pp. 42–43.
66. Blanchard, p. 175.
67. See Snowden, "From Triumph to Disaster," pp. 121–126.
68. *Ibid.*, pp. 127–129.
69. Snowden, "Fields of Death," p. 45.
70. Barry Sullivan, "More than meets the eye: The Ethiopian war and the Origins of the Second World War." In Gordon Martel ed., *The Origins of the Second World War Reconsidered* (London: Routledge, 1999), p. 193.
71. Snowden, "From Triumph to Disaster," p. 131.
72. *Ibid.*, pp. 130, 113, 115.
73. Erhard Geissler and Jeanne Guillemin, "German Flooding of the Pontine Marshes in World War II: Biological Warfare or Total War Tactic?" *Politics and the Life Sciences*, Vol. 29, No. 1 (Mar. 2010), p. 4.
74. See Snowden, "Triumph to Disaster," pp. 114–115.
75. On post-war anti-malarial measures, see Snowden, "Fields of Death," pp. 40–50, and Giancarlo Majori, "Short History of Malaria and its Eradication in Italy with Short Notes on the Fight Against the Infection in the Mediterranean Basin." *Mediterranean Journal of Hematology and Infectious Diseases*, Vol. 4, No. 1 (2012), doi: 10.4084/MJHID.2012.016.

Conclusion

1. On the Sofia Zago malaria case, see "Malaria girl's dad says feels 'impotent.'" *Redazione ANSA* (Sept. 8, 2017), retrieved from http://www.ansa.it/english/news/2017/09/08/malaria-girls-dad-says-feels-impotent-3_014b03af-ae12-45a5-baaa-a6d34301f97b.html; Amy Held, "In a Case that is 'Almost Impossible,' Girl Dies of Malaria in Italy. *NPR* (Sept. 5, 2017), retrieved from https://www.npr.

org/sections/thetwo-way/2017/09/05/548624097/in-a-case-that-is-almost-impossible-girl-dies-of-malaria-in-italy; and "Dead Girl got malaria in Trento hospital-ISS." *Redazione ANSA* (Nov. 9, 2017), retrieved from http://www.ansa.it/english/news/general_news/2017/11/09/girl-got-malaria-in-trento-hospital-iss-3_012d2d78-6461-46b4-82bd-2d6182a196d3.html.

2. For a second opinion, see R. Romi, D. Boccolini, M. Menegon, and G. Rezza, "Probable Autochthonous Introduced Malaria Cases in Italy 2009–2011 and the Risk of Local Vector-Borne Transmission." *Eurosurveillance,* Vol. 17, No. 48 (29 Nov. 2012).

3. See "Anopheles labranchiae." *European Centre for Disease Prevention and Control* https://ecdc.europa.eu/en/disease-vectors/facts/mosquito-factsheets/anopheles-labranchiae.

4. See Max Weber, *The Protestant Ethic and the "Spirit" of Capitalism and Other Writings,* Peter Baehr and Gordon C. Wells trans. (New York: Penguin, 2002).

5. See Kenneth Pomeranz, *The Great Divergence: China, Europe, and the Making of the Modern World Economy* (Princeton: Princeton University Press, 2000).

6. W. H. S. Jones, *Malaria and Greek History* (Manchester: University Press, 1909), pp. 107.

Bibliography

Primary Sources

The Annals of Fulda. Timothy Reuter trans. New York: Manchester University Press, 1992.
Barbarossa in Italy. Thomas Carson ed. and trans. New York: Italica Press, 1994.
Bede, *A History of the English Church and People*. Leo Sherley-Price trans. New York: Dorset Press, 1968.
Bernard de Clairvaux. *On Consideration*. George Lewis trans. Oxford: Clarendon Press, 1908.
Beste, John Richard Digby. *Transalpine Memoirs*. 2 vols. Bath: Richard Cruttwell, 1826.
Bettenson, Henry ed. Documents of the Christian Church. New York: Oxford University Press, 2011.
Beyle, Marie-Henri [Stendhal]. *Rome, Naples et Florence*. 3 vols. Paris: Delaunay, 1826.
Blainville, Monsieur de. *Travels through Holland, Germany, Switzerland, but Especially Italy*. 3 vols. London: John Noon, 1757.
Blessington, Marguerite. *The Idler in Italy*. 2 vols. London: Henry Colburn, 1839.
Bracciolini, Poggio. *Revival: The Facetiae of Poggio and Other Medieval Story-Tellers*. London: Routledge, 2018.
Bramsen, John. *Letters of a Prussian Traveller*. 2 vols. London: Henry Colburn, 1818.
Brewyn, William. *A XVth Century Guide-Book to the Principal Churches of Rome*. London: Marshall Press, 1933.
Brosses, Charles de. *Lettres Familières, Écrites d'Italie en 1739 & 1740*. 2 vols. Paris: Librarie Académique, 1869.
Butler, Alban. *Travels through France and Italy... During the Years 1745 and 1746*. Edinburgh: John Moir, 1803.
Caxton, William. *The Golden Legend; or Lives of the Saints*. 7 vols. London: J. M. Dent and Co., 1900.
Chaucer, Geoffrey. *The Canterbury Tales*. Edited by Michael Murphy. On-line at <http://academic.brooklyn.cuny.edu/webcore/murphy/canterbury/2genpro.pdf>
Ciampini, Joannis. *De Sacris Aedificiis a Constantino Magno Constructis: Synopsis Historica*. Rome, 1693.
Coëtlosquet, Charles Paul. *Souvenirs de Voyages*. Paris: Chez Waille, 1843.
Colomb, M. R. *Journal d'un Voyage en Italie et en Suisse*. Paris: Verdière, 1833.
Dante, Aligheri. *The De Monarchia of Dante Alighieri*. Aurelia Henry trans. New York: Houghton Mifflin, 1904.
_____. *The Inferno*. John Ciardi trans. New York: Penguin, 1982.
Defoe, Daniel. *Tour through the Eastern Counties of England in 1722*. London: Cassell and Company, 1888.
Dupaty, C. M. J. B. *Lettres sur l'Italie en 1785*. 3 vols. Paris: Depélafol, 1822.
Eaton, Charlotte Anne. *Rome, in the Nineteenth Century*. 3 vols. Edinburgh: Archibald Constable and Co., 1822.
Einhard. *The Life of Charlemagne*. Ann Arbor: University of Michigan Press, 1960.
The Essential Petrarch. Peter Hainsworth trans. Cambridge, UK: Hackett, 2010.
Eustace, John Chetwode. *A Classical Tour through Italy*. 2 vols. London: J. Mawman, 1815.
Forster, J. R. *Travels through Sicily and that Part of Italy Formerly Called Magna Graecia*. London: Edward and Charles Dilly, 1773.
Giegler, Jean-Pierre. *Manuel du voyageur en Italie, ou Nouvelle description de tout ce que ce pays offre*. Milan, 1818.
Glaser, F. L. ed. *Pope Alexander VI and His Court: Extracts from the Latin Diary of Johannes Burchardus*. New York: Nicholas L. Brown, 1921.
Goethe, Johan Wolfgang von. *Italian Journey*. New York: Penguin, 1962.
Gourdault, Jules. *Rome et la Campagne Romaine*. Paris: Hachette, 1885.
Gregory of Tours. *History of the Franks*, Ernest Brehaut ed. New York: Columbia University Press, 1916.
Guicciardini, Luigi. *The Sack of Rome*. James H. McGregor Trans. New York: Italica Press, 1993.
Harff, Arnold von. *The Pilgrimage of Arnold von Harff*, Malcolm Tetts trans. London: Hakluyt Society, 1949.
Henry VII. *Assertio Septem Sacramentorum, or Defense of the Seven Sacraments*. New York: Benziger Brothers, 1908.
History and Politics in Late Carolinian and Ottonian Europe: The Chronicle of Regno of Prüm and Adalbert of Magdeburg. Simon MacLean trans. New York: Manchester University Press, 2009.
Horace, *The Complete Odes and Epodes*. David West trans. New York: Oxford University Press, 1997.
Isabey, Jean Baptiste. *Voyage en Italie*. Paris: 1823.

Jacquot, Félix. *Lettres Médicales sur L'Italie, Comprenant L'Histoire Médicale du Corps d'Occupation des États Romains*. Paris: Librairie de Victor Masson, 1857.

James, Henry. *Daisy Miller*. London: Martin Secker, 1878.

Jameson, Anna. *Diary of an Ennuyée*. London: Henry Colburn, 1826.

Jansen, Katherine L., Joanna Dell, and Frances Andrew. *Medieval Italy: Texts in Translation*. Philadelphia: University of Pennsylvania Press, 2009.

John of Salisbury. *The Historia Pontificalis*. Marjorie Chinball trans. New York: Thomas Nelson and Sons, 1962.

Johnson, James. *Change of Air, or the Philosophy of Travelling*. New York: Samuel Wood and Sons, 1831.

Jordanes. *The Origin and Deeds of the Goths*. Charles C. Mierow trans. Princeton, NJ: Princeton University Press, 1908.

Julius Caesar. *The Commentaries of Caesar on His Wars in Gaul*. Dublin: John Cumming, 1844.

Kipling, Rudyard. *Debits and Credits*. New York: Charles Scribner's Sons, 1926.

Knight, Elizabeth. *Lady Knight's Letters from France and Italy, 1776–1795*. London: Arthur L. Humphreys, 1905.

Kylie, Edward ed. *The English Correspondence of Saint Boniface*. London: Chatto and Windus, 1911.

Lalande, Joseph Jérôme. *Voyage en Italie*. 8 Vols. Geneva: 1790.

Lassels, Richard. *The Voyage of Italy, Or a Compleat Journey through Italy*. London: John Starkey, 1670.

Liber Pontificalis. Louise Ropes Loomis trans. New York: Columbia University Press, 1916.

Lithgow, William. *Travels and Voyages through Europe, Asia, and Africa*. Edinburgh: J. Murray and J. Cochran, 1770.

Liudprand of Cremona. *The Complete Works of Liudprand of Cremona*. Paulo Squatriti trans. Washington, D.C.: The Catholic University of America Press, 2007.

Livy, *The History of Rome*. Canon Roberts trans. London: Everyman's Library, 1905.

Luther, Martin. *Against the Roman Papacy, an Institution of the Devil*. 1545.

_____. *The Life of Luther Written by Himself*. William Hazlitt trans. London: George Bell and Sons, 1904.

_____. "An Open Letter to the Christian Nobility of the German Nation Concerning the Reform of the Christian Estate." C. M. Jacobs ed. 1520.

Machiavelli, Nicolo. *The Prince*. W. K. Marriott trans. On-line at http://www.gutenberg.org/files/1232/1232-h/1232-h.htm.

Marindin, G. E., ed. *The Letters of John B. S. Morritt of Rokeby*. London: John Murray, 1914.

The Marvels of Rome. Francis Morgan Nichols trans. New York: Ithaca Press, 1986.

Michel, J. B. *Recherches Médico-Topographiques sur Rome et L'Agro Romano*. Rome: L'Imprimerie de Deromanis, 1811.

Montagne, Michel de. *The Journal of Montaigne's Travel in Italy by Way of Switzerland and Germany in 1580 and 1581*. 2 Vols. London: John Murray, 1903.

Montesquieu, Albert de. *Voyages de Montesquieu*. 2 vols. Paris: Alphonse Picard & Fils, 1895.

Moore, John. *A view of Society and Manners in Italy*. 2 vols. London: W. Strahan and T. Cadell, 1781.

Moryson, Fynes. *The Itinerary of Fynes Moryson*. 3 vols. London: J. Beale, 1617.

Munday, Anthony. *The English Romayne Lyfe*. Plaistow, UK: Curwen Press, 1925.

Myers, Henry A. ed. *The Book of Emperors: A Translation of the Middle High German Kaiserchronik*. Morgantown, WV: West Virginia University Press, 2013.

Otto of Freising. *The Deeds of Frederick Barbarossa*. Charles Christopher Mierow trans. New York: Columbia University Press, 2004.

Pelikan, Jaroslav, et al. eds. *Luther's Works*. 55 Vols. St. Louis, MO: Concordia Publishing House, 1955.

Pennington, Thomas. *A Journey into Various Parts of Europe*. 2 vols. London: George B. Whittaker, 1825.

Perac, Etienne du. *I Vestigi Dell'Antichità di Roma: Raccolti Et Ritratti In Perspettiva Con Ogni Diligentia*. Rome, 1621.

Pick, Bernhard. *The Apocryphal Acts of Paul, Peter, John, Andrew, and Thomas*. London: Kegan Paul, Trench, Trübner, 1909.

Procopius. *History of the Wars*. H. B. Dewing trans. 7 Vols. Cambridge, MA: Harvard University Press, 1919.

Roscoe, Thomas. *The Continental Tourist: Views of Cities and Scenery in Italy, France, and Switzerland*. London: Peter Jackson, 1850.

Rose, William Stuart. *Letters from the North of Italy*. 2 vols. London: John Murray, 1819.

Simond, Louis. *Voyage en Italie et en Sicile*. 2 vols. Paris: A. Sautelet, 1828.

Smith, Logan Pearsall. *The Life and Letters of Sir Henry Wotton*. 2 vols. Oxford: Clarendon Press, 1907.

Smyth, William Henry. *The Mediterranean: A Memoir*. London: John W. Parker, 1854.

Tacitus. *The Agricola and Germania*, R. B. Townshend trans. London: Methuen, 1894.

_____. *Annals*. Alfred John Church and William Jackson Brodribb trans. New York: Random House, 1942.

Terry, Charles. *Scenes and Thoughts in Foreign Lands*. London: William Pickering, 1848.

Thietmar of Merseburg. *Ottonian Germany: The Chronicon of Thietmar of Merseburg*, David A. Warner trans. New York: Manchester University Press, 2001.

Thomas, William. *The History of Italy*. Ithaca, NY: Cornell University Press, 1963.

Thomas of Marlborough, *History of the Abbey of Evesham*. Oxford, UK: Clarendon Press, 2003.

Villani, Giovanni. *Selections from the First Nine Books of the Croniche Fiorentine of Giovanni*

Villani. Rose E. Selfe trans. Westminster, UK: Archibald Constable, 1896.
Webb, William. *Minutes of Remarks ... Made in a Course along the Rhine, and During a Residence in Swisserland and Italy*. 2 vols. London: Baldwin, Cradock, and Joy, 1827.
Webbe, Edward. *His Trauailes*. London: Bloomsbury, no date.
Wicksteed, Philip H. ed. *Villani's Chronicle*. London: Archbald Constable, 1906.
Wright, Thomas ed. *Gesta Romanorum; or Entertaining Stories*. 2 Vols. London: John Camden Hotten, 1871.

Secondary Sources

Abulafia, David. *Frederick II: A Medieval Emperor*. New York: Oxford University Press, 1988.
_____. "The Italian South." In Michael Jones ed., *The New Cambridge Medieval History*, Vol. 6, pp. 488–514. Cambridge, UK: Cambridge University Press, 2015.
Aldrete, Gregory S. *Floods of the Tiber in Ancient Rome*. Baltimore: Johns Hopkins University Press, 2007.
Alexander, Paul J. "The Medieval Legend of the Last Roman Emperor and Its Messianic Origin." *Journal of the Warburg and Courtauld Institutes*, Vol. 41 (1978), pp. 1–15.
Almeida, E. Rodriguez, *Il Monte Testaccio, ambiente, storia, material*. Rome: Quasar, 1984.
Althoff, Gerd. *Otto III*. Phyllis G. Jestice Trans. University Park: Pennsylvania State University Press, 2003.
André, Jean-Marie. "La notion de "Pestilentia" à Rome: du tabou religieux à l'interprétation préscientifique." *Latomus*, Vol. 39, No. 1 (1980), pp. 3–16.
Angelluci, Emanuele, Nigel Burrows, Stefano Losi, Chris Bartiromo, and X. Henry Hu. "Beta-thalassemia (BT) Prevalence and Treatment Patterns in Italy: A Survey of Treating Physicians." *Blood*, Vol. 128 (2016). doi.org/10.1182/blood.V128.22.3533.3533
Bainton, Robert H. *Here I Stand: A Life of Martin Luther*. Peabody, MA: Hendrickson, 1950.
Barefoot, Brian. *The English Road to Rome*. Reading, UK: Images Publishing, 1993.
Baron, Christopher, and Christopher Hamlin. "Malaria and the Decline of Ancient Greece: Revisiting the Jones Hypothesis in an Era of Interdisciplinarity." *Minerva*, Vol. 53 (2015), pp. 327–358.
Barraclough, Geoffrey. *The Medieval Papacy*. New York: W. W. Norton, 1968.
Bayley, C. C. "Petrarch, Charles IV, and the 'Renovatio Imperii.'" *Speculum*, Vol. 17, No. 3 (July 1942), pp. 323–341.
Becher, Matthias. *Charlemagne*. New Haven, CT: Yale University Press, 2003.
Bertrand, Gilles. *Le Grand Tour Revisité: Pour Une Archéologie du Tourism: Le Voyage des Français en Italie (Milieu XVIIIe Siècle-Début XIX Siècle)*. Rome: École Français de Rome, 2008.
Birch, Debra J. *Pilgrimage to Rome in the Middle Ages: Continuity and Change*. Rochester, NY: Boydell Press, 1998.
Black, Jeremy. *Italy and the Grand Tour*. London: Yale University Press, 2003.
Blanchard, W. O. "Malaria as a Factor in the Italian Environment." *The Scientific Monthly*, Vol. 27, No. 2 (Aug., 1928), pp. 172–176.
Bolton, Brenda. "Papal Italy." In David Abulafia ed., *Italy in the Central Middle Ages*. New York: Oxford University Press, 2004, pp. 82–103.
Bonelli, Franco. "La malaria nella storia demografica ed economica dell'Italia: Prima lineamenti di una ricerca." *Studi Storici*, Vol. 7, No. 4 (Oct.-Dec., 1966), pp. 659–687.
Bono, P., and C. Boni. "Water Supply of Rome in Antiquity and Today." *Environmental Geology*, Vol. 27, No. 2 (1996), pp. 126–134.
Bowsky, William M. *Henry VII in Italy: The Conflict of Empire and City-State, 1310–1313*. Lincoln, NE: University of Nebraska Press, 1960.
Bray, R. S. *Armies of Pestilence: The Impact of Disease on History*. Cambridge, UK: James Clarke and Co., 1996.
Brion, Marcel. *Frédéric II de Hohenstaufen*. Paris: Librarie Jules Tallandier, 1978.
Brizay, François. "L'image de l'Italie dans les guides et les relations de voyage publiés en France au XVIIe siècle (1595–1713): sa construction et son évolution." Ph.D. thesis, University of Tours, 1996.
Brooke, Z. N. *The English Church and the Papacy: From the Conquest to the Reign of John*. Cambridge: Cambridge University Press, 1931.
Brown, Gordon S. *The Norman Conquest of Southern Italy and Sicily*. Jefferson, NC, and London: McFarland, 2003.
Bruce-Chwatt, Leonard Jan, and Julian de Zulueta, *The Rise and Fall of Malaria in Europe: A Historico-Epidemiological Study*. New York: Oxford University Press, 1980.
Bryce, James. *The Holy Roman Empire*. London: Macmillan, 1871.
Burgess, T. H. *The Climate of Italy in Relation to Pulmonary Consumption*. London: Longman, Brown, Green and Longmans, 1852.
Burke, Peter. "Rome as a Center of Information and Communication for the Catholic World, 1550–1650." In H. Jones and Thomas Worcester eds., *From Rome to Eternity: Catholicism and the Arts in Italy, ca. 1550–1650*. Boston: Brill, 2002, pp. 253–269.
Caferro, William. *John Hawkwood: An English Mercenary in Fourteenth-Century Italy*. Baltimore: Johns Hopkins University Press, 2006.
Carter, Richard, and Kamini N. Mendis. "Evolutionary and Historical Aspects of the Burden of Malaria." *Clinical Microbiology Reviews*, Vol. 15, No. 4 (2002), pp. 564–594.
Casillo, Robert. *The Empire of Stereotypes: Germaine de Stael and the Idea of Italy*. New York: Palgrave Macmillan, 2006.

Cassady, Richard F. *The Emperor and the Saint: Frederick II of Hohenstaufen, Francis of Assisi, and Journeys to Medieval Places.* DeKalb: Northern Illinois University Press, 2011.

Cauwenbergh, Étienne Van. *Les Pèlerinages Expiatoires et Judiciaires dans le Droit Communal de la Belgique au Moyen Âge.* Louvain: Bureaux du Recueil, 1922.

Celli, Angelo. *Malaria, According to the New Researches.* New York: Longmans, Green, 1900.

Champ, Judith. *The English Pilgrimage to Rome: A Dwelling for the Soul.* Leominster, UK: Gracewing, 2000.

Cheney, Christopher. *Pope Innocent III and England.* Stuttgart: Anton Hiersemann, 1976.

Cilli, Fiorenza. *Giubilei: Breve Storia Degli Anni Santi.* Rome: Olmata, 2016.

Cipolla, Carlo M. *Miasmas and Disease: Public Health and the Environment in the pre-industrial Age.* London: Yale University Press, 1992.

Clarke, M. L. "British Travellers to Rome in Tudor and Stuart Times." *History Today,* Vol. 28, No. 1 (Nov., 1978), pp. 746-750.

Collins, Roger. *Early Medieval Europe, 300-1000.* London: Macmillan, 1991.

———. *Keepers of the Keys of Heaven: A History of the Papacy.* New York: Basic Books, 2009.

Comyn, Robert. *History of the Western Empire from its Restoration by Charlemagne to the Accession of Charles V.* 2 Vols. London: William Allen, 1851.

Corp, Edward. *The Stuarts in Italy, 1917-1766: A Royal Court in Permanent Exile.* New York: Cambridge University Press, 2011.

Corradi, Alfonso. *Annali delle Epidemie Occorse in Italia dalle Prime Memorie Fino al 1850.* Bologna: Tipi Gamberini e Parmeggiani, 1865. 8 Vols.

Corti, Paola. "La Malaria nel Mezzogiorno tra Otto e Novecento." In F. Della Peruta ed., *Storia d'Italia,* Vol. 7. Einaudi, 1984, pp. 635-678.

Cowan, George. *The Most Fatal Distemper: Typhus in History.* Scotland, UK: Diadem Books, 2016.

D. Maffi et. al., "Glucose-6-phosphate dehydrogenase deficiency in Italian blood donors: prevalence and molecular defect characterization." *Vox Sang,* Vol. 106, No. 3 (2014), pp. 227-233.

Dales, Douglas. *Alcuin: His Life and Legacy.* Cambridge, UK: James Clark and Co., 2012.

Dandelet, Thomas James. *Spanish Rome, 1500-1700.* New Haven: Yale University Press, 2001.

Davies, Penelope J. E. "Pollution, Propriety, and Urbanism in Republican Rome." In Mark Bradley ed., *Rome, Pollution, and Propriety.* New York: Cambridge University Press, 2012, pp. 67-80.

Delogu, Paolo. "Lombard and Carolingian Italy." In Rosamond McKitterick ed., *The New Cambridge Medieval History,* Vol. 2. Cambridge, UK: Cambridge University Press, 2008., pp. 290-319.

Delumeau, Jean. *Rome au XVIe Siècle.* London: Hachette, 1975.

De Matthaeis, G. *Sul Culto Reso dagli Antichi Romani alla Dea Febbre.* Roma: Stamperia de Romanis, 1814.

d'Haenens, Albert. "Aller à Rome au Moyen Age." *Institut Historique Belge de Rome,* Vol. 50 (1980), pp. 93-129.

Dodwell, C. R. *Anglo-Saxon Art: A New Perspective.* Ithaca, NY: Cornell University Press, 1985.

Einstein, Lewis. *The Italian Renaissance in England.* New York: Columbia University Press, 1903.

Falkeid, Unn. *The Avignon Papacy Contested: An Intellectual History from Dante to Catherine of Siena.* London: Harvard University Press, 2017.

Faure, Eric. "The death of Alaric I (c. 370-410AD), the vanquisher of Rome: Additional arguments strengthening the possible involvement of malaria." *European Journal of Internal Medicine,* Vol. 37 (Jan., 2017), pp. e14-e15, doi: 10.1016/j.ejim.2016.06.021

Fornaciari, Gino, et al., "*Plasmodium falciparum* Immunodetection in Bone Remains of Members of the Renaissance Medici Family." *Transactions of the Royal Society of Tropical Medicine and Hygiene,* Vol. 104 (2010), pp. 583-587.

Fornasin, Alessio, Marco Breschi, and Matteo Manfredini. "Mortality Patterns of Cardinals (Sixteenth-Twentieth Centuries)." *Institut National d'Études Démographiques,* Vol. 65, No. 4 (2010), pp. 631-652.

Freed, John. *Frederick Barbarossa: The Prince and the Myth.* New Haven, CT: Yale University Press, 2016.

Frugoni, Arsenio. *Il Giubileo di Bonifacio VIII.* Rome: Editori Laterza, 1999.

Fuhrmann, Horst. *Germany in the High Middle Ages, c. 1050-1200.* Cambridge, UK: Cambridge University Press, 1986.

———. *Quis teutonicos constituit iudices nationum? The Trouble with Henry.* *Speculum,* Vol. 69, No. 2 (Apr., 1994), pp. 344-358.

Geissler, Erhard, and Jeanne Guillemin. "German Flooding of the Pontine Marshes in World War II: Biological Warfare or Total War Tactic?" *Politics and the Life Sciences,* Vol. 29, No. 1 (Mar., 2010), pp. 2-23.

Gething, Peter W., et al. "Climate Change and the Global Malaria Recession." *Nature,* Vol. 465 (20 May 2010), pp. 342-346.

Gilmour, David. *The Pursuit of Italy: A History of a Land, Its Regions, and Their Peoples.* New York: Farrar, Straus and Giroux, 2011.

Goldberg, Eric J. *Struggle for Empire: Kingship and Conflict under Louis the German, 817-876.* London: Cornell University Press, 2006.

Graf, Arturo. *Roma nella Memoria e nelle Immaginazioni del Medio Evo.* Torino: Giovanni Chiantore, 1923.

Greengrass, Mark. *Christendom Destroyed: Europe 1517-1648.* New York: Viking, 2014.

Gregorovius, Ferdinand. *History of the City of Rome in the Middle Ages.* Mrs. Gustavus W. Hamilton trans. 6 Vols. London: George Bell, 1906.

Gregory, Desmond. *Napoleon's Italy.* Teaneck, NJ: Fairleigh Dickinson University Press, 2001.

Grenon, Michel. *Charles d'Anjou: Frère Conquérant de Saint Louis.* Paris: L'Harmattan, 2012.

Grisar, Hartmann. *History of Rome and the Popes*

in the Middle Ages. 3 Vols. London: Kegan Paul, Trench, Trübner, and Co., 1911.

Grmek, Mirko. *Diseases in the Ancient Greek World.* Baltimore: Johns Hopkins University Press, 1991.

Hackett, L. W. *Malaria in Europe: An Ecological Study.* London: Oxford University Press, 1937.

Hall, Marcus. "Environmental Imperialism in Sardinia: Pesticides and Politics in the Struggle against Malaria." In Marco Armiero and Marcus Hall eds., *Nature and History in Modern Italy.* Athens: Ohio University Press, 2010, pp. 70–86.

Hamlin, Christopher. *More Than Hot: A Short History of Fever.* Baltimore: Johns Hopkins University Press, 2014.

Harper, Kyle. *The Fate of Rome.* Princeton: Princeton University Press, 2017.

Herde, Peter. "From Adolf of Nassau to Lewis of Bavaria, 1292–1347." In Michael Jones ed., *The New Cambridge Medieval History,* Vol. 6. Cambridge, UK: Cambridge University Press, 2015, pp. 515–550.

Hibbert, Christopher. *The Borgias.* London: Constable, 2009.

_____. *Rome: The Biography of a City.* New York: Penguin Books, 1985.

Hill, Joyce. "From Rome to Jerusalem: An Icelandic Itinerary of the Mid-Twelfth Century." *Harvard Theological Review,* Vol. 76, No. 2 (1983), pp. 175–203.

Hlaváček, Ivan. "The Luxemburgs and Rupert of the Palatinate, 1347–1410." In Michael Jones ed., *The New Cambridge Medieval History,* Vol. 6. Cambridge, UK: Cambridge University Press, 2015, pp. 551–571.

Hodgkin, Thomas. *Italy and Her Invaders.* 8 Vols. Oxford: Clarendon Press, 1880.

Holloway, Julia Bolton. *The Pilgrim and the Book: A Study of Dante, Langland, and Chaucer.* New York: Peter Lang, 1992.

Hook, Judith. *The Sack of Rome.* London: Macmillan, 1972.

Hoolihan, Christopher. "Health and Travel in Nineteenth-Century Rome." *The Journal of the History of Medicine and Allied Sciences,* Vol. 44 (1989), pp. 462–485.

Hopkins, John. "The 'Sacred Sewer': Tradition and Religion in the Cloaca Maxima." In Mark Bradley ed., *Rome, Pollution, and Propriety.* New York: Cambridge University Press, 2012, pp. 81–102.

Horden, Peregrine. "Disease, Dragons, and Saints: The Management of Epidemics in the Dark Ages." In Terence Ranger and Paul Slack eds., *Epidemics and Ideas.* London: Cambridge University Press, 1992, pp. 45–76.

Howard, Clare. *English Travellers of the Renaissance.* London: John Lane, 1914

Howard, Martin R. "Walcheren 1809: A Medical Catastrophe." *BMJ,* Vol. 310, No. 7225 (Dec 18, 1999), pp. 1642–1645.

Hughes, Donald. *Environmental Problems of the Greeks and Romans: Ecology in the Ancient Mediterranean.* Baltimore: Johns Hopkins University Press, 2014.

Jehel, Georges. *Les Angevins de Naples: Un Dynastie Européenne, 1246–1266–1442.* Paris: Ellipses, 2014.

Jones, W H S. *Malaria: A Neglected Factor in the History of Greece and Rome.* London: Macmillan, 1907.

_____. *Malaria and Greek History.* Manchester: University Press, 1909.

Keaveney, Raymond. *Views of Rome.* Scala Books, 1988.

Keevak, Michael. *The Pretended Asian: George Psalmanazar's Eighteenth-Century Formosan Hoax.* Detroit: Wayne State University Press, 2004.

Kendall, Alan. *Medieval Pilgrims.* London: Wayland Publishers, 1970.

Kertzer, David I. *The Pope Who Would Be King.* New York: Random House, 2018.

Kestner, Otto. ""Alpenpässe und Römische Malaria in der mittelalterlichen Kaiserzeit." *Historische Vierteljahrsschift,* Vol. 30 (1935), pp. 686–719.

Krautheimer, Richard. *Rome: Profile of a City, 312–1308.* Princeton, NJ: Princeton University Press, 2000.

La Due, William J. *The Chair of Saint Peter: A History of the Papacy.* Maryknoll, NY: Orbis Books, 1999.

Labande, Edmond René. "Recherches sur les pèlerins dans l'Europe des XIe et XIIe siècles." *Cahiers de Civilisation Médiévale,* Vol. 1, no. 3 (1958), pp. 339–347.

Lane, L. L. "Malaria, Medicine, and Magic in the Roman World." In David Soren and Noelle Soren eds., *A Roman Villa and a Late Roman Infant Cemetery.* Rome: L'Erma di Bretschneider, 1998, pp. 633–651.

Le Gall, Joël. *Le Tibre: Fleuve de Rome dans L'Antiquité.* Paris: Presses Universitaires de France, 1953.

Leighton, Albert C. *Transport and Communication in early Medieval Europe, AD 500–1100.* Newton Abbot, UK: David and Charles, 1972.

Lenkeith, Nancy. *Dante and the Legend of Rome.* London: Warburg Institute, 1952.

Llewellyn, Peter. *Rome in the Dark Ages.* London: Faber & Faber, 1971.

Loud, G. A. "Southern Italy in the Tenth Century." In Timothy Reuter ed., *The New Cambridge Medieval History,* Vol. 3. Cambridge, UK: Cambridge University Press, 1999., pp. 624–645.

Loy, Dorothy E., Weimin Liu, Yingying Li, Gerald H. Learn, Lindsey J. Plenderleith, Sesh A. Sundararaman, Paul M. Sharp, and Beatrice H. Hahn. "Out of Africa: Origins and Evolution of the Human Malaria Parasites *Plasmodium falciparum* and *Plasmodium vivax.*" *International Journal of Parasitology,* Vol. 47 (2017), pp. 87–97.

Lunt, William E. *Financial relations of the Papacy with England to 1327.* Cambridge, MA: Mediaeval Academy of America, 1939.

Macculloch, John. *Malaria: An Essay.* London: Longman, Rees, Orme, Brown, and Green, 1827.

Mackay, Alan L. *A Dictionary of Scientific Quotations.* Bristol, UK: IOP Publishing, 2001.

MacPhail, Eric. *The Voyage to Rome in French*

Renaissance Literature. Saratoga, FL: ANMA Libri, 1990.

Mączak, Antoni. *Travel in Early Modern Europe.* Cambridge, UK: Polity Press, 1995.

Magoun, Francis Peabody. "The Rome of Two Northern Pilgrims: Archbishop Sigeric of Canterbury and Abbot Nikolás of Munkathverá." *Harvard Theological Review,* Vol. 33, No. 4 (Oct., 1940), pp. 267–289.

Majori, Giancarlo. "Short History of Malaria and Its Eradication in Italy with Short Notes on the Fight Against the Infection in the Mediterranean Basin." *Mediterranean Journal of Hematology and Infectious Diseases,* Vol. 4, No. 1 (2012), doi: 10.4084/MJHID.2012.016.

Mallet, Michael, and Christine Shaw. *The Italian Wars, 1494–1559.* New York: Routledge, 2012.

Martin, Jean-Marie. *Italies Normandes: XIe–XIIe Siècles.* Paris: Hachette, 1994.

Matthaeis, G. de. *Sul Culto Reso degli Antichi Romani alla Dea Febbre.* Roma: Stamperia de Romanis, 1814.

McNees, Eleanor. "'Punch' and the Pope: Three Decades of Anti-Catholic Caricature." *Victorian Periodicals Review,* Vol. 37, No. 1 (Spring, 2004), pp. 18–45.

McNeill, William. *Plagues and Peoples.* New York: Anchor Books, 1976.

_____. *The Pursuit of Power.* Chicago: University of Chicago Press, 1982.

Moore, W. J. "The Saxon Pilgrims to Rome and the Schola Saxonum." Ph.D. diss., University of Fribourg, 1937.

Moorhead, John. "Ostrogothic Italy and the Lombard Invasions." In Paul Fouracre ed., *The New Cambridge Medieval History: I.* Cambridge, UK: Cambridge University Press, 2005, pp. 150–161.

Mordechai, Lee, Merle Eisenberg, Timothy P. Newfield, Adam Izdebski, Janet E. Kay, and Hendrick Poinar, "The Justinianic Plague: An inconsequential pandemic"? *Proceedings of the National Academy of Science USA,* Vol. 116, No. 51 (Dec, 2019), pp. 22546–25554. doi: 10.1073/pnas.1903797116

Mourret, Fernand. *The History of the Catholic Church.* 8 Vols. London: B. Herder, 1946.

Müller-Mertens, Eckhard. "The Ottonians as Kings and Emperors." In Timothy Reuter ed., *The New Cambridge Medieval History,* Vol. 3. Cambridge, UK: Cambridge University Press, 1999., pp. 234–266.

Munz, Peter. *Frederick Barbarossa: A Study in Medieval Politics.* Ithaca, NY: Cornell University Press, 1969.

Musto, Ronald G. *Apocalypse in Rome: Cola di Rienzo and the Politics of the New Age.* London: University of California Press, 2003.

Newfield, Timothy P. "Malaria and malaria-like disease in the early Middle Ages." *Early Medieval Europe,* Vol. 25, No. 3 (2017), pp. 251–300.

Nicassio, Susan Vandiver. *Imperial City: Rome Under Napoleon.* London: University of Chicago Press, 2005.

Noble, Thomas. F. X. "The Papacy in the Eighth and Ninth Centuries." In Rosamond McKitterick ed., *The New Cambridge Medieval History,* Vol. 2. Cambridge, UK: Cambridge University Press, 2008., pp. 563–586.

North, W[illiam]. *Roman Fever.* London: Sampson Low, Marston and Co., 1896.

Norwich, John Julius. *The Popes.* London: Vintage Books, 2011.

Ohler, Norbert. *The Medieval Traveller.* Caroline Hillier trans. Woodbridge, UK: The Boydell Press, 1989.

Oluwayemi, Oludare. "Cerebral Malaria." *Malaria Chemotherapy Control and Elimination,* Vol. 3, No. 116., 2014. doi:10.4172/2090-2778.1000116.

O'Sullivan, Lara, Andrew Jardine, Angus Cook, and Philip Weinstein. "Deforestation, Mosquitoes, and Ancient Rome: Lessons for Today." *BioScience,* Vol. 58, No. 8 (Sept., 2008), pp. 756–760.

Pacaut, Marcel. *Frederick Barbarossa.* London: Collins, 1970.

Packard, Randall. *The Making of a Tropical Disease: A Short History of Malaria.* Baltimore: Johns Hopkins University Press, 2007.

Parks, George B. *The English Traveler to Italy.* Stanford, CA: Stanford University Press, 1954.

Pemble, John. *The Mediterranean Passion: Victorians and Edwardians in the South.* London: Faber & Faber, 2009.

_____. *The Rome We Have Lost.* Oxford, UK: Oxford University Press, 2017.

Pomeranz, Kenneth. *The Great Divergence: China, Europe, and the Making of the Modern World Economy.* Princeton, NJ: Princeton University Press, 2000.

Prasad, Ram Naresh, and Kamal Jeet Virk. "Malaria as a cause of diarrhoea—a review." *PNG,* Vol. 36 (1993), pp. 337–341.

Puccinotti, Francesco. *Storia delle Febbri Intermittenti Perniciose di Roma,* 2 Vols. Napoli: Puzziello, 1838.

Retief, François, and Louis Cilliers. "Malaria in Graeco-Roman Times." *Acta Classica,* Vol. 47 (2004), pp. 127–137.

Reardon, Wendy J. *The Deaths of the Popes: Comprehensive Accounts, Including Funerals, Burial Places, and Epitaphs.* Jefferson, NC, and London: McFarland, 2004.

Reilly, Benjamin. "Cardinal Numbers: Changing Patterns of Malaria and Mortality in Rome, 494–1850." *Journal of Interdisciplinary History,* Vol. 49, Vol. 3 (2019), pp. 397–417.

_____. *Disaster and Human History: Case Studies in Nature, Society, and Catastrophe.* Jefferson, NC, and London: McFarland, 2009

_____. "Malaria, Protestants, and Google." *Environmental History,* Vol. 16 (April, 2011), pp. 312–321.

_____. "Northern European Patterns of Visiting Rome, 1400–1850." *Journal of Tourism History* (2019) DOI: 10.1080/1755182X.2019.1607571.

_____. "Seasons in Italy: Northern European Travelers, Rome, and Malaria." *Journal of Tourism and Cultural Change* (2020), DOI: 10.1080/14766825.2019.1693582.

_____. *Slavery, Agriculture, and Malaria in the Arabian Peninsula*. Athens: Ohio University Press, 2015.

Reuter, Timothy. *Germany in the Early Middle Ages*. New York: Longman, 1991.

Riché, Pierre. *The Carolingians: A Family Who Forged Europe*. Philadelphia: University of Pennsylvania Press, 1993.

Rinne, Katherine. "Urban Ablutions: Cleansing Counter-Reformation Rome." In Mark Bradley ed., *Rome, Pollution, and Propriety*. New York: Cambridge University Press, 2012, pp. 182–201.

_____. *The Waters of Rome: Aqueducts, Fountains, and the Birth of the Baroque City*. London: Yale University Press, 2010.

Roach, Levi. "Emperor Otto III and the End of Time." *Transactions of the Royal Historical Society*, Vol. 23 (2013), pp. 75–102.

Robinson, I. S. *Henry IV of Germany, 1056–1106*. New York: Cambridge University Press, 1999.

_____. "Innocent II and the Empire." In John Doran and Damien Smith eds., *Pope Innocent II: The World vs. the City*. New York: Routledge, 2016, pp. 27–68.

_____. "The Institutions of the Church, 1073–1216." In David Luscombe and Jonathan Riley-Smith eds., *The New Cambridge Medieval History*, Vol. 4 Part 1. Cambridge, UK: Cambridge University Press, 1999., pp. 368–460

_____. "The Papacy, 1122–1198." In David Luscombe and Jonathan Riley-Smith eds., *The New Cambridge Medieval History*, Vol. 4. Cambridge, UK: Cambridge University Press, 2004., pp. 317–383.

_____. "Reform and the Church: 1073–1122." In David Luscombe and Jonathan Riley-Smith eds., *The New Cambridge Medieval History*, Vol. 4 Part 1. Cambridge, UK: Cambridge University Press, 1999., pp. 268–334.

Rocco, Fiammetta. *Quinine: Malaria and the Quest for a Cure That Changed the World*. New York: HarperCollins, 2003.

Romi, R., D. Boccolini, M. Menegon, and G. Rezza. "Probable Autochthonous Introduced Malaria Cases in Italy 2009–2011 and the Risk of Local Vector-Borne Transmission." *Eurosurveillance*, Vol. 17, No. 48 (29 Nov., 2012).

Runciman, Steven. *The Sicilian Vespers: A History of the Mediterranean World in the Later Thirteenth Century*. Cambridge, UK: Cambridge University Press, 1958.

Russo-Mancuso, Giovanna, Maria Antonietta Romea, Vincenzo Guardabasso, and Gino Schiliro. "Survey of Sickle-Cell Disease in Italy." *Haematologica*, Vol. 83 (1998), pp. 875–881.

Saad, Neil J., Victoria D. Lynch, Marina Antillón, Chongguang Yang, John A. Crump and Virginia E. Pitzer, "Seasonal Dynamics of Typhoid and Paratyphoid Fever." *Scientific Reports*, Vol. 8 (2018). On-line at https://www.nature.com/articles/s41598-018-25234-w/.

Sallares, Robert. *Malaria and Rome: A History of Malaria in Ancient Italy*. New York: Oxford University Press, 2002.

Scheidel, Walter. "Death and the City: Ancient Rome and Beyond." R. Smith and E. A. Wrigley (eds.), publication of the conference on the fiftieth anniversary of the Cambridge Group for the History of Population and Social Structure. Cambridge, 2014.

_____. "Libitina's Bitter Gains: Seasonal Mortality and Endemic Disease in the Ancient City of Rome." *Ancient Society*, Vol. 25 (1994), pp. 151–175.

Scoresby-Jackson, R. E. *Medical Climatology: or, A Topographical and Meteorological Description of the Localities Resorted to in Winter and Summer by Invalids*. London: John Churchill, 1862.

Sedgewick, William T., and Charles-Edward A. Winslow. "Statistical Studies on the Seasonal Prevalence of Typhoid Fever in Various Countries and Its Relation to Seasonable Temperature." *Memoirs of the American Academy of Arts and Sciences*, Vol. 12, No. 5 (Aug., 1902), pp. 467, 469–470, 521–571.

Séguin, Philippe. *Louis Napoléon Le Grand*. Paris: Bernard Grasset, 1990.

Sergi, Giuseppe. "The Kingdom of Italy." In Timothy Reuter ed., *The New Cambridge Medieval History*, Vol. 3. Cambridge, UK: Cambridge University Press, 1999., pp. 346–371.

Shah, Sonia. *The Fever: How Malaria Has Ruled Humankind for 500,000 Years*. New York: Farrar, Straus and Giroux, 2010.

Shaw, Brent D. "Seasons of Death: Aspects of Mortality in Imperial Rome." *The Journal of Roman Studies*, Vol. 86 (1996), pp. 100–138.

Snowden, Frank M. "'Fields of Death': Malaria in Italy, 1861–1962." *Modern Italy*, Vol. 4, No. 1 (1999), pp. 25–57.

_____. "From Triumph to Disaster: Fascism and Malaria in the Pontine Marshes, 1928–1946." In John Kickie, Jonn Foot, and Frank M. Snowden eds., *Disastro: Disasters in Italy since 1860: Culture, Politics, Society*. New York: Palgrave, 2002, pp. 113–140.

Soren, David. "Can Archeologists Excavate Evidence of Malaria?" *World Archeology*, Vol. 35, No. 2 (2003), pp. 193–209.

_____. *Malaria, Witchcraft, Infant Cemeteries, and the Fall of Rome*. San Diego State: Gail A. Burnett Lectures in Classics, 2002.

Southern, R. W. *Western Society and the Church of the Middle Ages*. New York: Viking Penguin, 1992.

Squatriti, Paolo. "The Floods of 589 and Climate Change at the Beginning of the Middle Ages: An Italian Microhistory." *Speculum*, Vol. 85 (2010), pp. 779–826.

Sullivan, Barry. "'More than meets the eye': The Ethiopian war and the Origins of the Second World War." In Gordon Martel ed., *The Origins of the Second World War Reconsidered*. London: Routledge, 1999.

Sumption, Jonathan. *The Age of Pilgrimage: The Medieval Journey to God*. Mahwah, NJ: HiddenSpring, 2003.

Sweet, Rosemary. *Cities and the Grand Tour: The*

British in Italy, 1690–1820. Cambridge, UK: Cambridge University Press, 2012.
Symonds, J. A. *Sir Philip Sidney*. London: Macmillan, 1906.
Taussig, Gabriele. *The Roman Climate: Its Influence on Healthy and Disease, Serving as a Hygienical Guide*. Rome: Roman Typography, 1870.
Theilmann, John, and Frances Cate. "A Plague of Plagues: The Problem of Plague Diagnosis in Medieval England." *Journal of Interdisciplinary History*, Vol. 37, No. 3 (Winter, 2007), pp. 371–393.
Thurston, Herbert. *The Holy Year of Jubilee: An Account of the History and Ceremonial of the Roman Jubilee*. London: Sands and Co., 1900.
Tommasi-Crudeli, Corrado. *The Climate of Rome and the Roman Malaria*. London: J. & A. Churchill, 1892.
Tommasini, Anselo M. *Irish Saints in Italy*. J. F. Scanlan trans. London: Sands and Co., 1937.
Torelli, Luigi. *La Malaria D'Italia*. Roma: Stabilimento Tipografico Italiano, 1883.
Tournon-Simiane, Camille de. *Études Statistiques sur Rome*. Paris: Librarie de Firmin Didot Frères, 1855.
Travels of an English Gentleman from London to Rome. Anonymous. London: A. Bettesworth, 1718.
Tyler, J. E. *The Alpine Passes: The Middle Ages (962–1250)*. Oxford: Basil Blackwell, 1930.
Ullmann, Walter. *A Short History of the Papacy in the Middle Ages*. New York: Routledge, 2003.
Urban, William. *Medieval Mercenaries: The Business of War*. London: Greenhill Books, 2006.
Verhoeven, Gerrit. "Calvinist Pilgrimages and Popish Encounters: Religious Identity and Sacred Space on the Dutch Grand Tour (1598–1685)." *Journal of Social History*, Vol. 43, No. 3 (2010).
Vicchio, Stephen J. *The Legend of the Anti-Christ: A History*. Eugene, Oregon: Wipf and Stock, 2009.
Vidmar, John. *The Catholic Church Through the Ages: A History*. New York: Paulist Press, 2014.
Wace, Henry, and Philip Schaff. *Nicene and Post-Nicene Fathers of the Christian Church*. New York: Charles Scribner's Sons, 1912.
Warner, David A. "Ideals and Action in the Reign of Otto III." *Journal of Medieval History*, Vol. 25, No. 1 (1999), pp. 1–18.
Warner, Verner J. "Epithets of the Tiber in the Roman Poets." *The Classical Weekly*, Vol. 11, No. 7 (1917), pp. 52–54.
Watt, J. A. "The Papacy." In David Abulafia ed., *The New Cambridge Medieval History*. Vol. 5. Cambridge, UK: Cambridge University Press, 1999, pp. 107–163.
Webb, Diana. *Pilgrims and Pilgrimage in the Medieval West*. New York: I. B. Tauris, 1999.
Webb, James L. A. *Humanity's Burden: A Global History of Malaria*. New York: Cambridge University Press, 2009.
Weber, Max. *The Protestant Ethic and the "Spirit" of Capitalism and Other Writings*. Peter Baehr and Gordon C. Wells trans. New York: Penguin, 2002.
Whalen, Brett Edward. *The Medieval Papacy*. New York: Palgrave Macmillan, 2014.
White, Michael T., George Shireff, Stephan Karl, Arza C. Ghani, and Ivo Mueller. "Variation in Relapse Frequency and the Transmission Potential of Plasmodium vivax malaria." *Proceedings of the Royal Society B*, Vol. 283 (2016).
Wickham, Chris. *The Inheritance of Rome: Illuminating the Dark Ages, 400–1000*. New York: Penguin Books, 2009.
_____. *Medieval Rome: Stability and Crisis of a City, 900–1150*. Oxford, UK: Oxford University Press, 2015.
Wilson, Peter H. *Heart of Europe: A History of the Holy Roman Empire*. Cambridge, MA: The Belknap Press of Harvard University Press, 2016.
_____. *The Holy Roman Empire 1495–1806*. New York: Palgrave, 2011.
Winegard, Timothy C. *The Mosquito: A Human History of our Deadliest Predator*. New York: Dutton, 2019.
Wrigley, Richard. "Infectious Enthusiasms: Influence, Contagion, and the Experience of Rome." In Chloe Chard and Helen Langdon eds., *Transports: Travel, Pleasure, and Imaginative Geography, 1600–1830*. London: Paul Mellon Center for Studies in British Art, 1996, pp. 75–115.
_____. "Pathological Topographies and Cultural Itineraries: mapping 'mal'aria' in 18th- and 19th-century Rome." In Richard Wrigley and George Revill eds., *Pathologies of Travel*. Rodopi Bv Editions, 2000, pp. 207–228.
Ziegler, Michelle. "Malaria Landscapes in Late Antique Rome and the Tiber Valley." *Landscapes*, Vol. 17, No. 2 (2016), pp. 139–155.

Digital Resources

"Anopheles atroparvus." *European Centre for Disease Prevention and Control* https://ecdc.europa.eu/en/disease-vectors/facts/mosquito-factsheets/anopheles-atroparvus.
"Anopheles labranchiae." *European Centre for Disease Prevention and Control* https://ecdc.europa.eu/en/disease-vectors/facts/mosquito-factsheets/anopheles-labranchiae.
Miranda, Salvador. "The Cardinals of the Holy Roman Church." https://webdept.fiu.edu/~mirandas/cardinals.htm.

Index

A. gambiae 12, 14
A. labranchiae 14, 29, 48–49, 68, 179
A. sacherovi 41, 69
Aachen 64, 70, 75, 77, 85
Adrian IV, Pope 117
Adrianople, Battle of 38–39
Adriatic Sea 16, 19, 40, 79, 168
Africa 9, 11, 12, 27, 28, 40, 41, 43, 54, 69, 82, 173, 178–179, 181
Alaric 39, 40
Alban Hills 23, 86, 91, 98, 121, 123, 155, 170, 173
Albano 165, 170
Alcuin 50, 182
Alexander III, Pope 86–87
Alexander VI, Pope 132–133, 134
Algeria 29
Alps 24, 38, 50, 60, 65, 106
the "Anagni Slap" 126
Angevins 91–92, 95, 127, 128–129
Anopheles 9, 10, 12, 22, 25, 26, 49, 68, 98, 154, 155, 179, 175, 180, 181; *see also A. gambiae*; *A. labranchiae*; *A. sacherovi*
the Antichrist 1, 75, 84, 91, 140
anti-malaria campaigns 177–178, 180
Apennine Mountains 15, 18, 23, 24, 40, 42, 43, 45, 68, 70, 81, 86, 98, 121, 129, 130, 163, 176
appeals to the papacy 117, 119, 123–124, 143
Apulia 74, 89
aqueducts 20–21, 41, 43–44, 48–49, 68, 94, 131, 154–155
Arabian Peninsula 10–11
Arausio, Battle of 37
Archangel, Russia 11
aria cattiva 163, 164, 168, 170, 171, 175
Asia Minor 19
atabrine 180
Athens 16, 24, 168
Attila the Hun 40, 64
Augustus Caesar 19–20, 22, 36, 57, 84

Aventine Hill 17, 18, 22, 75, 98
Avignon papacy 95, 127–131, 132, 171

Babylon 140, 143, 169
The "Babylonian Captivity" 127, 131
"bad air" 3, 22, 23, 26, 41, 99, 151, 161, 163, 170, 171, 182; *see also aria cattiva*; *intempérance*
Baiae 138
Balkans 69, 179
Barbarossa *see* Frederick I
Bari 129
Bede 49, 50, 51
Bedouins 10
Belgium 105, 143, 149
Belisarius 41–42, 163
Benedict VII, Pope 74
Benedict IX, Pope 79–80
Benevento 43, 64, 74
Berengar II, King of Italy 72
Bernard of Clairvaux 123–124
Beste, John Richard Digby 161
Beyle, Marie-Henri 171
the Bible 57, 141
Biscop 50, 51, 52
Bishop of Rome 2, 44, 46–47, 84, 127; *see also* papacy
Black Death 111, 129
Blessington, Marguerite 164
Bologna 115, 138
Bolsena, Lake 163, 170
bonaficazione 178, 179
Bonaparte, Napoléon 168–169, 171
Boniface VIII, Pope 108, 109, 125–126
Borgia, Alexander *see* Alexander VI
Borgia, Cesare 133, 134
Borgo 52, 68, 69, 82, 148, 154
Bramsen, John 171
Brescia 91, 94, 181
Brindisi 89, 90
Brucella 8
bubonic plague 31, 45, 50, 138
Burgess, T.H. 163

Burgundy 70, 74
Butler, Alban 164
Byzantine Empire 41–42, 43, 74, 75, 88

Caesars of Rome 2, 68, 182
Calvin, John 142, 148
campagna of Rome 15, 23, 27, 28, 41, 42–43, 48, 60, 68, 71, 73, 77, 121, 127, 157, 163, 170, 172, 177, 179
Campus Martius 22, 23, 48, 68, 154, 164
Cannae, Battle of (216 BCE) 19, 37
Cannae, Battle of (1018 CE) 78
Canossa 81–82, 116,
Canterbury 48, 50, 115, 118, 121, 123, 132
Canterbury Tales 106, 108
Capitoline Hill 18, 21, 22, 37, 57, 58, 98
cardinals 3, 26, 31–33, 80, 86, 114, 115, 117–118, 121, 127, 128, 130–131, 132, 135, 136, 152, 153, 169
Cardinals of the Holy Roman Church 31
Carolingians 63–71, 75, 169
Carthage 19, 44
Castel Gandolfo 121
catacombs 46, 47, 52, 91, 164–165
Catholics 144–145, 147, 148–149, 153, 154, 172
Celestine III 117
Celli, Angelo 27
cerebral malaria 12, 181
Charlemagne 50, 64–66, 68, 69, 71, 72, 75, 77, 98, 169, 182–183
Charles IV, German Emperor 96, 97
Charles V, German Emperor 135, 138, 141
Charles VIII, French King 133
Charles Martel 63
Charles of Anjou 91–92
Chetwode, John 157

cholera 1, 90
Christian of Mainz 81, 115
Chrysopolis, Battle of 47
cinchona 151, 165–166, 182
Circus Maximus 22, 54
Clement II, Pope 79–80, 135
Clement V, Pope 127
Clement VII, Antipope 131
Clement VII, Pope 135, 137, 138
climate change 26–27, 33, 181
Cloaca Maxima 23
Coelfrid 51
Coëtlosquet, Charles 164
Colomb, M.R. 164
Colonna family 125–26, 127, 131
Colosseum 22, 40, 58, 149, 163, 166, 168
Conrad II, German Emperor 78–79
Conrad III, German Emperor 83–84
Conrad VI 91, 100
Conradin 92, 93, 95
Constantine, Roman Emperor 47, 59
Constantinople 36, 37, 42, 47, 48, 154, 168
"consumption" 163; see also tuberculosis
Corsica 29, 32, 109, 151
Cortenuova 91
Council of Constance 131
Council of Trent 143, 149
Council of Worms 83, 85
Count Cavour 174, 175
Counter-Reformation 151, 153
Cremona 85, 94
the Crusades 85, 88, 89, 90, 107

Dacia 38, 39
Daisy Miller 166, 176, 184
Damasus II, Pope 80, 135
Dante Alighieri 84, 93, 107; *De Monarchia* 84; *Divine Comedy* 84, 106
Danube River 15, 37, 38, 39, 40
Dark Ages 48, 103, 161
DDT 181
Dea Febris 23, 175
de Blainville, Monsieur 161
de Brosses, Charles 15, 23
deforestation 12, 23, 175
Desiderius, King of the Lombards 64
de Tournon, Camille 169–171
de Vere, Edward 159
diarrhea 14, 31, 70, 87, 88, 166
Dictatus Papae 116
Diet of Worms 141
Diocletian 36–37, 47
Divine Comedy 84, 106
divorce 70, 117, 121, 142
DNA 9, 25

Dog Star 87, 183
Donation of Constantine 116
dragons 59–62, 112, 173
Duffy negative antigen 11
Dupaty, C.M.J.B 157, 158

Eastern Roman Empire 36–37, 38, 40; see also Byzantine Empire
Eaton, Charlotte Anne 163
Einhard 63
Elizabeth I, Queen of England 148
England 1, 48, 50–51, 66, 67, 88, 96, 103, 116, 119, 123, 125, 129, 143, 145, 146, 147, 148, 149, 159, 163, 168, 171–172, 183–184
The English Traveler to Italy 45
epigraphy 26, 29–31
erosion 23, 175
Ethelbert, English King 48
Etruscans 18
the Eucharist 71, 95, 148
Eugenius III, Pope 117, 121, 123
Eusebius of Caesarea 103
Evesham Monastery 115–116, 119
excommunication 79, 89, 90–91, 125, 134, 135, 140

famine 37, 41, 183
favism 11, 65
the Fenlands 66, 67, 190*ch7n*10
Flaminian Gate 112, 193*n*50
Flavius Romulus Augustus 36, 40
flooding 22–23
Florence 95, 100, 130, 134, 138, 147, 148
Fontenay, Battle of 70
the Forum 21, 22–23, 58–60, 62, 149, 154, 168, 173
France 1, 19, 21, 25, 29, 37, 43, 48, 51, 65, 70, 74, 81, 88, 91, 93, 96, 103, 118, 125, 127, 129, 133, 135, 142, 143, 149, 150, 159, 169, 170, 172, 179
Franks 41, 43, 63–64, 69–70
Frederick I, German Emperor 85–88, 97, 98, 99, 101
Frederick II, German Emperor 89–91, 92, 97, 107
Frederick Barbarossa see Frederick I
French Revolution 144, 145
Frisians 52, 103–104

Garibaldi, Giuseppe 172
Gauls 37, 38
Geneva 146, 148
Geneva Protocol of 1925 179
German Empire 2, 72–74, 80–81, 85, 97–98, 118, 141, 169, 182–183; see also Holy Roman Empire
Germany 1, 4, 28, 43, 52, 66, 71, 72, 73, 74, 75, 77, 78, 80, 81, 83–84, 86, 87, 88, 89, 93, 95, 96–97, 117–118, 133–134, 139, 140–141, 142, 143, 144, 149, 169, 176, 179, 180, 183
Gesta Romanorum 4, 56–57, 58–59
Ghibellines 86, 91, 92, 93–94, 95, 129
Giegler, Jean-Pierre 171
global warming see climate change
Glorious Revolution 159
glucose-6-phosphate dehydrogenase deficiency see favism
Goethe, Johann Wolfgang von 157, 158, 160, 161, 186*ch*2*n*2
Golden Bull 96
The Golden Legend 59–60
gorillas 12, 185*n*8
Grand Tour 2, 143, 158–161, 163, 166, 168, 170, 171, 182
Grassi, Giovanni 177, 178
Greece 16, 19, 24, 62, 103, 179
Gregory I, Pope 47–48, 49
Gregory V, Pope 75
Gregory VII, Pope 81–83, 116, 121
Gregory IX, Pope 89, 90, 91
Gregory of Tours 25–26, 41, 52, 60
Guelfs 84, 92, 94, 95, 97, 129, 138

Habsburgs 97, 134, 136, 138
Hajj 1
Hadrian IV, Pope 85, 86
Hadrian VI, Pope 135, 146
Hannibal 19
Harff, Arnold von 112, 131
Hawkwood, John 129–130, 132, 138
hemoglobin 9, 10, 12, 165
hemozoin 10
Henry II, English King 119
Henry II, German Emperor 78
Henry III, German Emperor 79–80
Henry IV, German Emperor 81–83, 100, 101, 116, 134
Henry V, German Emperor 83
Henry VI, German Emperor 88–89, 101
Henry VII, German Emperor 93–96, 97, 100
Henry VIII, English King 142, 159, 184
Hippocrates 16
Hippolytus 46

Index

Hohenstaufen Emperors 86–92, 93
Holland *see* Netherlands
Holy Roman Empire 85, 101
honeysuckle *see* Lonicera carprifolia
Honorious of St. Augustine 121–123
Horace 23, 157
Hundred Years' War 125, 129
Hungarians 2, 72, 104, 109, 129
Huns 38, 39, 40, 43

Iberia 19, 32, 64, 114
Iliad 16
imperator 19, 20, 36, 72
Imperial Crisis 36
"infectious enthusiasms" 151–152
Innocent II, Pope 83
Innocent III, Pope 89, 103, 119, 121
Innocent IV, Pope 91
intempérance 15, 163, 197*n*33
intermittent fever 9, 10, 16, 25, 31, 49
investiture controversy 81–83, 116, 117, 118
Ireland 52, 105, 118
Iron Crown of Lombardy 64, 65, 96, 97, 138, 169
Islam 1, 56, 83
Istanbul 154, 168
Italian League 135, 136, 138
Italy 2, 11, 13, 15, 16, 18, 24, 26, 27, 28, 36, 40, 41, 43, 45, 48, 64, 65–66, 67–68, 69, 71, 72, 73, 74, 75, 77, 78, 81, 83, 85, 86, 88, 89, 91–92, 93, 95, 96–100, 101–102, 116, 121, 128, 129, 130, 132, 133–134, 139, 140, 142, 148, 149, 159, 160, 162, 163, 165, 168, 171, 175, 176, 177–178, 179, 180, 181–182, 183

Jacquot, Félix 28–29, 172–173
Jameson, Anna 160–161
Jerusalem 53, 75, 84, 85, 88, 90–91, 103, 107, 143
Jesus 46, 53, 55, 64, 84, 111, 112, 123
jinn 10
Joanna I, Queen of Naples 129
John, King of England 119
John VI, Pope 51
John VIII, Pope 69
John XII, Pope 72–73
John XXII, Pope 128
Johnson, James 163–164
Jones, W.H.S. 24, 184
Jubilee 2, 107–112, 113, 125, 128, 131, 143, 149, 160, 182
Julius II, Pope 134, 139, 142

Julius Caesar 19–20, 36, 37–38, 45, 56, 68, 84
Justinian I, Eastern Roman Emperor 41–42

Kaiserchronik 4, 56–57, 58–59, 60
Knight, Elizabeth 165

Lacus Curtius 58–59, 173
Lassels, Richard 58, 158–159
Last Emperor legend 75, 84–85, 91
the Lateran 53, 79, 95, 110, 128, 154, 164
Lateran Councils 118
Latina Province 177, 178, 179, 180
Latium 15–16, 17, 20, 23
lay investiture 81, 83
Lazio 99, 121, 179
Lechfeld, Battle of 72, 104
Leo III, Pope 65
Leo VII, Pope 72–73
Leo IX, Pope 80
Leo X, Pope 134–135
Leonine City 87, 95, 132
Leonine Walls 69, 82
Licinius, Eastern Roman Emperor 47
Limes Germanicus 38
Listeria 8
Lithgow, William 148
Little Ice Age 33
Liutprand, King of the Lombards 63–64
Liutprand of Cremona 73
Livy 22, 37
Lombard League 88, 91
Lombards 36, 42–43, 47, 48, 52, 63–64, 65, 68, 69, 74, 78, 81, 134, 155, 169
Lombardy 42, 86, 94, 96, 97, 111
London 1, 15, 49, 82, 162, 163, 168
Lonicera carprifolia 8–9
Lothair II, King of Italy 70–71
Lothair III, German Emperor 83, 85, 89
Louis II, King of Italy 70–71
Louis Napoléon, French Emperor 172–173
Louis of Anjou 129
Louis the Pius, Frankish King 69–70
Lucca 45, 163
Lugnano 8–9, 11, 14, 24, 36, 176
Lullus 51–52, 63
Luther, Martin 2, 4, 108, 132, 138, 139, 140–142, 143, 146, 147
Lutherans 142

MacCullough, John 171
Machiavelli 133

magister militium 39, 41
malaria: associated with monsters 59–62, 112, 173; confused with poisoning 95–96, 135, 192*ch9n*8; death rate 12, 14, 28, 30, 31, 67, 113–114, 172–173, 175, 177, 180; life cycle 9–14; and population density 26, 33, 49, 171, seasonality 25, 28, 30–33, 135, 152, 164, 172, 174, 182; *see also P. falciparum*; *P. malariae*; *P. vivax*; plasmodia
Malaria and Rome 1
Marcellus, Bishop of Paris 60
Marcus Aurelius, Roman Emperor 58, 59
the Maremma 71, 96, 170, 192*ch9n*10
Marengo, Battle of 169
Maria Santissima delle Febbri 23
Martin IV, Pope 128
Martin V, Pope 131
Mayors of the Palace 63
Mecca 1
Mediterranean Sea 4, 15, 16, 19, 20, 40, 42, 54, 163, 176, 179
Mellitus 49–50
Merovingians 41, 63
Messina 89
Michelangelo 134, 161
Milan 28, 78, 85, 86, 93, 94, 96, 97, 133, 134, 169
the Minotaur 24, 49, 59, 60–62, 98, 175
Mirabilia 4, 57–58, 59, 60
Mons Gaudii *see* Monte Mario
Moore, John 160
morbus Italicus 77
Morritt, John 168
Moryson, Fynes 147
mosquitoes 9, 10, 11, 15, 22, 27, 31, 49, 156, 157, 166, 175, 176–177, 181, 184; *see also A. gambiae*; *A. labranchiae*; *A. sacherovi*; *Anopheles*
Munday, Anthony 147, 148
Muslims 54, 63, 74, 107
Mussolini, Benito 174, 177–179

Naples 41, 88, 127, 129, 133, 134, 135, 138, 148, 168, 179
Napoléon III *see* Louis Napoléon
Napoleonic Wars 66, 168–169
Narses 42
Nero, Roman Emperor 112, 173
Netherlands 2, 52, 66, 70, 103, 142, 143, 146, 148, 146, 178, 183–184
Newfield, Timothy P. 25–26, 32–33

Index

Nicholas V, Pope 131
The Ninety-Five Theses 140
Normans 78, 81, 82–83, 86, 88, 101, 117
North, W. 175–176

Octavian *see* Augustus Caesar
Octavian of St. Cecilia 86–87, 117–118
Odoacer 36, 40
One Thousand and One Nights 56
Ontario, Canada 11
Open Letter to the Christian Nobility 140
Ostia 20, 163, 170
Ostrogoths 36, 40–43, 65, 81, 163
Otto I, German Emperor 72–74, 78, 97, 100
Otto II, German Emperor 74, 75, 81
Otto III, German Emperor 74–77, 78, 79, 84, 85, 100, 101
Otto IV, German Emperor 89
Ottonian Emperors 71–77, 93, 97

P. falciparum 1, 9, 12–14, 16, 22, 24, 26, 27–28, 29–30, 31, 33, 41, 43, 45, 9962, 68, 71, 73, 80, 88, 89, 90, 96, 98, 99, 112, 124, 127, 135, 138, 138, 172, 177, 180, 181, 182–183, 185n9
P. malariae 9–10, 11, 12, 14, 60, 62, 66, 139
P. vivax 11, 12, 14, 24, 28, 62, 66, 91, 99, 112, 139, 172, 177
Palatine Hill 17, 18, 21, 22
Palermo 91, 101
pallium 50, 118
the Pantheon 58
papacy 1, 2, 4, 46, 48, 50, 63–64, 65, 68–69, 70, 71, 72–73, 74, 75, 77, 79–83, 84, 86, 88, 89, 91, 95, 96, 101, 105, 107–108, 111, 116–120, 121, 123–124, 125, 127–128, 129, 130–132, 133–134, 139, 140–141, 146, 154–155, 169, 172, 174, 182
papal curia 2, 4, 117, 127
Papal States 129, 134, 174
Paris 1, 15, 29, 60, 62, 115, 125
patrician 36
Pavia 42, 64, 74, 78, 86, 135, 139
Peace of Westphalia 144,
penitential pilgrimage 105–106
Pennington, Thomas 171–172
Pepin, King of the Franks 63, 64, 69
Pepin, son of Charlemagne 69, 70, 72, 97, 100
persecution of Christians 46–47

Persia 37, 41, 42, 46
Petrarch 128
Philip the Fair, King of France 125, 127
Piazza de Popolo 112, 131, 170, 197n12
pilgrim numbers 107, 11, 113, 149
pilgrims 4, 24, 33, 44, 52, 53–54, 81, 103–109, 111–114, 119, 128, 132, 142, 143, 149, 153, 158, 159–160, 162, 171, 182
Pisa 95, 96
Pius V, Pope 154
Pius VII, Pope 169
Plague of Justinian 42, 50
Plagues and Peoples 68
plasmodia 1, 2, 4, 9–10, 12, 14, 25, 26, 28–29, 30, 49, 62, 65–66, 68, 96, 98, 111, 135, 140, 143, 146, 159, 165, 182, 184; *see also P. falciparum; P. malariae; P. vivax*
Plutarch 22
Po River 15, 27, 42–43, 67, 69, 85, 86, 139
Poland 39, 75, 75
Pontianus 46
Pontine Marshes 41, 163–164, 170, 177, 179
population of Rome 20, 22, 43, 68, 132, 151, 154, 171
Pozzuoli 133
The Protestant Ethic and the "Spirit" of Capitalism 183
Protestant Reformation 2–3, 4, 141–146, 147, 148, 149, 152–154, 159, 182, 183–184
Protestants 2–3, 4, 139, 142–146, 147–148, 149, 153–154, 159–160, 161, 183–184
Pseudo-Isidorian Decretals 116
Puccinotti, Francesco 176
Pyrrhus 19

quartan fever 10, 16, 23, 25, 60; *see also P. malariae*
quinine 165–166, 173–174, 175–176, 177, 180, 184

railways 162, 175
Raleigh, Sir Walter 104
Ravenna 40–41, 42, 69, 75
reform papacy 80–83
relics 52–53, 75, 106, 107, 112, 142, 165
Remus 15, 16, 17, 64
Renaissance 2, 45, 134, 140, 149, 150, 153, 154, 159
Revelation of Pseudo-Methodius 84
Revolutions of 1848 172
Rhine River 38, 39, 40, 66, 141
Rhône River 127, 130

the "Ridiculous Republic" 168–169
Robert Guiscard 82, 135
Robert of Naples 95
Rocca di Papi 121
Roger, Abbot of Evesham 115–116
Roger of Naples 127
Romagna 130, 132
Roman Empire 19–20, 36–37, 39, 40, 47, 56, 65, 96, 150, 175
"Roman Fever" 1, 3–5, 81, 82, 88, 96, 105, 109, 113, 116, 120, 121, 138, 146, 147, 153, 156, 159, 165, 166, 170, 171, 175–176, 177, 180, 182–184; *see also P. falciparum*
Roman Republic 18–19, 20, 24, 56
Romegedanke 1, 96
Romulus 15, 16, 17, 24, 36, 42, 57, 63, 154
Ross, Ronald 177

S-hemoglobin mutation 12
the Sack of Rome 135–138, 142, 149, 154
sacks of Rome 4, 36, 39, 40, 42, 43, 68–69, 82, 135–138, 168–169; *see also* the Sack of Rome
St. Angelo fortress 82, 95, 100, 131, 133, 136–137
St. Bernard Pass 106
Saint George 60–62, 112
Saint Peter 46, 47, 48, 49, 52, 59, 60, 79, 84, 85, 106, 112, 126, 127
Saint Peter's Basilica 45, 47, 65, 68, 87, 95, 107, 111, 131, 134, 140, 149, 164, 168
Sancta Maria de Inferno 59
Santiago de Compostela 104, 107
Sardinia 27, 109, 174
Saxony 65, 70, 72, 104
schola 52, 54, 68, 104
Scotland 43, 118, 142
the scrip 103, 104, 105, 106, 160
Seine River 15, 60
senate 17, 19, 40, 47, 75, 80
sewers of Rome 23, 43, 49, 68, 136, 138, 155–156
Shakespeare, William 159
the Sicilian Vespers 129
Sicily 19, 39, 41, 69, 74, 86, 88–89, 98, 101, 129, 179, 180
"Sickle-cell Eve" 12
sickle-cell trait *see* S-hemoglobin mutation
sieges of Rome 37, 39, 41, 42, 43, 48, 49, 82, 87, 91, 172
Siena 15, 95
Simond, Louis 171
simony 80, 81
Sistine Chapel 134, 161, 171

Index

Sixtus IV, Pope 132
Sol Invictus 47
Soren, David 8–9
Spoleto 43, 64, 64, 68, 71
"spring fever" 11, 139
steppe corridor 38, 39, 43, 71
Stilicho 39
Stilo, Battle of 74
Stuart, William Rose 165
the Stuarts 145, 159, 170
Subiaco 121–122
Suburra 22
Switzerland 134, 142, 143
Sylene 60–62
Sylvester I, Pope 59–60, 62, 173
Sylvester II, Pope 75
Sylvester III, Pope 79

Tacitus 22, 38
Tagliacozzo, Battle of 92
Tarentum 19
Tarquin 17–18
Taussig, Gabriele 166
Terry, Charles 164–165
tertian fever 14, 16, 23, 25, 171, 176; *see also P. falciparum; P. vivax*
Testaccio, Monte 20
thalassemia 65
Thames River 15
Theodoric, King of the Ostrogoths 40–41, 163
Theudebert, King of the Franks 41
Thirty Years' War 143, 144, 183
Thomas of Marlborough 115, 116, 120
Tiber Island 18
Tiber River 4, 8, 14, 15–17, 18, 20, 22–23, 42, 47, 48, 52, 54, 68, 95, 112, 121, 136, 154, 155, 157, 163
Tivoli 23, 75, 95, 121, 170
Torelli, Luigi 175, 176
Tortona 85, 99, 101
Totita, King of the Ostrogoths 42, 43
tourism 1, 158, 159, 162–163; *see also* Grand Tour
Tours, Battle of 63
Treaty of Verdun 70
Trento 181
tuberculosis 30, 163
Tuscany 18, 42, 71, 96, 111, 130, 170
Tusculum 121
typhoid 28, 31, 87, 80, 187n14
typhus 31, 195n60

Umbria 8
Unam Sanctam 125
United States 179
Urban IV, Pope 133
Urban VI, Pope 111, 130–131

Valens, Roman Emperor 38–39
Valerian, Roman Emperor 46
Vandals 39–40, 41, 43, 69, 134
Vatican City 69, 174
Vatican Hill 47, 49, 52, 82, 98, 132, 136, 154
Vatican Library 131
Veil of Veronica 107, 111
Velletri 123, 170
Venice 69, 134, 148, 160
Vercellae, Battle of 37
Victor IV, Pope 86, 87
Victor Emmanuel I, Italian King 174, 175
Victor Emmanuel III, Italian King 179
Vikings 43, 82
villeggiatura 87, 121, 125, 130, 134, 174, 176
Visigoths 39–40, 43, 63
Viterbo 120, 121, 173
von Platen-Hallermünd, August 77
Vosges, Battle of 37

Walcheren campaign 66–67
Wales 43
War of Spanish Succession 159
Webb, William 164
Webbe, Edward 148
Weber, Max 183
Welfs 84, 88, 89
Western Schism 111, 131, 132
the White Company 130, 138
Wighard 50
Wilfrid 50–51, 52, 54,
Willibald and Winnebald 45–46, 49, 50
World War II 20, 179
Wotton, Henry 147

Y. pestis 42, 112; *see also* Black Death; bubonic plague; Plague of Justinian

Zacharias, Pope 63, 69
Zago, Sofia 181–182
Zeno, Eastern Roman Emperor 40
Zwingli, Huldrych 142

www.ingramcontent.com/pod-product-compliance
Ingram Content Group UK Ltd.
Pitfield, Milton Keynes, MK11 3LW, UK
UKHW050528150426
5217IPUK00026B/1842